Color Atlas / Text of

EXCIMER LASER SURGERY

THE CORNEA

Color Atlas / Text of EXCIMER LASER SURGERY

THE CORNEA

Edited by

FRANK B. THOMPSON, M.D.
Associate Clinical Professor, Ophthalmology
Doheny Eye Institute
University of Southern California School of Medicine
Los Angeles, California

PETER J. McDONNELL, M.D.
Associate Professor, Ophthalmology
Director of Refractive Surgery
Doheny Eye Institute
University of Southern California School of Medicine
Los Angeles, California

IGAKU-SHOIN New York•Tokyo

Igaku-Shoin Medical Publishers, Inc. gratefully acknowledges the assistance of Alcon® Surgical Incorporated and VISX® Incorporated for their generous grant in support of this project.

Published and distributed by

IGAKU-SHOIN Medical Publishers, Inc.
One Madison Avenue, New York, New York 10010

IGAKU-SHOIN Ltd.,
5-24-3 Hongo, Bunkyo-ku, Tokyo

Library of Congress Cataloging-in-Publication Data
Color atlas/text of excimer laser surgery : the cornea / edited by
Frank B. Thompson, Peter J. McDonnell.
p. cm.
Includes bibliographical references and index.
1. Cornea—Laser surgery. 2. Excimer lasers. I. Thompson, Frank
B. (Frank Brown), 1934– . II. McDonnell, Peter J.
[DNLM: 1. Cornea—surgery—atlases. 2. Laser Surgery—methods—
atlases. WW 17 C71982]
RE86.C65 1993
617.7′19—dc20
DNLM/DLC
for Library of Congress 92-1551
CIP

ISBN: 0-89640-225-8 (New York)
ISBN: 4-260-14225-9 (Tokyo)

Printed and bound in the U.S.A.

10 9 8 7 6 5 4 3 2 1

To my wife, Joan, and to our children,
Steven, Kyra, and Doug

(F. B. T.)

To Jan, Laura, Peter, and Emma

(P. J. M.)

Foreword

New technology, driven by innovators, quickly generates a confusing debate as detractors and supporters vie to declare their own versions of its worth. Since the first description of the interaction of excimer laser light with the corneal surface, many people recognized its enormous surgical potential for both therapeutic and refractive applications. Yet early clinical reports, driven by commercial interests, often failed to clarify the uncertainties that persisted and allowed the fog of confusion to spread. While animal experimentation confirmed that extremely small and well-defined amounts of corneal tissue could be removed and that the animal eye would heal with a transparent, optically smooth anterior surface, the clinical applications of the simple surgical premise derived from these observations were far more complex.

This book reflects the experiences of innovators, all of whom played a significant role in the clinical development of the excimer laser. Ronald Krueger worked with me in 1984 as a medical student and did extensive work studying the qualitative and quantitative nature of the corneal tissue interaction for all the excimer wavelengths. Theo Seiler used a prototype system and was the first to excise diseased tissue from the corneal surface and the first to explore refractive applications by creating laser relaxing incisions. Marguerite McDonald verified the theoretical underpinnings of photorefractive keratectomy in an extensive series of experiments involving rabbits and primates that led to the first successful application in a normally sighted eye in May 1988. Francis L'Esperance fostered commercial development of excimer technology and did early studies with a breadboard prototype on blind human eyes. Walter Stark pioneered the surgical techniques of large-area ablation for therapeutic purposes and produced the clinical evidence that showed corneal transplantation could be avoided in many cases by using the laser to remove superficial tissue in scarred and dystrophic eyes. Roger Steinert was an early investigator of the excimer tissue interaction and demonstrated the best way to smooth the irregular surfaces of diseased human corneas. The importance of corneal topography in planning excimer laser applications was proved by Stephen Klyce, working with Marguerite McDonald. Peter McDonnell pioneered surface ablation for astigmatism and stayed the course from plastic, through rabbits, blind eyes, and postsurgical eyes into otherwise entirely normal eyes with idiopathic astigmatism.

This book shows us why, in many parts of the world, photorefractive keratectomy using the excimer laser has become the preferred refractive surgical technique. James Salz, a radial keratotomy pioneer, has studied the comparative safety, efficacy, and simplicity of excimer laser photorefractive keratectomy. The intense interest in this technology is traced in this book from primates through the first groups of patients with limited vision, both in the United States and Europe to the current broad status of applications including diseased corneas and the full range of refractive errors.

Clearly, we are all comfortable with therapeutic applications of this laser because the risks and uncertainties can be justified more readily in view of the usual alternatives. Nonetheless, the accuracy and precision of refractive control that all investigators have shown in initial studies have focused the debate and produced evidence to allow claims and counterclaims to be tested.

Does controversy remain? Of course. All refractive technology has historically generated conflict. Historically, this includes spectacles, contact lenses, and all surgical applications. To many of us, the excimer is an incremental achievement that has substantially improved any alternative technology for lamellar keratectomy. The strongest lingering uncertainty has to do with long-term effects on these treated eyes, many of which will be in young patients. Only time and very large numbers of patients can make us comfortable with all aspects of this.

Will this be the last word in surgical technology to alter the refractive power of the eye? Of course not, but each technique must be evaluated against extremely high standards of accuracy, precision, and safety that the excimer laser has set in its first 4 years of clinical use. We look forward to the future with confidence but are left with enormous responsibility. The many questions about excimer laser surgery that linger, and the new applications that are suggested, point to studies that must be undertaken so that we can understand not only how to do it but how to do it best.

Stephen L. Trokel, M.D.
Professor of Ophthalmology
Harkness Eye Institute
Columbia University
New York, New York

Acknowledgment

Excimer laser refractive surgery has evolved so rapidly since its development that it has not been possible to publish a text that encompasses our accumulated knowledge and experience with this procedure until now. This book is an attempt to consolidate the information available and to describe the present state of corneal refractive surgery.

The continued rapid development of this procedure necessitated publication of this book within a very short period of time. This would not have been possible without the extraordinary efforts of Igaku-Shoin Medical Publishers and our editor, Terry-lynn Grayson.

Dr. Thompson would like to express his appreciation to Karen Frankfurt, whose effort in collating the materials and whose follow-up work with the contributing editors brought everything together; Dr. Michael Pritchard, who helped to proofread the manuscripts and has contributed his time, ideas, and eloquence of language to many of these chapters; and Mr. William Ludwick, F.O.B.S., C.O.T., who helped with many of the beautiful photographs that contribute so much to this volume. Dr. McDonnell wishes to acknowledge the generous support of Mr. Herbert Hoover III and Mr. and Mrs. Gene Autry. Dr. McDonnell is grateful to the Doheny Eye Institute and, in particular, Drs. Stephen Ryan and Ronald Smith, Ms. Barbara Baker, and Ms. Jenny Garbus.

Without the total cooperation and timely completion of their manuscripts by the contributing authors, this book would not be available to you, the reader, at this time. Their collaboration and good humor during times of stress are much appreciated by both of us.

Frank B. Thompson, M.D.
Peter J. McDonnell, M.D.

Preface

THE EXCIMER LASER CHALLENGE

Ophthalmologists pride themselves on being members of a specialty that is quick to bring technological advances to the clinic. The excimer laser has been added to the list of high-technology items being explored for the better care of our patients. We live in an exciting time!

Every so often in ophthalmology, we are forced to confront and critically evaluate fundamental "truths." With the advent of vitrectomy, we were required to discard our assumption that the vitreous humor is a vital structure, the surgical violation of which will greatly increase the chances of subsequent complications, such as retinal detachment. With the excimer laser, we must reexamine the role of Bowman's membrane in the physiology and pathophysiology of the cornea. Will violation of Bowman's membrane lead inevitably to corneal scarring? Will surgical disruption of this membrane, suggested by some to be a primary event in the pathogenesis of keratoconus, result in eventual corneal ectasia and an iatrogenic form of keratoconus? Will removal of Bowman's membrane, thought to represent at least a partial barrier to superficial infections, predispose to stromal infiltration and scarring in cases of herpes simplex and other forms of keratitis? If refractive surgery in general and excimer laser in particular do nothing else, they will have stimulated a whole generation of intellectually curious ophthalmologists and vision scientists to challenge old assumptions about the cornea, make new and fundamental observations about corneal physiology and pathophysiology, and develop new instruments (such as topographic measuring devices) that have applications well beyond refractive surgery alone.

Innumerable patients world-wide with refractive errors might benefit from photorefractive keratectomy. Because the vast majority of refractive errors are treatable with glasses or contact lenses, with small attendant risks, a careful and complete analysis of the risks and benefits of excimer laser surgery is appropriate. The U.S. Food and Drug Administration (FDA) has determined that 5-year results of human clinical trials will be reviewed as this agency determines whether or not to approve photorefractive keratectomy. Thus, we are engaged in an exciting and precedent-setting undertaking, as this regulatory agency contemplates whether to approve surgery for ametropias in otherwise normal eyes. What criteria will be used in this approval process? What percentage of eyes will be allowed to lose best-corrected visual acuity? What level of precision will the FDA expect from this procedure before it will grant approval? Physicians and potential patients will watch the review process with a mixture of curiosity and excitement as these questions and many others are addressed.

What will happen if the FDA grants approval for photorefractive keratectomy? Outside the United States, in countries most of which have regulatory bodies considered lax in comparison with the FDA, a marked proliferation of laser sites has occurred. Does this mean that this procedure will be readily and widely accepted by physicians and patients as an alternative to spectacles and contact lenses? How will market pressures influence the distribution and use of these lasers? When will ophthalmologists, their families, and their staffs start having this procedure in significant numbers?

Each month, new journal articles describe an additional small piece of the excimer laser story, but where does one obtain an overall view of the body of work in this area? In a rapidly changing field, no book is totally current for long, but we have endeavored to gather in one source a review of excimer laser corneal surgery as performed in late 1992. The contributors to this book include many of the internationally recognized and most respected individuals in the field of refractive surgery. It was not possible to include all of the men and women who are making significant contributions to the study of excimer laser corneal surgery, but we have assembled a collection of perspectives with differing backgrounds and expertise. We have done our best to give the reader a history of the excimer story, a detailed look at the current state of the art, and a feel for what we might encounter in the future.

Excimer laser corneal surgery is in its infancy. During this decade, we will continue to look to dedicated and open-minded clinicians and basic scientists to explore its potential and determine its limitations. If an updated version of this book were to be written 10 years from now, it would include more "hard data" and less speculation, but it would not likely convey a stronger sense of the excitement than we believe is reflected on these pages.

Peter J. McDonnell, M.D.

Contributors

Dimitri T. Azar, M.D.
Assistant Professor, Ophthalmology
Wilmer Eye Institute
Johns Hopkins University
Baltimore, Maryland

Mauro Campos, M.D.
Cornea Fellow
Doheny Eye Institute
University of Southern California School of Medicine
Los Angeles, California

Wallace Chamon, M.D.
Cornea Fellow
Wilmer Eye Institute
Johns Hopkins University
Baltimore, Maryland

Cheryl L. Enger, M.S.
Assistant Professor, Ophthalmology
Wilmer Eye Institute
Johns Hopkins University
Baltimore, Maryland

Mary T. Kamp, M.S.
Senior Research Program Coordinator
Wilmer Eye Institute
Johns Hopkins University
Baltimore, Maryland

Stephen D. Klyce, Ph.D.
Professor of Ophthalmology
Louisiana State University Eye Center
New Orleans, Louisiana

Ronald R. Krueger, M.D.
Cornea Fellow
Doheny Eye Institute
University of Southern California School of Medicine
Los Angeles, California

Gerhard K. Lang, M.D.
Professor and Chair, Ophthalmology
Universität Ulm
Ulm, Germany

David H. Leach, M.D.
Cornea Fellow
Louisiana State University Eye Center
New Orleans, Louisiana

Francis A. L'Esperance, Jr., M.D.
Professor of Clinical Ophthalmology
Columbia Presbyterian Medical Center
New York, New York

Marguerite B. McDonald, M.D.
Professor of Ophthalmology
Louisiana State University Eye Center
New Orleans, Louisiana

Peter J. McDonnell, M.D.
Associate Professor, Ophthalmology
Director of Refractive Surgery
Doheny Eye Institute
University of Southern California School of Medicine
Los Angeles, California

Gottfried O.H. Naumann, M.D.
Professor and Chair, Ophthalmology
Erlangen—Nürnberg
Nürnberg, Germany

James J. Salz, M.D.
Clinical Professor of Ophthalmology
University of Southern California
Los Angeles, California

Theo Seiler, M.D., Ph.D.
Professor of Ophthalmology
Freie Universität Berlin
Berlin, Germany

Walter J. Stark, M.D.
Professor of Ophthalmology
Johns Hopkins University School of Medicine
Baltimore, Maryland

Roger F. Steinert, M.D.
Professor of Ophthalmology
Tufts University School of Medicine
Center for Eye Research
Ophthalmic Consultants of Boston
Boston, Massachusetts

Frank B. Thompson, M.D.
Associate Clinical Professor, Ophthalmology
Doheny Eye Institute
University of Southern California School of Medicine
Los Angeles, California

Contents

FOREWORD vii
Stephen L. Trokel, M.D.

PREFACE xi
Peter J. McDonnell, M.D.

CHAPTER **1. HISTORY AND DEVELOPMENT OF THE EXCIMER LASER** 1
Francis A. L'Esperance, Jr., M.D.

CHAPTER **2. CORNEAL TOPOGRAPHY IN REFRACTIVE KERATECTOMY** 19
Stephen D. Klyce, Ph.D.

CHAPTER **3. MYOPIC PHOTOREFRACTIVE KERATECTOMY: U.S. EXPERIENCE** 37
Marguerite B. McDonald, M.D., and
David H. Leach, M.D.

CHAPTER **4. PHOTOREFRACTIVE KERATECTOMY: EUROPEAN EXPERIENCE** 53
Theo Seiler, M.D., Ph.D.

CHAPTER **5. RADIAL KERATOTOMY VERSUS PHOTOREFRACTIVE KERATECTOMY** 63
James J. Salz, M.D.

CHAPTER **6. PHOTOREFRACTIVE KERATECTOMY: HIGH MYOPIA** 77
Frank B. Thompson, M.D.,
Mauro Campos, M.D., and
Peter J. McDonnell, M.D.

CHAPTER **7. PHOTOREFRACTIVE KERATECTOMY: ASTIGMATISM** 93
Mauro Campos, M.D., and
Peter J. McDonnell, M.D.

CHAPTER **8. THERAPEUTIC KERATECTOMY: CORNEAL OPACITIES** 105
Walter J. Stark, M.D., Wallace Chamon, M.D.,
Dimitri T. Azar, M.D., Mary T. Kamp, M.S., and
Cheryl L. Enger, M.S.

CHAPTER **9. THERAPEUTIC KERATECTOMY: CORNEAL SMOOTHING** 121
Roger F. Steinert, M.D.

CHAPTER **10. CORNEAL TREPHINATION WITH THE EXCIMER LASER FOR PENETRATING KERATOPLASTY** 131
Gerhard K. Lang, M.D., and
Gottfried O. H. Naumann, M.D.

CHAPTER **11. NEW DIRECTIONS IN EXCIMER LASER SURGERY** 137
Ronald R. Krueger, M.D., and
Peter J. McDonnell, M.D.

INDEX 153

CHAPTER 1

History and Development of the Excimer Laser

FRANCIS A. L'ESPERANCE, JR.

HISTORICAL ASPECTS*

The history of laser development in physical science has been embellished with many instances in which the physicist, through pure genius, evolved a laser principle that worked and eventually led to another brilliant concept. For every stroke of genius, there were scores of hunches that went wrong, some that were correct, multiple cases of trial and error, and many "what if" scenarios. The development of the excimer laser was fraught with a multiplicity of avenues that deserved pursuit, some of which proved to be of great benefit, although most were totally useless. The excimer laser was not invented with one pure stroke of brilliance but rather was the result of an evolution of events that read much like a fascinating science novel.

First, it must be realized that *excimer* is a word from organic molecular physics. It is a contraction of the words *excited dimers,* and it is compact and easy to pronounce. *Dimers* means two of the same thing, such as two atoms of xenon, or krypton, or fluorine that form Xe_2, Kr_2, or F_2 molecules, respectively. The word *excimer,* as it is now considered in laser physics, is definitely a misnomer because we refer to mixed molecular combinations such as argon fluoride or krypton fluoride as excimers. According to many physicists, the correct name for these molecular configurations would be an *exciplex* structure. But one realizes immediately that the term *exciplex laser* is difficult to pronounce and does not sound as correct or as mellifluous as *excimer laser*. Therefore, the term *excimer laser,* despite its incorrectness, has been adopted by everyone much in the way that the word *laser,* coined by Gordon Gould, was adopted from the classic terminology *optical masers,* even though Bell Telephone Laboratories refused to use the word *laser* and, in effect, discouraged others from using the term for a considerable period of time.

The concept of rare gas dimers such as Xe_2 and Kr_2 had been suggested by individuals such as James Keck at the Avco Everett Research Laboratory in the late 1960s, when he was considering the use of hydrogen as a pure gas dimer.[1] Houtermans[2] had the concept of using mercury molecules as the laser medium during the latter part of that decade. Later, Charles Rhodes, then at Livermore Labora-

The author acknowledges the exceptional assistance of Linda Kampley and Elizabeth Mooney.

*Portions excerpted from an account in Jeff Hecht, *Laser Pioneers* (Academic Press, Boston, 1992).

tories, was working on the principle of using the pure rare gas excimers such as Xe_2, Kr_2, and Ar_2 gas molecules[1] as the laser medium. There was also rare gas dimer experimentation at the Sandia Corporation and Northrop Corporation, and work was evolving in the Soviet Union in the early 1970s. However, it was Charles Brau at Avco who reportedly was the first to say, "Excimer lasers, that is something to go after."[3]

The first studies in impure rare gas dimers, that is, with rare gas–halide dimers, began with the work of Donald Setser, then a professor at Kansas State University. It was his observation of fluorescence from the xenon chloride molecule that led Hao-Lin Chen, Brau, and Robert Center from Avco to collaborate with James Ewing to start working extensively on the rare gas halides in an attempt to produce laser action. With a tremendous amount of work from various groups, all contributing small parts of the puzzle of laser action with the so-called excimers, it was Stuart Searles who bombarded a medium of xenon bromide with an electron beam gun and produced the first excimer laser action in early May of 1975. Two weeks later, Ewing and his team succeeded in creating laser action in a xenon fluoride mixture, and 1 week later in a xenon chloride mixture. Within several weeks, Ewing and his team succeeded in producing a krypton fluoride laser, which seemed enormously powerful at that time. During the months of May and June 1975 the excimer laser, as a rare gas–halide molecular combination, was introduced to the world.

It is interesting that although Setser's brilliant work on fluorescent emissions of the xenon chloride molecule stimulated so many people throughout the world to the possibility of laser action in the rare gas–halide combinations, it was really Golde and Thrush in England who, working with argon chloride emissions of 172 nm before Setser's work, realized that the combination of a rare gas and a halogen could produce a fluorescent emission. However, they did not consider the possibility of laser action. It was not until the winter of 1975–1976 that the physicists and engineers at the Sandia Corporation were successful in making an argon fluoride mixture laser, producing approximately 100 J of energy from this laser action. During this initial attempt, when the argon fluoride spectrum was recorded for the first time, an enormous amount of energy was produced at inception. This event was truly a historic and outstanding accomplishment.

HISTORICAL MEDICAL DEVELOPMENT

As the cavity designs, pumping modules, and basic physical components of various excimer laser systems improved, it became apparent to Charles Brau, in a 1979 publication edited by Charles Rhodes,[4] that the excimer laser should be used for micromachining and processing and could extend into the field of biological materials. In the same year, Huestis[5] noted that the world of the physical sciences was indeed entering "an excimer age," and that the excimer laser would be applied to many different materials including certain biological structures. Also in 1979,[6] Warren Ruderman was the first to directly state that the excimer laser could have an enormous place in medicine and that its application in the field of medicine should be investigated.

Despite these visionary proddings by extremely knowledgeable physicists, the excimer laser was relegated to publications in the physical sciences, but I found it interesting to review the physics abstracts at the Columbia University physics library on a monthly basis. It was evident to me that the excimer laser was emerging as a more powerful laser during the beginning of the 1980s, and experimentation and evaluation of the various excimer rare gas–halide combinations were being conducted in many countries. However, it was not until a meeting of the Aero-Space Medical Association in May 1981 that John Taboada[7] reported that threshold damage determinations with the argon fluoride laser had produced a strange indentation of the epithelium of the cornea, which he attributed initially to dehydration. Both this presentation and Taboada's article concerning the interaction of the krypton fluoride excimer laser with the epithelium, published the following month in *Health Physics*,[8] indicated that a new laser–tissue interaction, which was enigmatic and perplexing, had taken place. At this time, Taboada and his coworkers[7,8] felt that either the anatomic configuration of the rabbit epithelium or a thermal process could possibly explain the unusual epithelial indentation or dimpling that occurred.

From June 1981 until September 1982, a myriad of reports in the physics literature concerning excimer lasers were published. The most significant article was a report by R. Srinivasan and coworkers in *Applied Physics Letters* in September 1982.[9] This report and a subsequent report in the December 1982 issue of the *Journal of the Americal Chemical Society*[10] indicated that the argon fluoride excimer laser is capable of removing extremely small particles of plastic substances such as polyethylene terephalate films without thermal deformation in a manner that would be highly desirable for the construction of electronic elements such as integrated circuits.

At the end of 1982 and into the early months

of 1983, Linsker, Srinivasan, and their coworkers[11] began to test the potential of the argon fluoride excimer laser on biological substances and found that "photoablative decomposition," as Srinivasan called it, of various tissues occurred with a precision that was equal to that found with plastic compounds. The work of Srinivasan, Linsker, Wynne, and Blum, which began in early 1983 and was published partially in May 1983[12] and completely in 1984,[11] established the fact that biological materials such as cartilage, aorta, bone, and hair can be micromachined in a nonthermal fashion with extraordinary precision. This single discovery led to the application trials of excimer lasers in many fields of medicine.

During the interval from 1979 to 1983, the progress of the excimer laser had become very exciting, and it became apparent to me that a new laser–tissue interaction had occurred. Similarly, IBM researchers realized that Srinivasan's "photoablative decomposition" could be applied to tissues, and in 1982 they applied for (and later received) a patent on this biological process.

During the period between 1982 and 1983, it occurred to me that corneal tissue could be removed in a manner similar to that demonstrated and reported by the IBM group in plastics in 1982[8,9] and in other animal tissues in May 1983.[12] It seemed reasonable that, if the excimer laser energy were properly deployed over the surface of the cornea, the shape of the cornea could be recontoured or reprofiled in order to correct myopia, hyperopia, and astigmatism (Figs. 1.1–1.4). In essence, the anterior cornea would assume the curvature of the anterior surface of a contact lens that would be used to render a particular eye emmetropic. To this end, I submitted the first patent application in the ophthalmic (and medical) field on November 17, 1983;

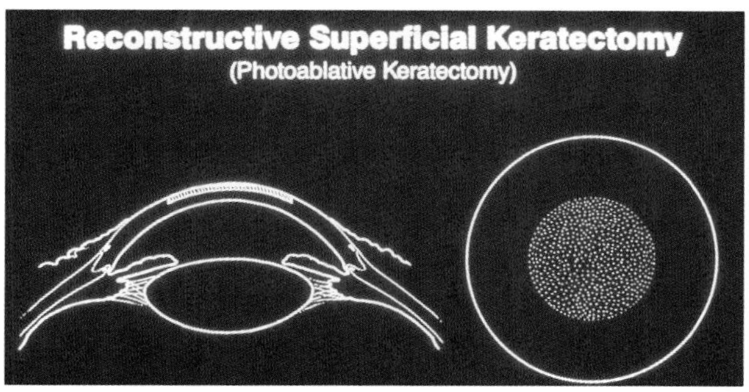

FIGURE 1.1. Diagram of excimer laser superficial lamellar (phototherapeutic) keratectomy to ablate or remove superficial scar tissue from the cornea, thereby permitting optimal clearing of the underlying cornea. (Reproduced from L'Esperance FA Jr: *Ophthalmic Lasers,* 3rd ed. St. Louis, Mosby-Year Book, 1989, p. 891.)

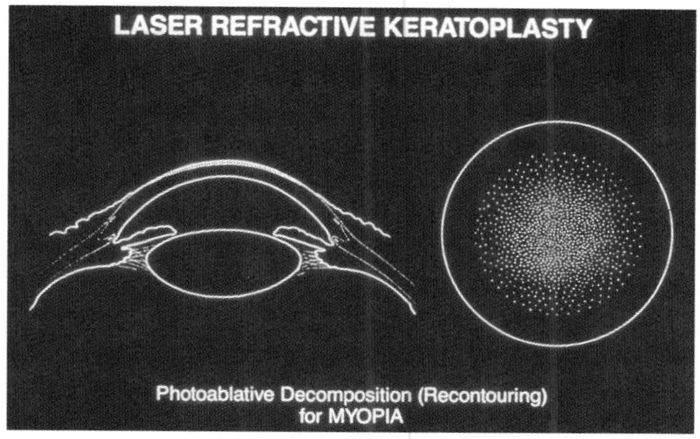

FIGURE 1.2. Diagram of excimer laser recontouring, sculpting, or reprofiling of the anterior corneal structures (photorefractive keratectomy) in order to increase the radius of curvature and flatten the anterior corneal curvature for correction of myopic refractive errors. (Reproduced from L'Esperance FA Jr: *Ophthalmic Lasers,* 3rd ed. St. Louis, Mosby-Year Book, 1989, p. 891.)

the patent covered the various aspects of corneal sculpting, recontouring, or reprofiling (U.S. Patent 4,665,913 issued May 19, 1987).

In July 1983, Stephen Trokel began a collaboration with Srinivasan at the IBM Thomas J. Watson Research Center in Yorktown Heights, New York. This work culminated in December 1983 in a publication in the *American Journal of Ophthalmology*[13] that showed that the cornea of a bovine eye responded to excimer laser radiation in a manner similar to that of cartilage, aorta, and so forth[11,12] and could be incised precisely, and that tissue could be

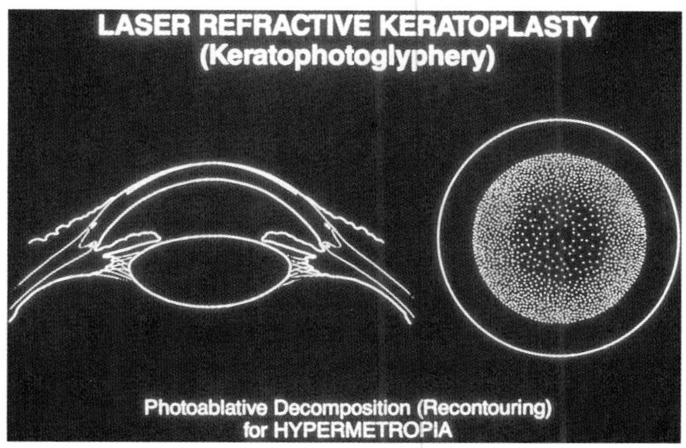

FIGURE 1.3. Diagram of excimer laser recontouring of the anterior surface of the central cornea (photorefractive keratectomy) in order to decrease the radius of curvature and steepen the curvature of the cornea in order to correct hyperopic refractive errors. (Reproduced from L'Esperance FA Jr: *Ophthalmic Lasers,* 3rd ed. St. Louis, Mosby-Year Book, 1989, p. 892.)

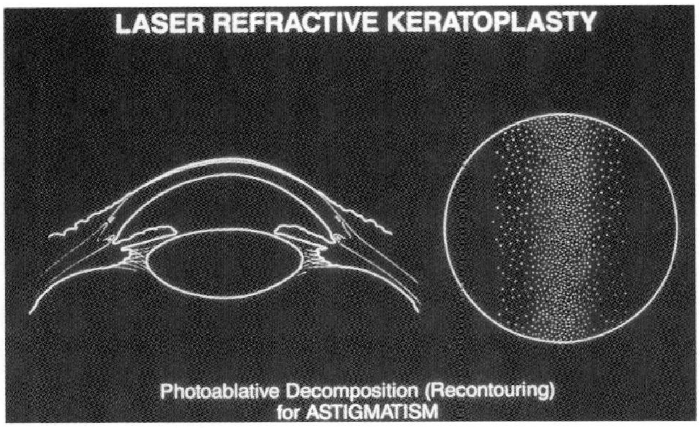

FIGURE 1.4. Diagram of excimer laser recontouring of the anterior surface of the central cornea (photorefractive keratectomy) along a particular axis of the cornea for correction of astigmatism. (Reproduced from L'Esperance FA Jr: *Ophthalmic Lasers,* 3rd ed. St. Louis, Mosby-Year Book, 1989, p. 892.)

removed in a nonthermal manner. On December 15, 1983, Trokel also applied for a patent based on his argon fluoride excimer laser work with the bovine cornea. A Lambda Physic excimer laser was later installed at the Edward S. Harkness Eye Institute at the Columbia-Presbyterian Medical Center, and numerous experiments concerning the effect of repetition rate and energy per pulse, and work on the short- and long-term light and electron microscopic histopathology of rabbit and monkey eyes, were conducted.

It became apparent that the utilization of the excimer laser for definitive experimental and clinical evaluation with sophisticated instrumentation was a multimillion dollar commitment involving investors, multiple patents, and the recruitment of a highly capable team of physicists, engineers, businesspeople, and medical personnel. In 1984, following the recommendation of Eugene Gordon, a former executive at Bell Telephone Laboratories, I discussed the possibility of forming a joint venture with Tropel, which was a division of the Geophysical Corporation of America (GCA). The Tropel company was refining lenses and lens units used to produce integrated circuits to an accuracy of 1/100 of the wavelength of visible light, and were using techniques that, interestingly, were analogous to those that would be employed for corneal recontouring. This association appeared to be highly advantageous, and during our preliminary discussions it was decided that the Alcon company would be the marketing arm of the company, while Tropel would be involved with the design and eventual manufacturing. Because of a tremendous influx of integrated circuits from Japan and its adverse effect on GCA, our discussions were terminated, although Alcon remained in place as our marketing partner.

I then turned to the optical division of the Perkin-Elmer Corporation and found six individuals who were brilliant managers, optical designers, and engineers as well as laser experts. Together with this former Perkin-Elmer team, I formed a new company called Taunton Technologies, with the purpose of designing and constructing an excimer laser system for the correction of myopic, hyperopic, and astigmatic refractive errors. At the first installation, in Monroe, Connecticut, the "bread-

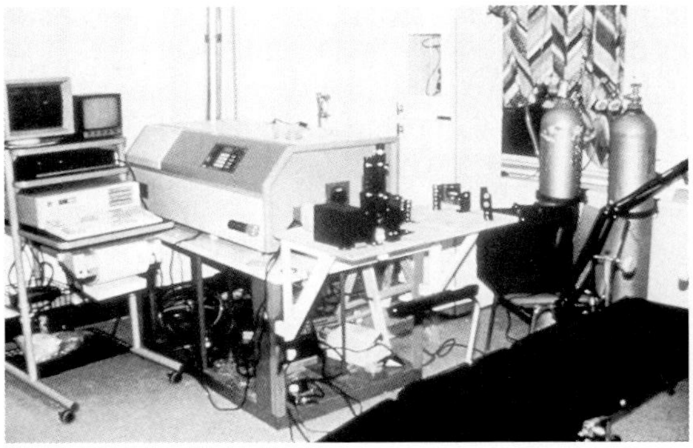
A

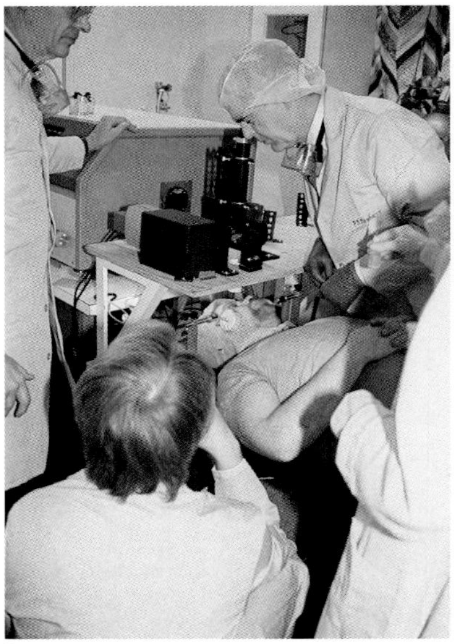
B

FIGURE 1.5. (A) The "breadboard" argon fluoride excimer laser system with laser and optical components arranged to deliver 193 nm of laser radiation precisely to the eye, but with less concern for the ergonomic or packaging requirements of the final instrument version. (B) Alignment of the central cornea of the first human patient with the axis of the breadboard excimer laser beam in order to ensure proper centration and energy distribution.

board" version (the version in which the components were spread out, although integrated, over a medium-sized room) was completed in 1986 (Fig. 1.5). This excimer laser instrument worked exceedingly well on a large series of monkey eyes on which Daniel Taylor directed extensive light and electron microscopic histopathologic evaluations at the University of Connecticut.[14] During this time, negotiations with the Food and Drug Administration were very productive, and Taunton Technologies received the first investigational device exemption from the FDA to establish clinical trials in phase I studies on humans. This study was conducted on blind eyes or eyes scheduled for enucleation. On February 6, 1987, I treated the first of three human eyes in a series of 11 patients in the phase I study and created the first human wide-area superficial lamellar keratectomy (Figs. 1.6 and 1.7). The spot size was 3.0 mm in diameter, and approximately 35 μm of Bowman's membrane and superficial stroma was removed. I treated two additional eyes in this series, and all three eyes were then enucleated within a period of 2 weeks because of choroidal malignant melanomas (Figs. 1.8 and 1.9). This first use of the argon fluoride excimer laser for human wide-area superficial lamellar keratectomy was designed to provide corneal tissue samples for light and electron microscopy to evaluate the acute phase of the excimer laser interaction.[15] Interestingly, the third patient was the first one with a sighted eye that was treated with an excimer laser superficial lamellar keratectomy; his vision was 20/20 without correction before the treatment, and 20/20 with correction following the keratectomy, although his eye was removed 12 days after treatment, due to a nasally located choroidal malignant melanoma. The fourth patient in this phase I series had sustained a traumatic leukoma of the central cornea and was treated by Dr. Taylor; the eye was allowed to heal for a 4-month period before Dr. Taylor performed a corrective corneal transplant to remove the leukoma and the area of excimer laser irradiation. Therefore, both short-term and relatively long term light and electron microscopic specimens (Figs. 24–29) were obtained in order to guide our design efforts during future improvements of the Taunton Technologies excimer laser instrument.[16–18]

Toward the end of 1987, the "brass-board" instrument (Fig. 1.10), in which the components of the system were grouped together in a fashion similar to the placement in a prototype machine (Fig. 1.11), was produced, and soon thereafter the first

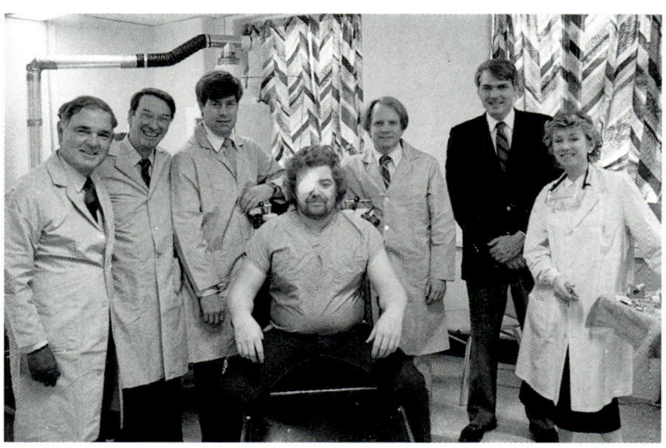

FIGURE 1.6. The first human patient treated with wide-area superficial lamellar keratectomy (center), and the Taunton Technologies team of physicists and medical personnel, on February 6, 1987.

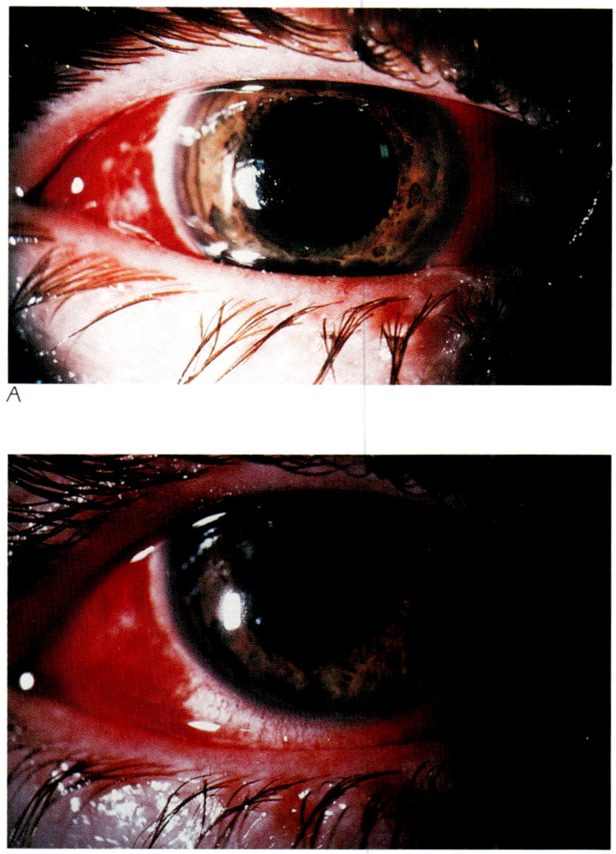

A

B

FIGURE 1.7. (A) The first human patient to be treated with the excimer laser in order to produce a superficial keratectomy—1 day after laser treatment. The 3 mm diameter circular, 35 μm deep treatment area is slightly eccentric to the optical axis toward the 8 o'clock position. (B) Healing of the epithelium was complete in 64 hours. The cornea remained perfectly clear prior to enucleation. (Copyright Taunton Technologies, Inc.)

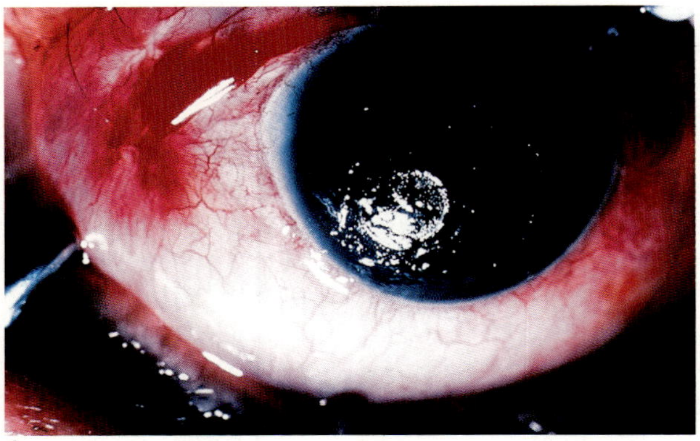

A

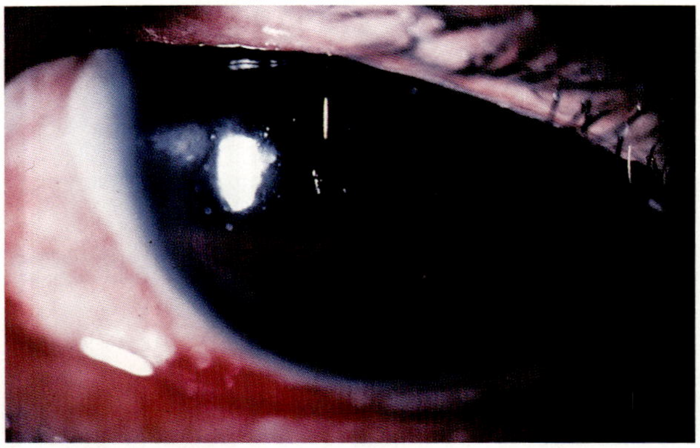

B

FIGURE 1.8. The second human to be treated with excimer laser keratectomy was a 68 year-old man with a malignant melanoma of the iris and ciliary body in the right eye, for which enucleation had been recommended. His intraocular pressure was 51 mm Hg, and he presented with an anterior chamber that was half-filled with blood. (A) Appearance of the eye 1 day after 4 mm circular, 40 μm deep excimer laser keratectomy. (B) The epithelium re-epithelialized within 68 hours after the treatment, and the cornea remained perfectly clear at the time of enucleation 12 days after laser irradiation. (Copyright Taunton Technologies, Inc.)

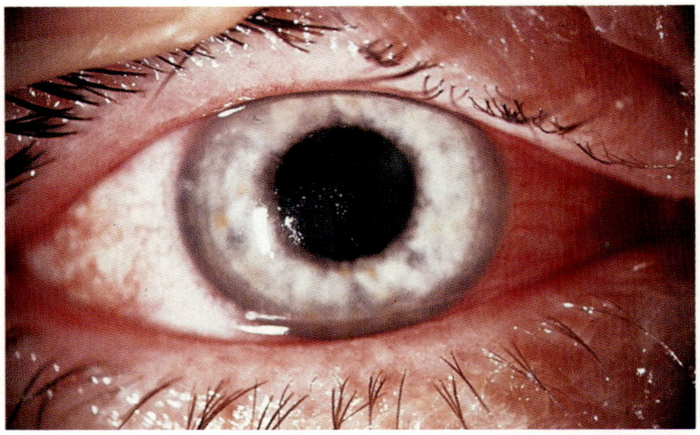

A

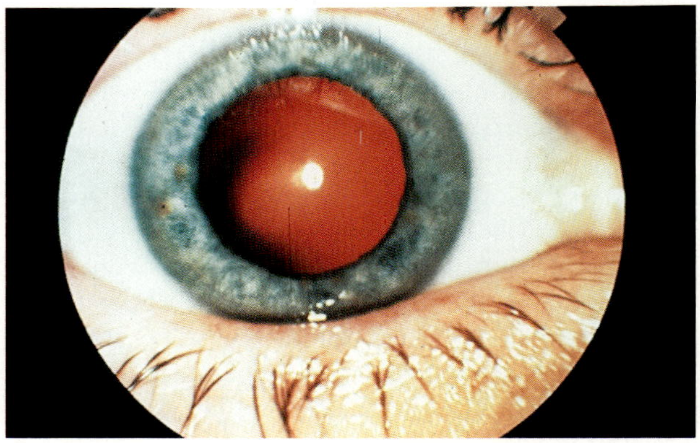

B

FIGURE 1.9. The third patient was a 44 year-old man with a choroidal melanoma impinging on the right optic nerve. (A) Appearance of the eye 1 day after excimer laser keratectomy was performed to a depth of approximately 45 μm from the surface of Bowman's membrane in a 4 mm excision area. (B) The epithelium and eye healed with perfect clarity, leaving an oil-drop reflex in the area of ablation at the time of enucleation 7 days following the laser treatment. (From L'Esperance FA Jr, Taylor DM, and Warner JW: Human excimer laser keratectomy: Short term histopathology, *J Refract Surg* 4:118, 1988.)

patients in phase IIA of the FDA investigation were enrolled. Eventually Taunton Technologies moved their operation to a 12,000-ft^2 facility in Monroe, Connecticut, and created the final version of their excimer laser instrument (Fig. 1.12). With this device, the remainder of the phase II studies were completed and the phase III studies commenced.

During late 1986 and 1987, Summit Technology embarked on their design and construction of an ophthalmic excimer laser system, although they had considerable experience with excimer laser investigations in other fields of medicine. The Summit Technology group produces their own excimer lasers and has had an active international marketing staff as well as the important scientific input of John Marshall at the University of London and Theo Seiler at the University of Berlin. Other laser experts in the United States have been instrumental in conducting many of the FDA studies for Summit Technology in the fields of glaucoma therapy, control of astigmatism by various forms of peripheral corneal slits, and the removal of superficial corneal scars, in addition to the correction of myopia.

In 1986 the Cooper Surgical division of Cooper Laboratories also started a project to design and construct an ophthalmic excimer laser system under the direction of Charles Munnerlyn prior to the sale of the Cooper Surgical division to the Alcon

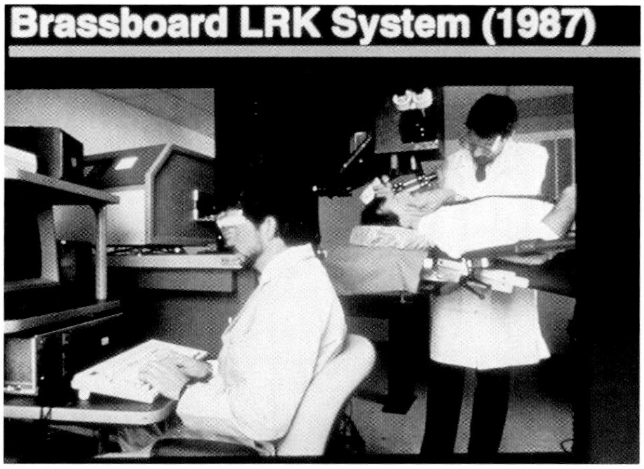

FIGURE 1.10. The "brass-board" argon fluoride excimer laser system with optical components in a nearly final position for the more ideal treatment of patients enrolled under the auspices of the FDA at the Danbury Hospital in Danbury, Connecticut. (Copyright Taunton Technologies, Inc.)

Corporation. The excimer laser project was sequestered and taken as a private entity apart from its parent company. This new entity then became a public company under the name of VISX and proceeded to develop its instrumentation leading to the progression through the various stages of FDA approval. Trokel joined the staff of VISX, and during the years between 1987 and 1989, three companies—Summit Technology, Taunton Technologies, and VISX—were racing toward premarket approval to use the argon fluoride excimer laser for the removal of superficial scars and opacifications

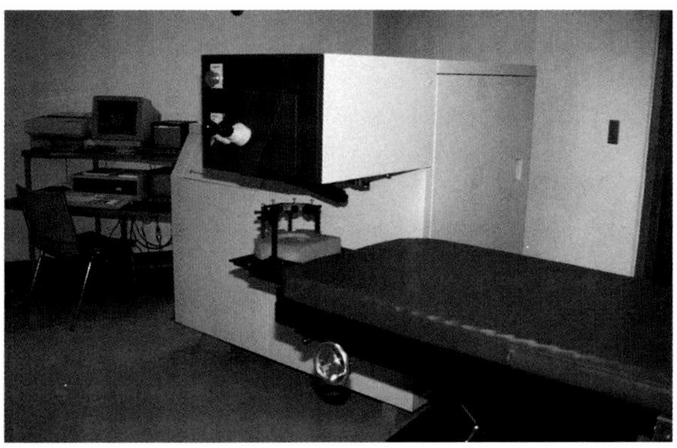

FIGURE 1.11. A prototype excimer laser instrument designed for the precise volumetric removal of the anterior corneal structures to produce a reconstructive superficial lamellar (phototherapeutic) keratectomy or a photorefractive keratectomy. (Copyright Taunton Technologies, Inc.)

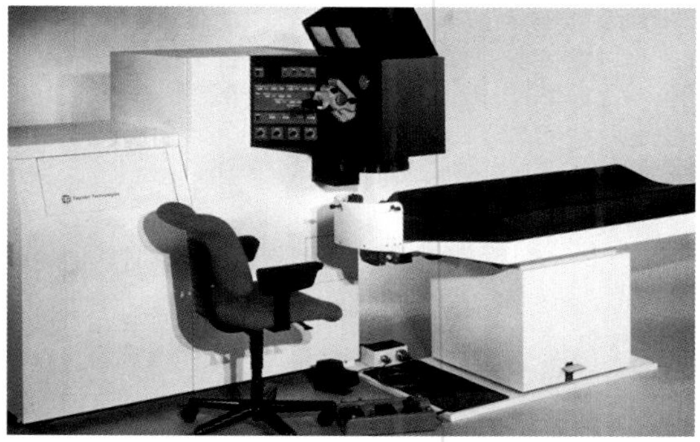

FIGURE 1.12. An extremely sophisticated excimer laser instrument designed as a production model with a "cockpit" display for the surgeon. This system was used in stages II and III of the phototherapeutic keratectomy and photorefractive keratectomy FDA-sponsored human trials. (Copyright Taunton Technologies, Inc.)

of the cornea (phototherapeutic keratectomy) and for the correction of myopia, hyperopia, and astigmatism (photorefractive keratectomy).

In 1990, Taunton Technologies, after significant negotiations, acquired VISX and then changed its name to VISX in such a way that the VISX parent company still retained its identity for the purposes of the FDA regulations as VISX, California. In this manner, Taunton Technologies, now VISX, was allowed to proceed with their FDA investigations, and VISX was allowed also to proceed with their investigations in a separate, but obviously closely combined fashion. At the present time, both VISX and Summit Technology have entered the 700-patient FDA phase III study with an eventual cohort of 500 eyes; this will be followed for a 2-year period in order to evaluate the safety and efficacy of the excimer laser phototherapeutic and photorefractive keratectomy procedures.

In the meantime, excimer lasers are being placed in various locations throughout the world, and a host of new medical and ophthalmic applications are being developed for this extraordinary new laser–tissue interaction.

DEVELOPMENTAL ASPECTS

INSTRUMENTATION

Argon Fluoride Excimer Laser

Although the frequency-quadrupled and frequency-quintupled neodymium–yttrium-aluminum-garnet (yag) lasers, as well as frequency-double organic dye lasers, and several other families of ultraviolet lasers, were available to produce laser outputs in the far-ultraviolet spectrum, it was the excimer family of lasers that seemed to be most easily applicable to corneal incision, excision, or reprofiling. Theoretically, the extremely short pulse duration of the excimer laser (10–20 ns) would decrease thermal effects to infinitesimal levels because of the apparent lack of time for thermal diffusion. Second, the pulse-to-pulse energy level is reproducible within acceptable limits, and the repetition rate (Hz) of the pulses can be varied over a relatively large range, typically 1 to 50 Hz. Third, sufficient energy is available (typically up to 450 mJ) so that a large beam can be produced to ablate or reprofile a 4 to 7 mm diameter portion of the central cornea without energy limitations. Despite these apparent advantages, the available excimer lasers in 1984 and 1985 were extremely crude when compared with other existing conventional ophthalmic lasers, and extensive modifications were required for clinical application.

Beam Delivery System

Several versions of beam delivery apparatus with progressively improved capability were developed to permit precise amounts or thicknesses of tissue to be ablated at exact locations on the anterior corneal surface without involving normal adjacent or deeper corneal tissue. Various systems were utilized, ranging from a blocking contact lens mask to a system of variable apertures that were projected onto the cornea for the correction of refractive errors. All the excimer laser delivery systems operated under computer control, and the apertures used for the correction of myopia and hyperopia were adjusted with great precision so that the required number and density of photons impacted the anterior cornea and removed the correct amount of tissue in specific areas. The general configurations of beam delivery systems were similar in the various excimer laser ophthalmic instruments that were being developed in the mid to late 1980s.

Laser Subsystem

Both the VISX and the Taunton Technologies excimer laser instruments used the Questek Series 2000 argon fluoride excimer lasers as the source of intense pulses of 193 nm radiation. All functions of these lasers were controlled by computer software, and the lasers had automatic gain compensation, automatic gas replenishing, and other features that were controlled by internal microprocessors. Gases and cooling water were obtained from external sources, and sensors that constantly monitored temperature, gas pressure, coolant flow, hardware status, and microprocessor function were integrated into the system. The Summit Technology, laser and the Meditec laser utilized excimer lasers of their own design and manufacture, but all were similar in many details.

Optical Subsystem

The optical subsystem of most of the excimer lasers was similar to the Taunton Technologies diagram shown in Figure 1.13. With most excimer lasers, the raw laser beam that entered the optical subsystem was rectangular, with dimensions of approximately 11 × 22 mm. The intensity profiles, in the short and long directions, were essentially Gaussian and "top hat," respectively, as indicated in Figure 1.14. Significant "hot spots" at the edges of the beam were eliminated by passing the laser beam

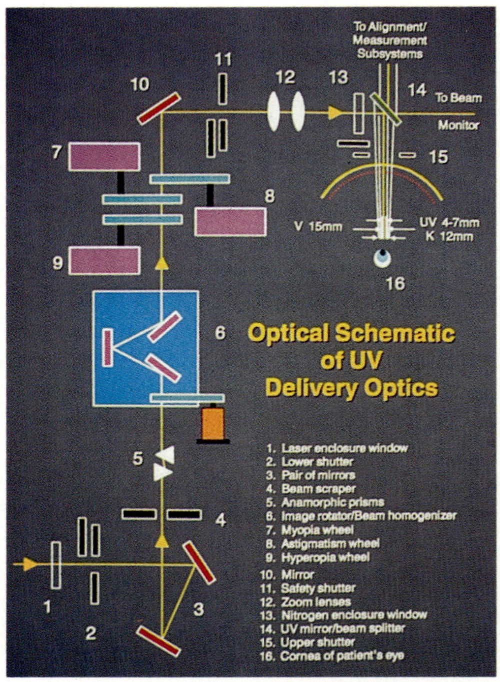

FIGURE 1.13. Diagram of the optical design of the overall excimer laser instrument including anamorphic prisms, a beam-homogenizing system, aperture wheels, and a beam-monitoring device. (1) Laser-enclosure window; (2) lower shutter; (3) pair of mirrors; (4) beam scraper; (5) anamorphic prisms; (6) image rotator–beam homogenizer; (7) myopia wheel; (8) astigmatism wheel; (9) hyperopia wheel; (10) mirror; (11) safety shutter; (12) zoom lenses; (13) nitrogen-enclosure window; (14) ultraviolet mirror–beam splitter; (15) upper shutter; (16) cornea of patient's eye. (Copyright Taunton Technologies, Inc.)

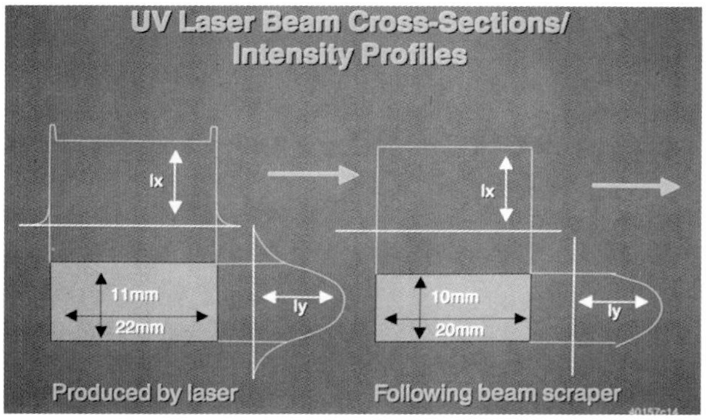

FIGURE 1.14. Diagram of the excimer laser beam as it is manipulated after exiting from a specially designed excimer laser, so as to clip away the "wings" of the partially Gaussian beam. (Copyright Taunton Technologies, Inc.)

through a 10 × 20 mm aperture mask. The beam was then expanded anamorphically in order to form a square 20 × 20 mm beam.

Because the expanded laser beam still had different intensity profiles in the principal directions after expansion, it was necessary to pass the beam through a "K-mirror" type beam rotator to time-average the multipulse energy delivered to the cornea (Figs. 1.15 and 1.16).

The rotating square beam, having time-averaged axially symmetric intensity profiles, was then passed through a set of three aperture wheels spaced along the axis of the beam in the Taunton Technologies instrument (Fig. 1.13). The various decreasing-diameter aperture wheels were used for the correction of myopia, and annular apertures of decreasing radial width were used for the correction of hyperopia (Figs. 1.17 and 1.18). The mechanism was developed to allow each aperture to remain in

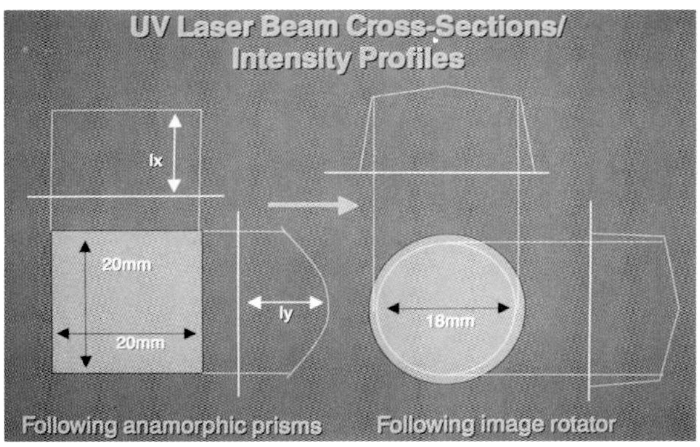

FIGURE 1.15. Anamorphic prisms convert the rectangular beam to a square beam, which is then homogenized in a beam image rotator that converts the beam to a circular configuration. (Copyright Taunton Technologies, Inc.)

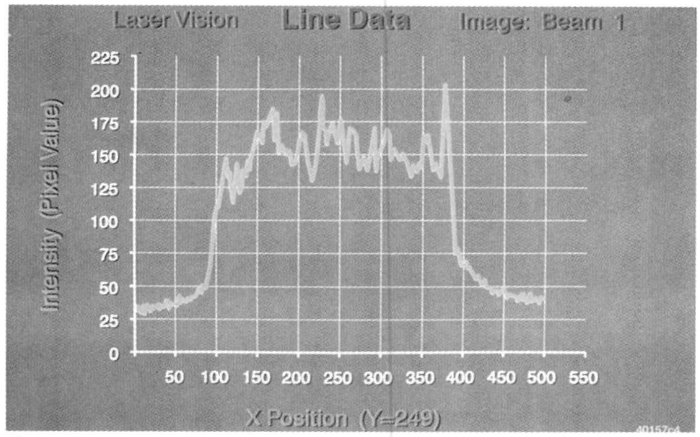

A

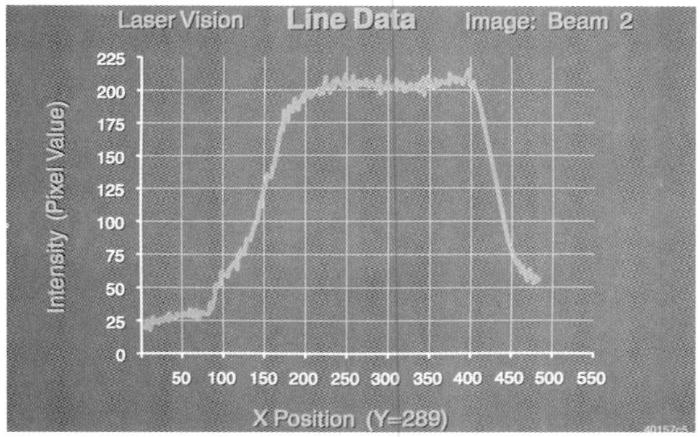

B

FIGURE 1.16. The essentially ragged beam that exits from the excimer laser (A) is restructured by multiple manipulations into a flat "top hat" beam configuration (B) that can then be applied to the cornea so that the excimer laser energy is equally distributed over the corneal impact zone. (Copyright Taunton Technologies, Inc.)

position for the appropriate number of pulses to be delivered to the cornea for the removal of a precise amount of corneal tissue as determined by a "recipe" previously entered into the computer. With the VISX system, a similar removal of tissue was accomplished by an iris diaphragm of decreasing diameter that allowed more photons to strike the central portion of the cornea than the peripheral portions, and therefore to ablate the precise amount of tissue to produce the correct flattening of the curvature of the cornea for the correction of the myopia.

The astigmatism wheel (Fig. 1.19), which was included in later models of the Taunton Technologies and VISX systems, had a series of slit-shaped apertures of varying width. Means were provided to adjust the slit orientation about the laser beam axis so as to align the cylindrical ablation axis with the proper astigmatism axis of the patient's eye, as previously determined by the appropriate measure-

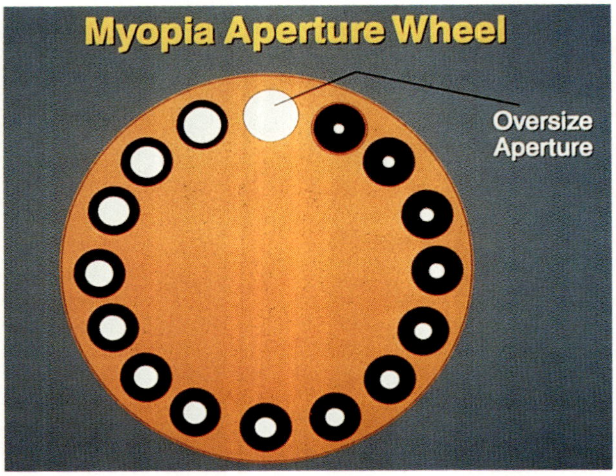

A

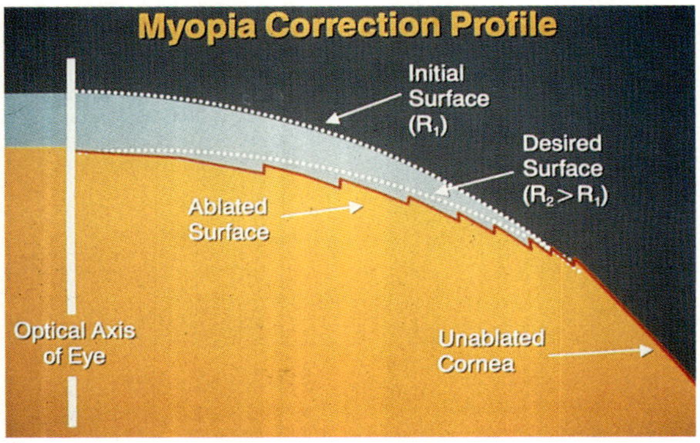

B

FIGURE 1.17. Diagram of the myopia aperture wheel (A) that removes more of the central cornea than the peripheral cornea (B) in order to flatten the corneal curvature by a series of stepwise enlargements of the beam impacting on the cornea. The length of time that the aperture opening remains at each of these stations is controlled by a computer whose "recipe" can change for various myopic corrections. (Copyright Taunton Technologies, Inc.)

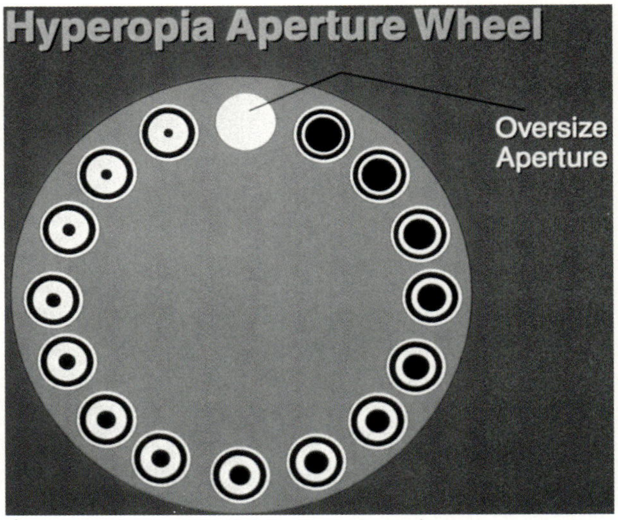

A

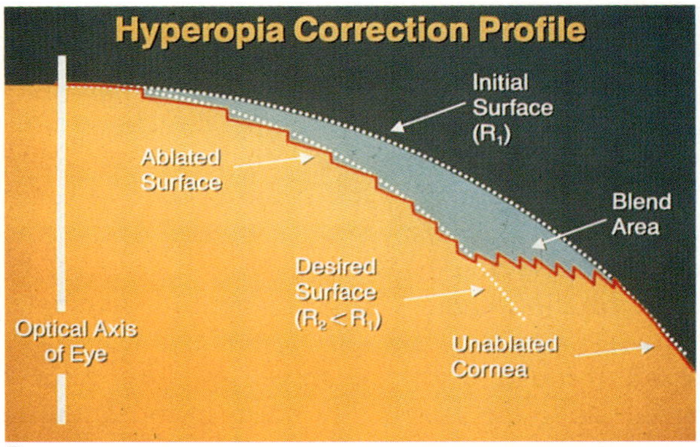

B

FIGURE 1.18. Diagram of the hyperopia aperture wheel constructed so that progressively enlarging annuli (A) remove a greater amount of peripheral corneal tissue than central corneal tissue to steepen the curvature of the cornea (B) in order to correct the hyperopic refractive condition. (Copyright Taunton Technologies, Inc.)

ments. Exposure of the cornea through a series of slits recontours the original toroidal surface into a more nearly spherical one. If the resulting optical power of this ablated surface is then not optimal, the above-discussed myopia- or hyperopia-reducing procedures can be followed to reshape the spherical surface to the desired contour.

The last optical device in the delivery system of most excimer lasers is a lens that focuses the collimated beam as received through the aperture, or diaphragm, to a point in front of the cornea. The diverging beam then falls upon the cornea and selectively ablates tissue in accordance with the recipe controlled by the computer located in the instrument.

Alignment Subsystem

It has been noted by all clinical investigators that the cornea of the patient's eye must be accurately located along the ultraviolet laser beam axis. The reference for positioning of the eye is a microscope that allows the ophthalmologist to look along the axis of the ultraviolet beam through a beam splitter and see a magnified frontal view of the eye. A cross-hair reticle pattern in the microscope, seen superimposed on the image of the eye, can be boresighted to the ultraviolet beam so alignment of the eye to this pattern ensures proper centering of the ablation (Fig. 1.20). In this manner, constant moni-

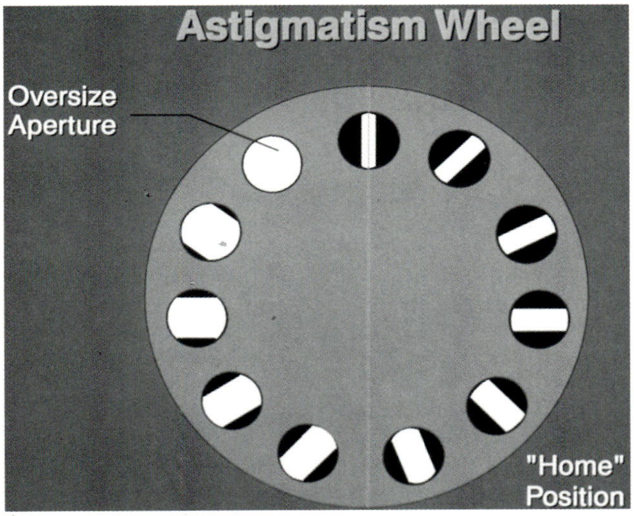

A

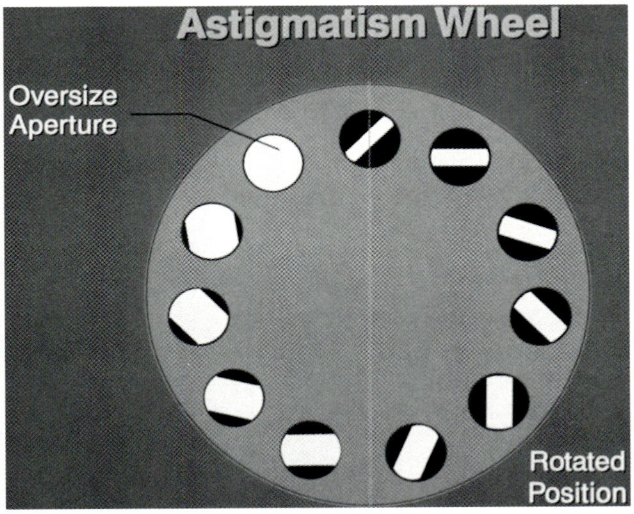

B

FIGURE 1.19. The astigmatism aperture wheel incorporating a series of enlarging rectangles that can be aligned and rotated to coincide with the axis of the astigmatism. (A) The "Home position" and (B) the "rotated" position. (Copyright Taunton Technologies, Inc.)

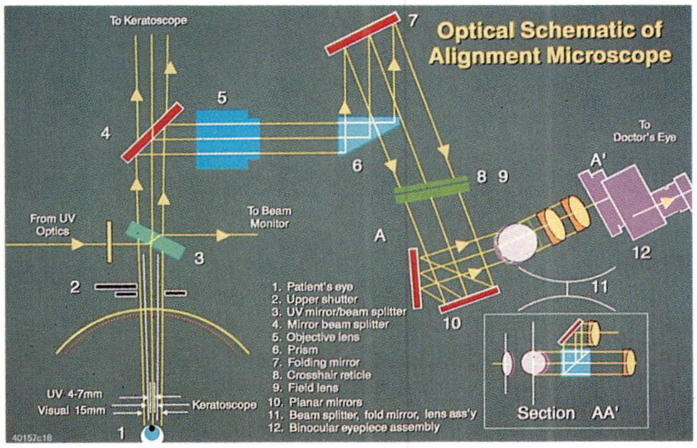

FIGURE 1.20. Diagram of the alignment microscope that tracks and monitors the corneal photoablation process while part of the beam travels to the keratoscope television monitor. (1) Patient's eye; (2) upper shutter; (3) ultraviolet mirror–beam splitter; (4) mirror beam splitter; (5) objective lens; (6) prism; (7) folding mirror; (8) cross-hair reticle; (9) field lens; (10) planar mirrors; (11) beam splitter, fold mirror, lens assembly; (12) binocular eyepiece assembly. (Copyright Taunton Technologies, Inc.)

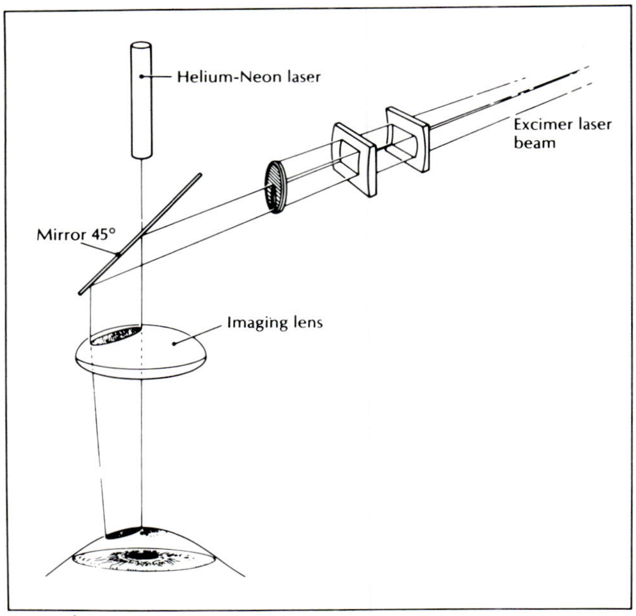

FIGURE 1.21. Diagram of the rotating-slit delivery system for argon fluoride excimer laser nonuniform lamellar keratectomy for myopic correction. (From Hanna KD et al: *Arch Ophthalmol* 106:245, 1988. Copyright 1988, American Medical Association.)

toring throughout the ablation procedure is possible with all existing ophthalmic excimer laser instruments.

Instrumental Variations

Hanna and others[19,20] developed a rotating-slit delivery system for nonuniform lamellar keratectomies that could be used for the correction of myopia, hyperopia, and myopic and hyperopic astigmatism (Fig. 1.21). The laser beam was shaped by a slit rotating at 0.033 Hz that, because each pulse was of 23 ns duration, was effectively stationary during each pulse but shifted to another area with subsequent pulses, thereby allowing less energy to dissipate from the corneal surface between pulses. Because the shape of the slit was predetermined, for myopic correction the central part of the ablated zone would be deeper than the peripheral part, and for hyperopic correction the peripheral part of the ablated zone would be deeper than the central part. This rotated-slit configuration reportedly produced a smooth ablation utilizing 4.5 mJ per pulse delivered to the cornea at a repetition rate of 20 Hz. The fluence of the cornea was reported to be 200 mJ/cm^2, and astigmatic corrections could be obtained by varying the laser repetition rate with the angular position of the slit.[21]

In 1987 Loertscher and associates,[22] working with a pulsed hydrogen fluoride laser (Fig. 1.22), and Serdarevic and associates,[23] working with the argon fluoride excimer laser, investigated the feasibility of laser corneal trephination. Using the argon fluoride excimer laser, Serdarevic achieved noncontract corneal trephination that was distinctly more precise than that obtained by mechanical devices.[23] Her delivery system included rotating circular slits that allowed the projection of a hollow circular beam onto the cornea (Fig. 1.23). Pulse energies at the cornea were between 4.0 and 6.6 mJ, and the repetition rates were 15 to 20 Hz. The trephination diameter could be varied from 4 to 8 mm, depending on the distance of the cornea from the spherical lens. This unique trephination instrument will certainly complement our armamentarium of excimer laser uses in the future.

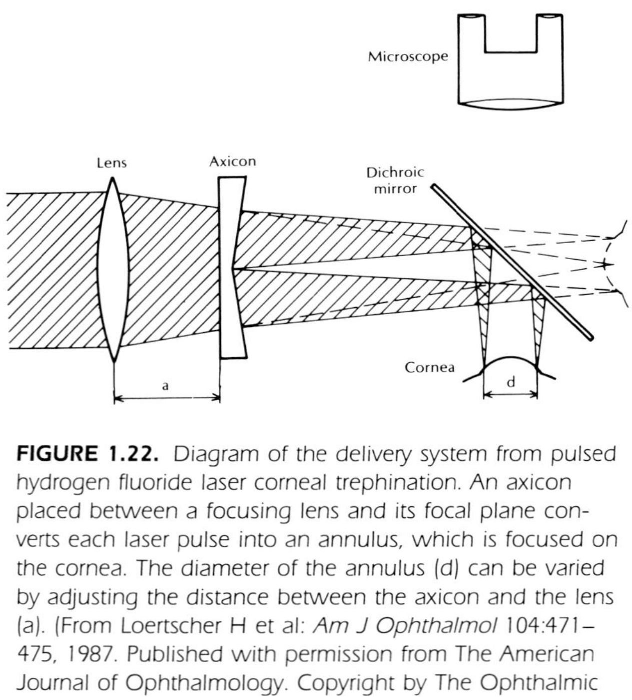

FIGURE 1.22. Diagram of the delivery system from pulsed hydrogen fluoride laser corneal trephination. An axicon placed between a focusing lens and its focal plane converts each laser pulse into an annulus, which is focused on the cornea. The diameter of the annulus (d) can be varied by adjusting the distance between the axicon and the lens (a). (From Loertscher H et al: *Am J Ophthalmol* 104:471–475, 1987. Published with permission from The American Journal of Ophthalmology. Copyright by The Ophthalmic Publishing Company.)

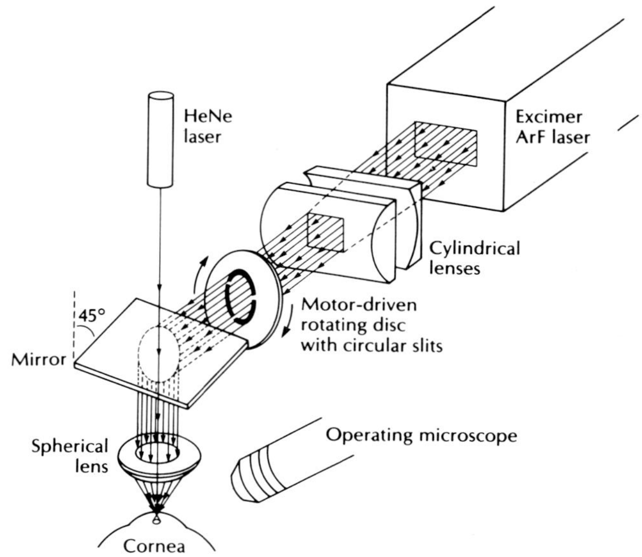

FIGURE 1.23. Diagram of the rotating-slit delivery system for argon fluoride excimer laser corneal trephination. (From Serdarevic ON et al: *Ophthalmology* 95:493–505, 1988. Published by permission of *Ophthalmology*.)

LASER–CORNEAL INTERACTIONS

The excimer laser–corneal interaction was investigated for the first time in 1981 by Taboada and others who studied the response of the corneal epithelium to the 248 nm krypton fluoride[8] and the 193 nm argon fluoride[7] excimer lasers. In 1983 Trokel and associates[13] achieved precise sharply controlled cutting with the argon fluoride excimer laser using masks with narrow slits to ablate bovine corneas, in order to observe the type of laser damage that was created. In addition to finding that there were no thermal effects at that wavelength, they noted that the sides of the laser incisions were parallel and straight and showed little disorganization. They also determined that the tissue ablation rate was approximately 1 μm of corneal tissue removed at a fluence of 1 J/cm^2. A study that compared 193 and 248 nm excimer laser photoablation of freshly enucleated human and bovine eyes was performed by Puliafito and his coworkers[24]; they varied the total number of pulses, the pulse rate, and the fluence (mJ/cm^2) in order to determine the minimal amount of energy per unit area that was required for ablation. They found that a higher amount of radiation is required for the krypton fluoride 248 nm wavelength to produce incisional depths equal to those at the argon fluoride 193 nm wavelength (58 mJ/cm^2 vs. 46 mJ/cm^2 for a human eye). In addition to a higher fluence required for ablation at the 248 nm radiation band, it was also noted by this group that the stromal damage at the edge of the 248 nm incision was wider than that of the 193 nm incision (2.5 vs. 0.3 μm), and greater disorganization and disruption of the corneal tissue were observed at the longer wavelength. Additional work by Krueger and others[25,26] on the quantitative aspects of excimer laser corneal ablation, utilizing various energy densities per pulse at different wavelengths, determined the most efficient wavelengths for ablation of the cornea where a specific amount of impinging energy is converted to the greatest amount of corneal tissue removal. They found that 200 mJ/cm^2 at 193 nm (argon fluoride), 1000 mJ/cm^2 at 248 nm (krypton fluoride), and 1500 mJ/cm^2 at 308 nm (xenon chloride) were the fluences per pulse that were most efficient for ablation at those wavelengths. These particular observations all correspond with the respective absorption coefficients of the various wavelengths, namely, 2700 cm^{-1} at 193 nm, 210 cm^{-1} at 248 nm, and 200 cm^{-1} at 308 nm.

The threshold values at various pulse rates necessary to ablate corneal tissue were also determined by Krueger and his associates.[26] His findings indicated there was no significant production of heat at 193 nm, since the threshold at that wavelength was constant for different pulse rates. At 248 and 308 nm their studies indicated that there is an increase in the threshold at a lower pulse rate, and slight coagulation and vacuolization of the walls of the tissue incision were noted at 248 nm, while extensive corneal coagulation was observed at 308 nm. Thermal mechanisms appear to be increasingly prominent with longer wavelengths, particularly in the ultraviolet portion of the spectrum.

The apparent superiority of the 193 nm argon fluoride excimer laser for photoablative decomposition of the cornea may be explained by several different observations. It is a well-known phenomenon that decreased thermal effects occur at shorter exposure times throughout the visible and near-infrared spectrum. This concept can be conveyed to the exposure at 193 nm whereby not only is the exposure time short, thereby decreasing the thermal deposition or production capabilities, but also the absorption length of the 193 nm wavelength in corneal tissue is extremely short (3.7 μm). Therefore, the laser radiation at 193 nm incurs a minimal amount of heat diffusion beyond the targeted region due to the short pulse duration (10–20 ns) and to the inherent high absorption coefficient and thereby minimal absorption length. With these factors alone, it would be an ideal wavelength for ablation of corneal tissue regardless of any other inherent properties. However, the sufficiently high photon energy (6.4 eV at 193 nm) is more than adequate to disrupt the peptide bonds, which require approximately 3.0 eV, and the carbon–carbon bonds, requiring 3.5 eV for bond disruption, in the polypeptide chains such as seen in the collagenous corneal stroma. Furthermore, the glycosaminoglycans absorb 193 nm radiation highly, are interspersed throughout the collagen of the stroma, and in combination with the inherent peptide intramolecular bond breakage would create a condition for excellent tissue removal with minimal energy density requirements at the argon fluoride 193 nm wavelength.

ANIMAL STUDIES

In 1984, Serdarevic and her associates[27] were the first to apply argon fluoride excimer laser radiation to create a therapeutic lamellar keratectomy in rabbit corneas that had been inoculated with the *Candida albicans* fungus, to produce an inflamed, necrotic cornea. A precise lamellar keratectomy was produced with the argon fluoride excimer laser in these rabbit corneas, and healing progressed with minimal scarring. The fact that the cornea healed with minimal surface irregularities and scarring stimulated further intensive investigation into the use of lamellar keratectomies (uniform and nonuniform) for therapeutic and refractive procedures.[15,16,18-21,28-42]

Radial laser incisions, simulating those found in radial keratotomy, were made by Cotliar and others[43] on enucleated human eyes utilizing argon fluoride excimer laser radiation. Considerable flattening of the cornea (up to 5.35 D) was produced, and the degree of corneal flattening appeared to be a function of the laser energy and incisional depth achieved. Steinert and Puliafito[44] utilized a slit lamp biomicroscope to perform the first in vivo argon fluoride excimer laser radial keratotomy on a rabbit, in a manner similar to that performed by Cotliar. Marshall and his associates[35] produced wide-area keratectomies in living rabbit and monkey corneas with fluences ranging from 140 to 310 mJ/cm^2 per pulse and dosages approximating levels between 50 and 600 pulses per cornea. These investigators noted extremely smooth surfaces, similar to the early findings of Serdarevic,[27] with excimer laser radiation at 193 nm. Puliafito, working with monkey corneas in vivo found that opacification of the treated area occurred within 1 week using 500 pulses, 20 Hz, and 160 mJ/cm^2 per pulse.[24] These divergent findings necessitated the analysis of the beam structure in order both to ensure its homogeneity and to create a beam with a flat surface configuration. The remarkable instrumental changes that were created to modify the beam, have been enumerated in the instrumentation section.

Marshall and associates[45] continued their work with an argon fluoride excimer instrument and ablated 3 mm diameter discs in monkey corneas to depths of 40 to 130 μm. Postoperatively, most of the corneas were clear for several weeks, but then became hazy and showed opacification. By electron microscopy, Marshall and his associates[45] showed that a "pseudomembrane" covered the surface of the keratectomy area, much like Bowman's membrane, and reconstituted the deeper epithelial layer until a natural basement membrane could form. The concept of the pseudomembrane is still perceived as a transitional phase, between the irradiated stromal bed and the overlying new epithelium. Del Pero and his associates,[14] using the calculations of Munnerlyn to determine the ablation diameters and depths necessary to correct spherical refractive errors,[38] ablated 4 to 7 mm diameter zones of monkey corneas in order to produce myopic and hyperopic corrections of approximately 6 D. Slit lamp examinations showed at the epithelial–stromal interface in all monkey corneas a mild granular haze that gradually decreased with the passage of time. For the first time, regression of the original dioptric corneal correction was noted, so that at 18 months a considerable amount of the original myopic flattening and the hyperopic steepening had been lost. McDonald and her associates[46] treated a series of monkeys with energy densities of 160 mJ/cm^2 per pulse and utilized 5 pulses per second with a finely regulated slowly closing iris diaphragm. Five-mm-diameter nonuniform keratectomy zones were produced at depths intended to correct 1.50 and 3.00 D of myopia. Although an early fibrillar haze was reported with all the monkey corneas, it was noted that the corneas were clear at 17 weeks and remained through an interval of 1 year. Goodman and her associates[47] utilized an argon fluoride excimer laser system that produced small pulsed steps of 0.25 μm and demonstrated from their studies that keratectomies of 50 μm or less showed no haze at 8 weeks, although those keratectomies extending to 100 μm revealed opacification at the same time interval. The rationale to explain the increased opacification at 100 μm has still not been explained satisfactorily. Therefore, regression of the intended dioptric power change and faint haze at the stromal–epithelial interface have remained persistent, although extremely subtle, problems.

HUMAN STUDIES

Following the development of the argon fluoride excimer laser clinical instruments, L'Esperance in 1987[15,16] and Taylor in 1988[17,48] performed the first photorefractive keratectomy trial on humans using the Taunton Technologies argon fluoride excimer laser instrument. These first human wide-area lamellar keratectomies were conducted under the auspices of the first FDA investigational device exemption granted in the United States for the correction of refractive errors by the excimer laser and were restricted to excimer laser keratectomies in blind eyes or those eyes scheduled for enucleation (Figs. 1.5–1.9). Parameters of 80 to 125 mJ/cm^2 per pulse at a repetition rate of 10 Hz were used, which produced superficial keratectomies that were 3 to 4.5 mm in diameter and ranged in depth from 30 to 150 μm. The early clinical and histopathologic findings (Figs. 1.24–1.29) were similar to those found during the animal studies and confirmed the fact that a fine fibrillar haze existed in the area of excimer laser treatment and disappeared with the passage of time. Regression of the intended dioptric power also occurred and corresponded with findings documented in the animal studies. In 1988 Seiler and others[49] published the results of their use of the excimer laser to create linear corneal T excisions in order to correct astigmatism in a series of blind and some sighted human eyes. In 1990 Seiler[50]

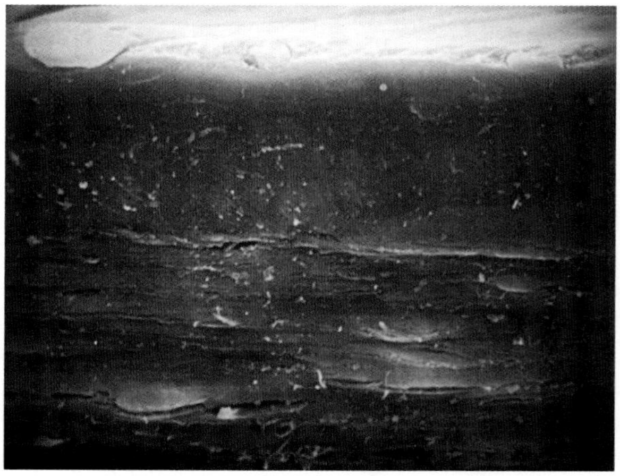

FIGURE 1.24. Scanning electron micrograph (short term) showing absence of Bowman's membrane, and the epithelium in direct contact with the irradiated and excised anterior stroma in the treated corneal zone. (Copyright Taunton Technologies, Inc.)

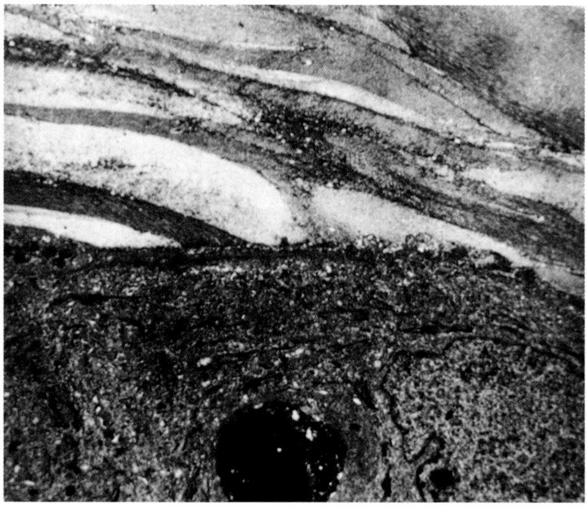

FIGURE 1.25. Transmission electron micrograph (short term) showing a large epithelial cell in direct apposition to the ablated corneal lamellae with a suggestion of a slightly electron-dense epithelial–stromal interface layer. (Copyright Taunton Technologies, Inc.)

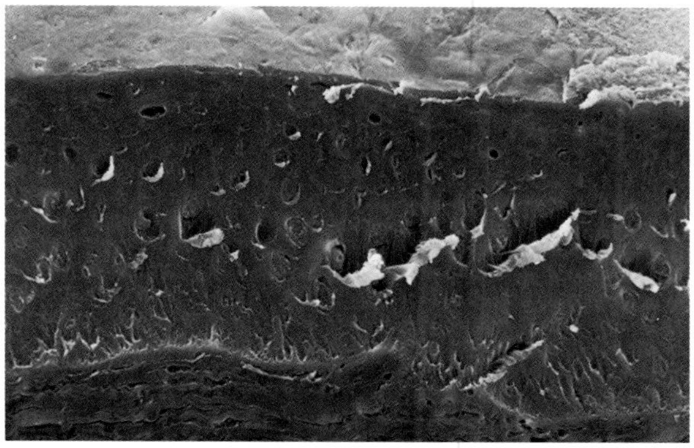

FIGURE 1.27. Scanning electron micrograph (long term) of the corneal button that was excised at the time of corneal transplantation 4 months after excimer laser keratectomy. The micrograph shows somewhat hyperplastic epithelium lying directly on the keratectomy site in firm apposition to the stromal layers without evidence of Bowman's membrane. (Copyright Taunton Technologies, Inc.)

reported on his results with photorefractive keratectomy on blind and sighted human eyes. Using a laser fluence of 180 mJ/cm^2 at 10 pulses per second, they were able to treat 4.5 mm diameter areas for the correction of axial myopia, ranging from -2.00 to -6.00 D. In some cases, patients with as much as -10.00 D of myopia were treated utilizing 3.5 mm diameter keratectomies in order to decrease the depth of the keratectomy required to correct this degree of myopia. In most eyes, they reported an early overcorrection that generally reversed, while several of the eyes regressed beyond 1.00 D of the intended initial correction.

In a study reported in 1990, McDonald and oth-

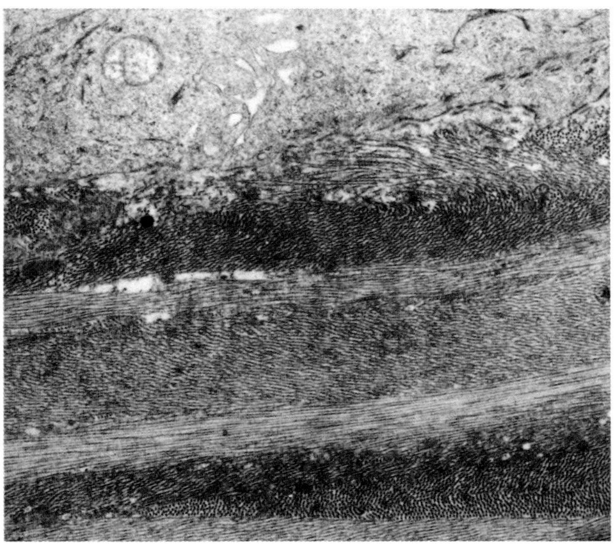

FIGURE 1.26. Transmission electron micrograph (short term) of the epithelial–stromal interface, showing direct adhesion of the overlying epithelium to the underlying ablated stroma. (Copyright Taunton Technologies, Inc.)

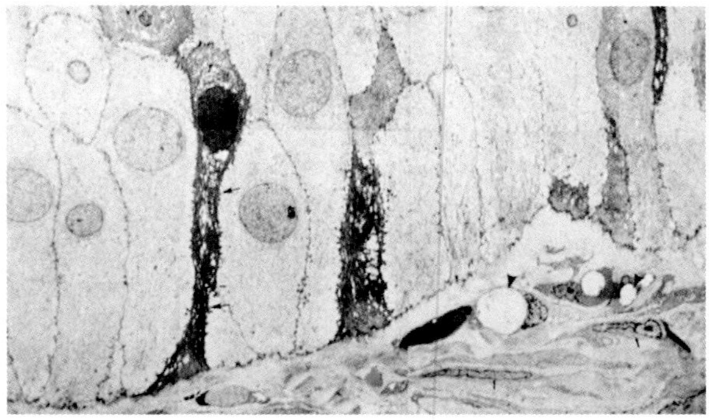

FIGURE 1.28. Transmission electron micrograph (long term) of the corneal button removed 4 months after laser–corneal tissue interaction, showing the periphery of the portion that underwent excimer laser keratectomy. The corneal epithelium in the ablated area is firmly adherent to the underlying corneal stroma. Numerous extremely elongated basal epithelial cells indicated by arrows are noted; Bowman's layer is absent, although there is an increased number of spindle-shaped fibroblasts, noted by arrows present in the subepithelial tissue. Some of the cells, particularly toward the periphery, contain numerous vacuoles indicated by the arrowheads, and some are extracellularly evident. (Copyright Taunton Technologies, Inc.)

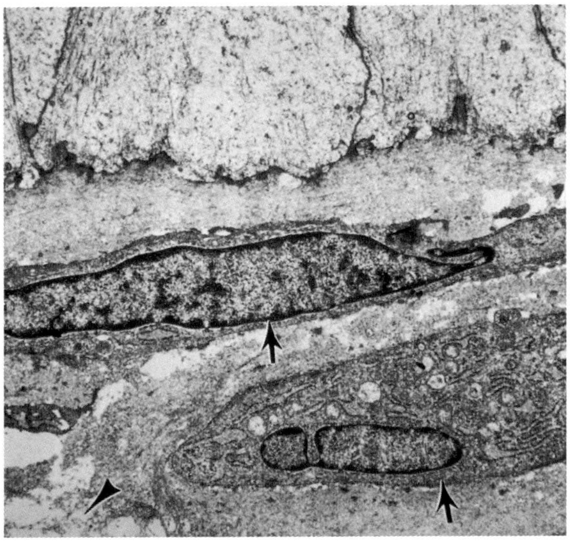

FIGURE 1.29. Transmission electron micrograph (long term) of the central portion of the laser keratectomy region, showing a firm adherence of the corneal epithelium to the underlying stroma, and presence of numerous elongated basal cells. Higher magnification of two fibroblasts, noted by the arrows, in close proximity to each other can be seen in the subepithelial tissue. An abundant amount of electrolucent material is also noted in the extracellular spaces indicated by the arrowhead. (Copyright Taunton Technologies, Inc.)

ers[51] performed photorefractive keratectomy on nine blind eyes, using a VISX ophthalmic excimer laser instrument that utilized laser energy density and pulsing parameters similar to those used by Seiler and his coworkers.[50] Two-thirds of the corneas treated showed a residual fibrillar haze and regression of the intended refractive correction, seen to be greater with a greater intended dioptric change in a particular eye. These changes were also corroborated by the results of previous animal studies.

In 1990 Zabel, working with the University of Minnesota Group,[52] reported a study of six sighted eyes that underwent photorefractive keratectomy for myopic corrections of −5.50 to −12.00 D. Using a Taunton Technologies ophthalmic excimer laser instrument with energy parameters of 100 mJ/cm^2 per pulse and repetition rates of 5 Hz, they utilized the 15 apertures to create 5 mm diameter circular keratectomies. A fine reticular haze was reported in all patients at 1 week; this haze decreased remarkably by 6 weeks, and a high percentage of patients achieved excellent vision at 6 weeks. The importance of using 0.1% fluorometholone was reinforced because these patients remained within 1.00 D of their intended correction during the duration of the investigation. The exact strength or duration of therapy with the anti-inflammatory agents or other pharmaceuticals that may enhance the healing process is still under significant study.

Recently, McDonnell and coworkers[53] utilized excimer laser photorefractive keratectomy to perform toric ablations designed to correct cylindrical astigmatic errors. An expanding slit was used to flatten the cornea in the steep meridian. In each of four patients, surgery reduced the regular component of the astigmatism, although all patients experienced a shift in the spherical equivalent toward hyperopia. Toric ablations with the excimer laser show great promise and appear to represent a strategy for the correction of compound myopic astigmatism.[53]

In a multicenter study Sher and his associates[54] performed photorefractive keratectomy utilizing the argon fluoride excimer laser on 31 sighted myopic eyes ranging from −12.00 to −4.00 D. All patients returned to a corrected visual acuity within one line of their preoperative visual acuity. At 6 months, 68% of the eyes were corrected within 2.00 D of the intended result, and 55% within 1.00 D of the attempted correction. There was no significant change in astigmatism, contrast sensitivity, corneal sensation, or endothelial cell counts.[54]

This chapter has been intended to be a review of the history and development of the excimer laser for corneal surgery, especially phototherapeutic keratectomy and photorefractive keratectomy. The number of brilliant research endeavors that have not been mentioned in this narrative is considerable, and these teams should all be commended for their interest, innovation, and perseverence.[55-76] The use of short-wavelength ultraviolet, high-photon-energy laser radiation should ultimately prove to be one of the great technologic advances in ophthalmology and other fields of medicine.

REFERENCES

1. In *Laser Pioneer Interviews,* 1st ed. Torrance, CA, High Tech Publications (*Lasers and Applications* issues), 1985, p. 181.
2. Houtermans FG: *Helv Phys Acta* 33:933, 1969.
3. In *Laser Pioneer Interviews,* 1st ed. Torrance, CA, High Tech Publications (*Lasers and Applications* issues), 1985, p 182.
4. Rhodes CK: *Excimer Lasers: Topics in Applied Physics.* Berlin, Springer-Verlag, 1979, vol 30, pp 130, 180.

5. Huestis DL: The excimer age. Lasing with the new breed. *Optical Spectra* 13:51–55, 1979.
6. Ruderman W: Excimer lasers in photochemistry. *Laser Focus* May 1979, pp 68–69.
7. Taboada J, Archibald CJ: An extreme sensitivity in the corneal epithelium to far UV-ArF excimer laser pulses. In *Proceedings of the Aero-Space Medical Association, 52nd Annual Meeting*. Washington, DC, Aerospace Medical Association, 1981, pp 8–9.
8. Taboada J, Mikesell GW, Reed RD: Response of the corneal epithelium to KrF excimer laser pulses. *Health Phys* 40:766, 1981.
9. Srinivasan R, Mayne-Banton V: Self-developing photoetching of poly(ethylene terephthalate) films by far-ultraviolet excimer laser radiation. *Appl Phys Lett* 41:576–578, 1982.
10. Srinivasan R, Leigh WJ: Ablative photodecomposition: Action of far-ultraviolet (193 nm) laser radiation on poly(ethylene terephthalate) films. *J Am Chem Soc* 104:6784, 1982.
11. Linsker R, Srinivasan R, Wynne JJ, et al: Far-ultraviolet laser ablation of atherosclerotic lesions. *Lasers Surg Med* 4:201–206, 1984.
12. Srinivasan R, Wynne JJ, Blum SE: Far-UV photoetching of organic material. *Laser Focus* 19:62, 1983.
13. Trokel SL, Srinivasan R, Braren B: Excimer laser surgery of the cornea. *Am J Ophthalmol* 96:710–715, 1983.
14. Del Pero RA, Gigstad JE, Roberts AD, et al: A refractive and histopathologic study of excimer laser keratectomy in primates. *Am J Ophthalmol* 109:419–429, 1990.
15. L'Esperance FA Jr, Taylor DM, Warner JW: Human excimer laser keratectomy: Short term histopathology. *J Refract Surg* 4:118, 1988.
16. L'Esperance FA Jr, Taylor DM, Del Pero RA, et al: Human excimer laser corneal surgery: Preliminary report (presented at the American Ophthalmological Society Meeting, Hot Springs, May 22–25, 1988). *Trans Am Ophthalmol Soc* 86:208–275, 1988.
17. Taylor DM, L'Esperance FA, Del Pero RA, et al: Human excimer laser lamellar keratectomy: A clinical study. *Ophthalmology* 96:654–664, 1989.
18. L'Esperance FA Jr, Warner JW, Telfair WB, et al: Excimer laser instrumentation and technique for human corneal surgery. *Arch Ophthalmol* 107:131–139, 1988.
19. Hanna K et al: A rotating-slit delivery system for excimer laser refractive keratoplasty. *Am J Ophthalmol* 103:474, 1987.
20. Hanna KD et al: Corneal wound healing after excimer laser keratomileusis in rabbits. *Invest Ophthalmol Vis Sci* 29:390, 1988.
21. Hanna KD, Chastang JC, Pouliquen Y, et al: Excimer laser keratectomy for myopia with a rotating-slit delivery system. *Arch Ophthalmol* 106:245, 1988.
22. Loertscher H et al: Noncontact trephination of the cornea using a pulsed hydrogen fluoride laser. *Am J Ophthalmol* 104:471, 1987.
23. Serdarevic ON et al: Excimer laser trephination in penetrating keratoplasty: Morphologic features and wound healing. *Ophthalmology* 95:493, 1988.
24. Puliafito CA, Steinert RF, Deutsch TF, et al: Excimer laser ablation of the cornea and lens: Experimental studies. *Ophthalmology* 92:741–748, 1985.
25. Krueger RR, Trokel SL: Quantitation of corneal ablation by ultraviolet laser light. *Arch Ophthalmol* 103:1741, 1985.
26. Krueger RR, Trokel SL, Schubert HD: Interaction of ultraviolet laser light with the cornea. *Invest Ophthalmol Vis Sci* 26:1455, 1985.
27. Serdarevic ON et al: Excimer laser therapy for experimental *Candida* keratitis. *Am J Ophthalmol* 99:534, 1985.
28. Berlin M, Bende T, Seiler T: Corneal resurfacing by excimer laser photoablation. *Invest Ophthalmic Vis Sci* 29:310, 1988.
29. Burstein N: Corneal epithelial, stromal and endothelial response to excimer laser ablation. Paper presented at the Laser Symposium, CLAO-ISRK. Annual Meeting, Las Vegas, Jan 16, 1988.
30. Del Pero RA et al: Human excimer laser lamellar refractive keratectomy: A clinical study. *Invest Ophthalmol Vis Sci* 29:281, 1988.
31. Fantes F et al: Excimer radiant exposure and quality of surface ablation. *Invest Ophthalmol Vis Sci* 29:309, 1988.
32. Gaster et al: Excimer laser ablation and wound healing of superficial cornea in rabbits and primates. *Invest Ophthalmol Vis Sci* 29:309, 1988.
33. Kerr-Muir MG et al: Ultrastructural comparison of conventional surgical and argon fluoride excimer laser keratectomy. *Am J Ophthalmol* 103:448, 1987.
34. Mandel ER et al: Excimer laser large area ablation of the cornea. *Invest Ophthalmol Vis Sci* 28:275, 1987.
35. Marshall J, Trokel SL, Rothery S, et al: Photoablative reprofiling of the cornea using an excimer laser: Photorefractive keratectomy. *Lasers Ophthalmol* 1:21, 1986.
36. McDonald MB et al: Refractive surgery with the excimer laser. *Am J Ophthalmol* 103:469, 1987.
37. McDonald M et al: Excimer laser surface shaping of the primate cornea for the correction of myopia. *Invest Ophthalmol Vis Sci* 29:310, 1988.
38. Munnerlyn CR, Koons SJ, Marshall J: Photorefractive keratectomy: A technique for laser refractive surgery. *J Cataract Refract Surg* 14:46, 1988.
39. Pouliquen Y: Wound healing after excimer laser keratomileusis. Paper presented at the International Cornea Laser Society Meeting, Dallas, Nov 7, 1987.
40. Renard G et al: Excimer laser experimental keratectomy: An ultrastructural study. *Cornea* 6(4):269, 1987.
41. Tuft S, Zabel R, Marshall J: Corneal remodeling following anterior keratectomy. *Invest Ophthalmol Vis Sci* 29:310, 1988.
42. Zabel R, Tuft S, Marshall J: Excimer laser photorefractive keratectomy: Endothelial morphology following area ablation of the cornea. *Invest Ophthalmol Vis Sci* 29:390, 1988.

43. Cotliar AM, Schubert HD, Mandel ER, et al: Excimer laser radial keratotomy. *Ophthalmology* 92:206, 1985.
44. Steinert RF, Puliafito CA: Corneal incisions with the excimer laser. In Sanders DR, Hofmann RF, Salz JJ (eds): *Refractive Corneal Surgery*. Thorofare, NJ, Charles Slack, 1986, pp 401–410.
45. Marshall J, Trokel SL, Rothery S, et al: Long-term healing of the central cornea after photorefractive keratectomy using an excimer laser. *Ophthalmology* 95:1411, 1988.
46. McDonald MB, Frantz JM, Klyce SD, et al: One-year refractive results of central photorefractive keratectomy for myopia in the nonhuman primate cornea. *Arch Ophthalmol* 108:40, 1990.
47. Goodman GL, Trokel SL, Stark WJ, et al: Corneal healing following laser refractive keratectomy. *Arch Ophthalmol* 107:1799–1803, 1989.
48. Taylor DM, L'Esperance FA, Warner JW, et al: Experimental corneal studies with the excimer laser. *J Cataract Refract Surg* 15:384, 1989.
49. Seiler T, Bende T, Wollensak J, et al: Excimer laser keratectomy for correction of astigmatism. *Am J Ophthalmol* 105:117, 1988.
50. Seiler T, Kahle G, Kriegerowski M: Excimer laser (193 nm) myopic keratomileusis in sighted and blind human eyes. *Refract Corneal Surg* 6:165, 1990.
51. McDonald MB, Frantz JM, Klyce SD, et al: Central photorefractive keratectomy for myopia: The blind eye study. *Arch Ophthalmol* 108:799, 1990.
52. Zabel RW, Sher NA, Ostrov CS, et al: Myopic excimer laser keratectomy: A preliminary report. *Refract Corneal Surg* 6:329, 1990.
53. McDonnell PJ, Moreira H, Clapham TN, et al: Photorefractive keratectomy for astigmatism. *Arch Ophthalmol* 109:1370–1373, 1991.
54. Sher NA et al: The use of the 193-nm excimer laser for myopic photorefractive keratectomy in sighted eyes—A multicenter study. *Arch Ophthalmol* 109: 1525–1530, 1991.
55. Aron Rosa DS, Boerner CF, Gross M, et al: Wound healing following excimer laser radial keratotomy. *J Cataract Refract Surg* 14:173, 1988.
56. Bende T, Seiler T, Wollensak J: Side effects in excimer corneal surgery. Corneal thermal gradients. *Graefes Arch Clin Exp Ophthalmol* 226:277, 1988.
57. Berns MW, Liaw L-H, Oliva A, et al: An acute light and electron microscopic study of ultraviolet 193-nm excimer laser corneal incisions. *Ophthalmology* 95: 1422, 1988.
58. Dehm EJ, Puliafito CA, Adler CM, et al: Corneal endothelial injury following excimer laser ablation at 193 and 248 nm. *Arch Ophthalmol* 104:1364, 1986.
59. Fantes FE, Hanna KD, Waring GO, et al: Wound healing after excimer laser keratomileusis (photorefractive keratectomy) in monkeys. *Arch Ophthalmol* 108:665, 1990.
60. Fantes FE, Waring GO: Effect of excimer laser radiant exposure on uniformity of ablated corneal surface. *Lasers Surg Med* 9:533, 1989.
61. Hanna KD, Pouliquen YM, Waring GO, et al: Corneal stromal wound healing in rabbits after 193-nm excimer laser surface ablation. *Arch Ophthalmol* 107:895, 1989.
62. Hanna KD, Pouliquen YM, Savoldelli M, et al: Corneal wound healing in monkeys 18 months after excimer laser photorefractive keratectomy. *Refract Corneal Surg* 6:340, 1990.
63. Lieurance RC, Patel AC, Wan WL, et al: Excimer laser cut lenticules for epikeratophakia. *Am J Ophthalmol* 103:475, 1987.
64. Liu JC, McDonald MB, Varnell R, et al: Myopic excimer laser photorefractive keratectomy: An analysis of clinical correlations. *Refract Corneal Surg* 6:321, 1990.
65. Malley DS, Steinert RF, Puliafito CA, et al: Immunofluorescence study of corneal wound healing after excimer laser anterior keratectomy in the monkey eye. *Arch Ophthalmol* 108:1316–1322, 1990.
66. McDonnell PJ, Moreira H, Garbus J, et al: Photorefractive keratectomy to create toric ablations for correction of astigmatism. *Arch Ophthalmol* 109:710, 1991.
67. Peyman GA, Kuszak JR, Weckstrom K, et al: Effects of XeCL excimer laser on the eyelid and anterior segment structures. *Arch Ophthalmol* 104:118, 1986.
68. Puliafito CA, Stern D, Krueger RR, et al: High-speed photography of excimer laser ablation of the cornea. *Arch Ophthalmol* 105:1255, 1987.
69. Puliafito CA, Wong K, Steinert RF: Quantitative and ultrastructural studies of excimer laser ablation of the cornea at 193 and 248 nanometers. *Lasers Surg Med* 7:155, 1987.
70. Seiler T, Wollensak J: Myopic photorefractive keratectomy with the excimer laser. *Ophthalmology* 98:1156–1163, 1991.
71. Sher NA, Bowers RA, Zabel RW, et al: Clinical use of the 193-nm excimer laser in the treatment of corneal scars. *Arch Ophthalmol* 109:491, 1991.
72. Thompson KP, Barraquer E, Parel J-M, et al: Potential use of lasers for penetrating keratoplasty. *J Cataract Refract Surg* 15:397, 1989.
73. Thompson KP, Hanna K, Waring GO: Emerging technologies for refractive surgery: Laser adjustable synthetic epikeratoplasty. *Refract Corneal Surg* 5:46, 1989.
74. Thompson KP: Will the excimer laser resolve the unsolved problems with refractive surgery? *Refract Corneal Surg* 6:315–317, 1990.
75. Tuft SJ, Zabel RW, Marshall J: Corneal repair following keratectomy: A comparison between conventional surgery and laser photoablation. *Invest Ophthalmol Vis Sci* 30:1769–1777, 1989.
76. Waring GO: Development of a system for excimer laser corneal surgery. *Trans Am Ophthalmol Soc* 87:854, 1989.

CHAPTER 2

Corneal Topography in Refractive Keratectomy

STEPHEN D. KLYCE

The use of the argon-fluoride 193 nm excimer laser for photorefractive keratectomy (PRK) has spawned renewed interest in keratorefractive surgery, particularly because this technology offers the potential for a more precise correction of myopia than might be possible with alternative surgical techniques. The efficacy of this approach will be reviewed and, where appropriate, compared with radial keratotomy (currently the most prevalent form of refractive surgery) using the powerful new technology of computerized analysis of corneal topography.

The author is indebted to his collaborators in corneal topography for their many contributions reviewed in this chapter. Particular recognition is due to Dr. Herbert E. Kaufman for his foresight in directing me to explore the avenue of corneal topography to help with the improvement of keratorefractive surgery and to Dr. Marguerite B. McDonald, whose excimer patients form the population from which the data and conclusions presented in this chapter are drawn.

The work reported in this chapter was supported in part by Public Health Service grants EY03311, EY08101, and EY02377 from the National Eye Institute, National Institutes of Health, Bethesda, Md., and by research grants and equipment donations from Computed Anatomy, Inc., New York, N.Y.

Dr. Klyce has been a paid consultant to Computed Anatomy, Inc.; he has no financial or proprietary interests in any other devices or treatments mentioned in this chapter.

The outcome of refractive surgery has been best evaluated by comparing the induced change in refraction with the desired change; this comparison provides a measure of predictability for a specific procedure. Although this correlation seems justified by the goals of keratorefractive surgery—to optimize visual acuity and eliminate the need for corrective appliances—in fact, evaluation of a keratorefractive surgical procedure (which aims to modify corneal curvature) is most objectively accomplished by measuring the alteration of corneal shape. It is necessary to measure the change in refraction, but this clinical parameter alone does not describe the induced change in corneal curvature without confounding variables. During postoperative evaluations, refractions cannot identify those eyes that may have experienced a change in axial length or accommodation. The best assessment tool would measure corneal curvature directly without being subject to the potential errors of interference caused by simultaneous extracorneal changes.

Keratorefractive procedures have undergone substantial development and use in the United States since 1979; this was the stimulus for the evolution of the modern principles of corneal topographic analysis. In this chapter the background of this evolution will be reviewed, and the progress made in applying these principles to the evaluation and improvement of the technique of excimer laser area ablation will be presented.

EARLY METHODS FOR ANALYSIS OF CORNEAL TOPOGRAPHY

While the keratometer (Fig. 2.1) is one of the most accurate tools available for measuring corneal contours, this device measures the curvature of the cornea from only four positions separated by 3 to 4 mm on the paracentral cornea and is specifically designed to measure only spheres and any associated regular or uniform cylinder such as would be represented by the side of an ellipsoid. For fitting rigid contact lenses, keratometer readings are an essential first step in the trial-and-error avenue to success, but the number of trial lenses used is testimony to the woeful inadequacy of the keratometer in this application; corneas are flatter in the periphery than in the paracentral region measured by keratometry, and while the normal cornea may be classified geometrically as having the general shape of the end of an ellipsoid, each person's corneal contours are as unique as his or her fingerprints.[1,2] Keratometry is even less applicable to surgical corneas. Given the fact that keratorefractive surgical procedures do not alter corneal curvature globally from limbus to limbus, and that each type of procedure may produce a different optical zone* diameter of modified corneal surface power, it becomes clear that clinical keratometer readings are insufficient to characterize corneal curvature, at least for post-surgical corneas. Small treatment zone diameter, unintended decentration of treatment, nonuniform effect of treatment and/or preexisting irregular astigmatism often produce misleading keratometer readings, particularly when the measuring mires fall on or beyond the perimeter of the optical zone. Additionally, the change in refraction produced by refractive surgery often is not accurately measured

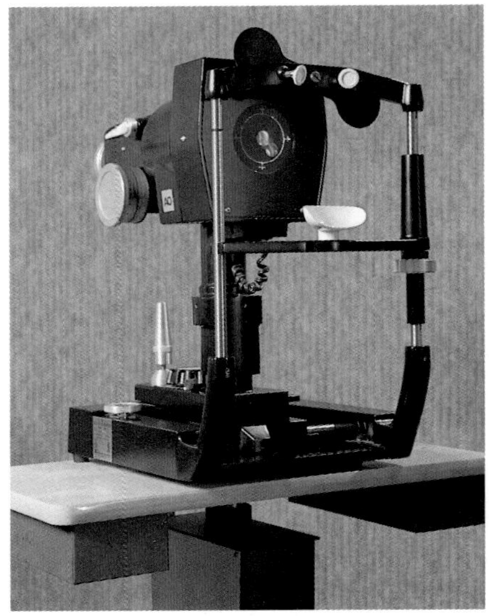

FIGURE 2.1. The American Optical clinical keratometer (CLC Ophthalmometer, Model 11750).

with the keratometer because of keratometer calculational assumptions that neglect corneal thickness change and altered position of the major refracting surface relative to the retina.[3] In sum, the keratometer is generally a highly accurate, reliable, and useful clinical tool, but for the surgical eye or for the eye with congenital or acquired shape anomalies, the keratometer cannot be relied upon for consistently meaningful readings.

In order to add to the curvature information provided by clinical keratometers, photokeratoscopes were developed that enable the photographic capture of Placido disc mires reflected from the surface of the cornea. Using early photokeratoscopes, such as the Nidek model PKS-1000 (Fig. 2.2) or the Kera Corneascope, clinicians were able to appreciate, on a qualitative basis, distortions inherent in individual corneal shapes. For example, moderately advanced keratoconus, high corneal cylinder, and moderate degrees of irregular astigmatism can be easily appreciated from simple visual inspection of photokeratoscope mire patterns (Fig. 2.3). This is done using simple guidelines based on the principles of convex mirror reflections. A highly curved mirror (analogous to a steep cornea) minifies images more than a flatter convex mirror. Hence, with keratoscopy, when the mires appear larger in diameter, broader, or more widely separated than normal, they must arise from regions of the underlying cornea with lower-than-normal surface power. The converse is true for steep areas of the cornea. With this approach, regular corneal cylinder is diagnosed

*In a keratorefractive surgical procedure, the optimal and purely theoretical result would be an alteration of corneal curvature over all of the corneal surface from limbus to limbus. The operation that would achieve this result has not yet been discovered and would necessitate a direct alteration of the purse-string anatomic nature of the limboscleral junction. Rather, keratorefractive procedures have confined themselves to methods that lead to a change in curvature within a confined, generally circular, region of the corneal surface. Most commonly, this circular area of altered corneal curvature or power is dubbed the *optical zone*. It can be loosely defined as that circular region of the corneal surface whose curvature has been altered in a moderately uniform fashion by the surgery.

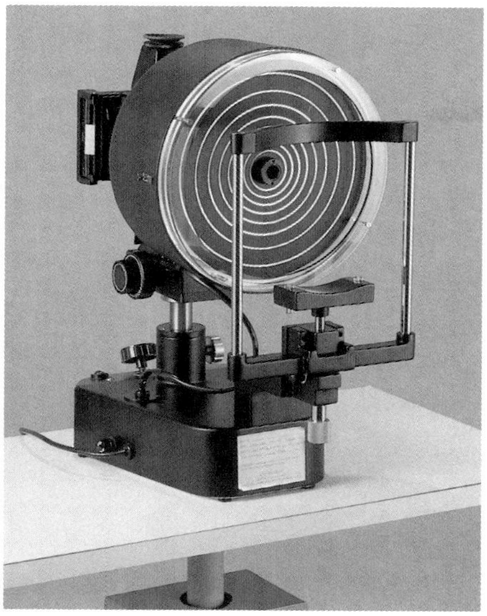

FIGURE 2.2. The Nidek PKS-1000 photokeratoscope.

from the elliptical characteristic of the mires, with the short axis of the ellipse corresponding to the axis of high cylindrical power. Irregular corneal astigmatism is evidenced by nonelliptical distortion of the mires.

Similar visual inspection techniques are currently used with intraoperative keratometers during surgery to reduce the amount of postoperative astigmatism following corneal transplantation.

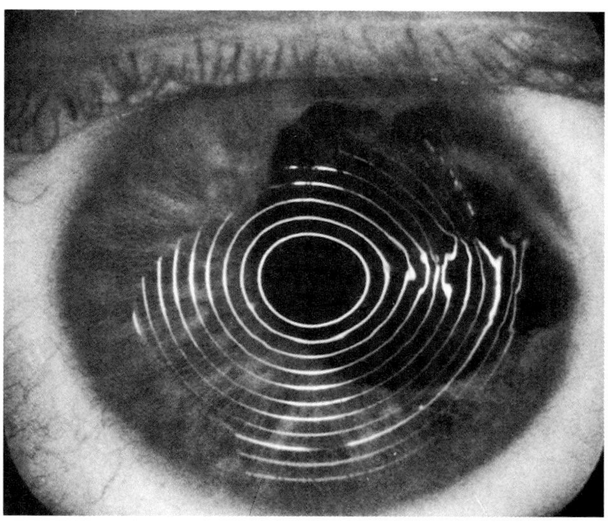

FIGURE 2.3. Keratoscope photograph (made with the Nidek PKS-1000) of an eye recovering from ocular trauma. Using the visual inspection technique, one can observe the severe central astigmatism as well as the peripheral irregular astigmatism in the temporal quadrant of this cornea.

However, the average amount of regular corneal cylinder obtained with corneal transplantation is about 4 D in the experienced corneal surgeon's practice. Unfortunately, the use of current intraoperative keratoscopy does not permit the appreciation or realization of amounts of corneal cylinder less than about 3 D, which constitutes a clinically significant astigmatism. More devastating to spectacle-corrected visual acuity following corneal transplantation is irregular astigmatism, which can have an enormous impact on visual performance; a judgment can be made on the severity of irregular astigmatism by inspecting mire distortion, but keratoscope mires can look remarkably distortion-free even in the presence of severe corneal topographic alterations.[4]

Despite the pioneering efforts of Rowsey to teach the visual inspection method in keratoscopy,[5] there was a clear need for improvements in clinical corneal topography analysis that went beyond the limited information that could be gleaned from reading keratoscope photographs. Four separate technological approaches, each using distinct basic principles, have been attempted to automatically measure corneal shape:* (1) Direct measurement of optical sections through the cornea using both coherent and normal light sources has been tried with both conventional and confocal microscopy. This approach is limited in the accuracy of curvature measurement and does not lend itself to rapid measurement of curvature over a broad corneal surface area. (2) The use of interferometry principles has captured a great deal of interest because of the phenomenal sub-wavelength-of-light precision of measurement promised. While this approach has proven potential for measuring small distortions in optical surfaces, current interference techniques do not have the ability to measure the broad range of surface powers encountered in the clinical corneal practice. (3) Rasterstereography, which uses a direct measurement of corneal shape from a pattern obtained from the fluorescein-stained tear film, has the advantage of being able to measure grossly distorted surfaces (e.g., advanced keratoconus and early postoperative corneal transplants) with good accuracy. The somewhat low sensitivity of the method, however, makes it unsuitable for ascertaining more subtle corneal abnormalities such as the detection of early keratoconus. (4) Finally, computer-automated video keratoscopy has the necessary sensitivity and range (0.25 D or better

*Waring provides an excellent review of the specific instruments, both experimental and commercially available, in his recent textbook.[6]

over 10–100 D) to provide a clinically complete data set. Only this approach has been successful in widespread clinical application.

THE MODERN COMPUTER-AUTOMATED VIDEO CORNEAL TOPOGRAPHIC ANALYSIS SYSTEM

To provide curvature data that would be more useful for clinical diagnosis and application,* a number of advances have been made in the development of computerized keratoscopy;[11-19] these advances permit the analysis of corneal contour over a fairly broad region of the corneal surface. Early approaches to the computerization of corneal topography analysis relied on manual digitization of keratoscope photographs,[11,12] a costly, labor-intensive effort begging for automation. In the mid-1980s, modern digital video image capture and image-processing techniques provided powerful and cost-effective technology to support automatic digitization of mire patterns. At this writing, at least three corneal topography analyzers based upon video keratoscopy are available; purchase prices range from $25,000 to $30,000.[8]

These systems share several features. They all employ circular mire patterns that are projected onto the cornea, where their positions are detected electronically. Each utilizes a reconstruction algorithm of a proprietary nature and of specific design that permits the transformation of the two-dimensional mire shapes to the three-dimensional shape of the individual cornea from which the mire pattern was reflected. The basic principles for creating reconstruction algorithms are readily available from the literature.[11,12,20] The cardinal rule for the algorithms is similar to that given above for the determination of corneal shape from the visual inspection of keratoscope mire distortion: Mires that become larger than normal in diameter arise from a surface that is flatter, and mires that become smaller than normal arise from a surface that is steeper. Between 256 and 360 positions on each mire are determined automatically, and these form the raw data set that is used for surface reconstruction. Each of these reconstruction algorithms necessarily makes approximations[21] as there is no known exact analytic solution, and, in general, such estimates lead to errors in corneal surface power that are greatest in the corneal periphery.[20] Conversely, these implementations lead to generally precise estimates of corneal contour in the central cornea, which is appropriate since this is the most important area for good visual acuity. Nevertheless, comparisons of available devices have appeared in the literature,[22,23] and the accuracy of individual instruments has been assessed. Such determinations can be referred to for an appreciation of instrument capability and reliability. One caveat in the interpretation of such studies is their use of spheres rather than aspheric models resembling corneal topography; when spheres are used for evaluation of accuracy, the results may mask the errors that can arise when the shape of the radially asymmetric, aspheric cornea is measured.[20,24]

A guide to selection of a corneal topography device has been published,[25] but as time passes, the similarities among the instruments increase. However, a major important difference lies in the area of coverage and in the graininess or density (not total number) of points collected and analyzed from the corneal surface. The greater the number of points analyzed per unit area without oversampling, the finer will be the texture or detail provided by the device. Oversampling occurs when points are so close together that the same individual video pixel is sampled multiple times.

In this chapter, the video keratoscope called the Topographic Modeling System (TMS-1, Computed Anatomy, New York, N.Y.)[14,15] is used for purposes of illustration (Fig. 2.4). This device uses a conical 26-ring Placido disc mire pattern to obtain information concerning the degree of distortion in individual corneas (Figs. 2.5 and 2.6). Other measuring cones are available for special applications such as animal studies and contact lens fitting; these

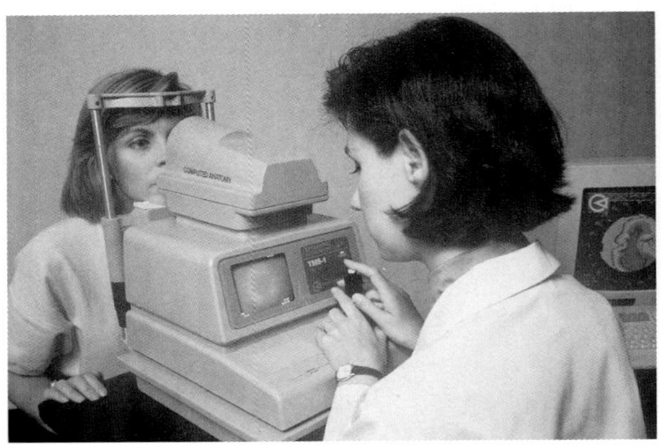

FIGURE 2.4. Topography modeling system (TMS-1).

*The number of clinical applications of computerized corneal topographic analysis has grown explosively over the last few years. A thorough survey of these is beyond the scope of this chapter, but broader overviews of the utility of this clinical test are available.[6-10]

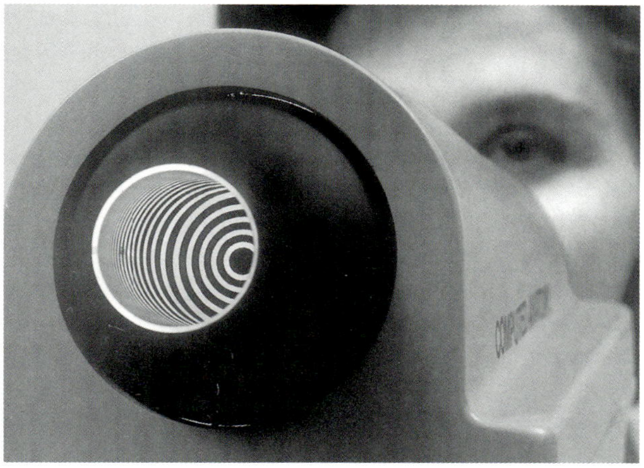

FIGURE 2.5. View of the TMS-1 cone-shaped Placido illuminator. The small size of the cone prevents data loss that normally occurs with other keratoscopes.

additional cones are interchangeable, are internally coded, and are recognized electronically. The conical design has the potential to permit analysis of the entire corneal surface. The normally used cone has 26 rings ranging in diameter on the corneal surface from 0.3 to 9 mm (these are estimates; their actual size is a function of individual corneal curvature). A cone used for contact lens fitting, on the other hand, measures an area 10.5 mm in diameter or more on the cornea.

Perhaps the most important common feature among the new video keratoscopes is the primary method they use for presentation of their data—the color-coded contour map of corneal surface power developed at Louisiana State University (LSU) Eye Center in New Orleans.[13] The video keratoscope gathers corneal curvature information from more than 8000 points on the corneal surface. A discrete data set in a computer printout of all these values would not be particularly easy to use for diagnosis. Hence, we developed and proposed the use of a color-coded contour map of corneal surface powers wherein cool colors (violets, blues) represent low corneal power and warm colors (orange, reds) represent high corneal powers.[13] The so-called *international standard scale* is detailed in Figure 2.7. With this approach to the clinical presentation of corneal surface shape distortions, it has become clear that all the clinically relevant information can be obtained when the interval between the contours of these power plots is set to 1.5 D. A finer, higher-resolution contour interval can be selected; doing so will often reveal topographic features that are not of consequence to visual acuity, but their depiction may be used to inspect the details of a refractive procedure. A specific palette of colors was selected so that one could easily associate the power of an interval with a region of identifiable color. For this reason, monochrome versions or color coding that employs a hue series of one color are limited in their utility. In order to cover the entire range of powers that could be encountered in one cornea, the lower and higher ends of the scale were originally assigned 5 D power intervals. A more popular scale uses 1.5 D intervals over the range of 28.0 to 65.5 D. This graphic design—the color-coded contour map of corneal power—has become the norm

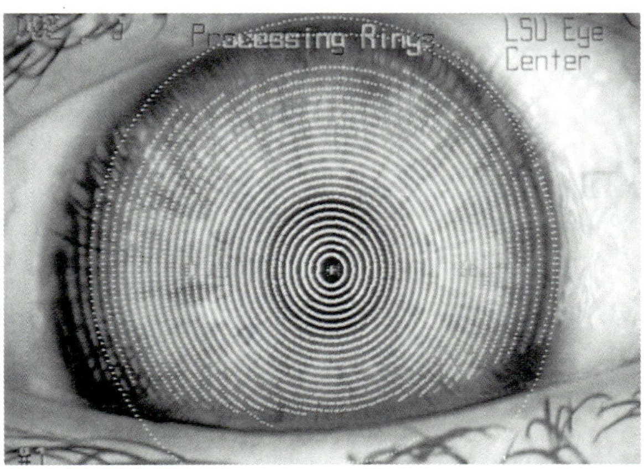

FIGURE 2.6. The mire pattern produced by the standard cone of the TMS-1 video keratoscope. Note the more extensive coverage of the mires by comparison with the keratoscope photograph shown in Figure 2.3.

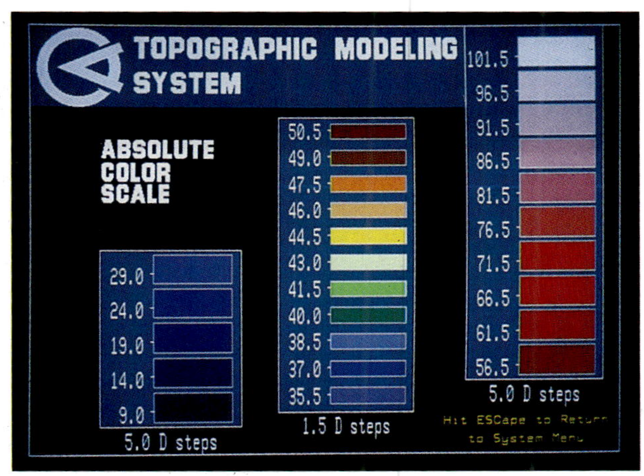

FIGURE 2.7. Absolute color scale (also called the international standard scale) as implemented on the TMS-1 video keratoscope.

in the industry because it permits the diagnosis of extremely subtle corneal shape distortions at a glance. In fact, the modern instrumentation, with its graphic diagnostic aids, has become a standard and necessary clinical tool in keratorefractive surgical practice.

Alternative displays available for use present diopter-at-a-point plots, astigmatism overlays, and isometric presentation, to name a few. Importantly, all of the data can be presented in the form of either corneal power (diopters) or radius of curvature (millimeters); the selection is based on the application. For example, to evaluate corneal topography for keratorefractive surgery, diopters are often selected; for contact lens fitting, radius of curvature in millimeters is often easier to use. Keratoscope reconstruction algorithms provide anterior surface curvatures. To maintain familiarity with the traditional units of the clinical keratometer, *total* corneal power, C_p, in diopters (not corneal *surface* power) is generally calculated directly from radius of curvature, R_c, in millimeters using the keratometric index (337.5):

$$C_p = \frac{337.5}{R_c}$$

The limitations and assumptions made with keratometry calculations are discussed elsewhere;[3] importantly, modern video keratoscopes generally report corneal power. If an application calls for knowledge of corneal *surface* power, one can accurately obtain the original curvature information using the above equation plus Snell's Law.

While the color maps have been quite useful for clinical diagnosis, they are limited to a great extent to descriptive analysis. In order for corneal topography to become a practical tool in clinical trials where numerical values are required to permit comparisons of corneal surface topography, it was necessary to develop quantitative descriptors of corneal surface optical qualities.[26,27] These have taken several forms, but the most useful appear to be descriptors that simulate keratometry values (called SimK) and an index of the corneal surface regularity (abbreviated SRI), both derived from topographic analysis data. The SRI is particularly useful; it was derived from a clinical correlation between the best spectacle-corrected visual acuity of eyes with 20/20 or better visual potential determined by rigid contact lens acuity measurement and a measure of the optical quality (smoothness) of the corneal area over the entrance pupil. The full details of its current implementation are available;[27] however, while the correlation coefficient for this relation was strong (0.8) and highly significant ($P < .001$), work in the area of correlating individual corneal shape with visual performance continues. Improvements in contrast sensitivity tests will most certainly play a part in the process of developing stronger numerical correlates between corneal shape and optical performance.

MINISURVEY OF CORNEAL TOPOGRAPHY WITH THE COLOR-CODED MAP

The display of information from the measurement of corneal shape has taken the form of a color-coded contour map of corneal surface power, as described above. A brief atlas of corneal topography will provide an introduction to the analysis of excimer laser alterations of corneal shape.

With the video keratoscope, the characteristics of the normal cornea can be ascertained (Fig. 2.8).[2] First, the normal cornea is nearly always steeper in the center than in the periphery. Second, a person's corneas often appear to be nonsuperimposable mirror images of each other, or enantiomorphs. Finally, the color-coded contour map of corneal surface powers appears to be unique for each individual cornea. It is quite clear from this type of analysis that the normal cornea has an aspheric and radially asymmetric topography.

One form of commonly encountered corneal topographic distortion is that of regular astigmatism. A with-the-rule regular corneal cylinder often takes the form of a vertically aligned bow-tie-shaped pattern easily visible on the color-coded contour map (Fig. 2.9). Similarly, against-the-rule corneal astigmatism takes the form of a horizontally aligned bow-tie pattern with the higher-power axis running along the meridian at 180° (Fig. 2.10). Irregular corneal astigmatism is displayed as irregularly arrayed contours of varying power distributions (Fig. 2.11); this kind of corneal surface distortion often can be overcome only with the use of rigid contact lenses.

The color-coded contour map is extremely useful for the detection of early keratoconus.[28,29] A typical example is the patient who complains of blurred vision with spectacles but has no other clinical symptoms that might underlie the complaint. Such a patient often has spherical keratometry readings. However, with the color-coded contour map, one can easily detect patterns associated with early keratoconus (Fig. 2.12). In our clinic at LSU, the diagnosis *keratoconus suspect* is no longer written in patient medical records.

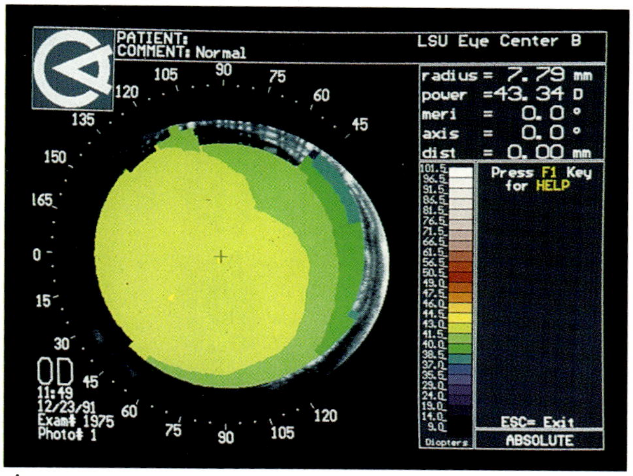

A

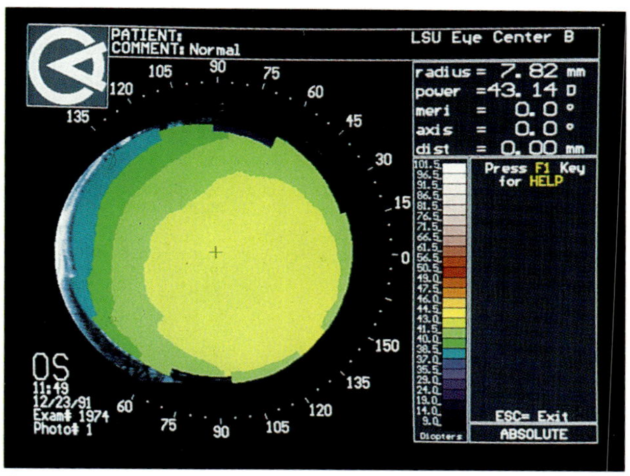

B

FIGURE 2.8. Color-coded contour map of corneal surface powers of a normal eye. (A) Right eye. (B) Left eye. Note the presence of enantiomorphism in the pattern of power distribution in these two video keratographs from the same individual. The cross hairs at the center of the color-coded map can be moved to any position for the purpose of reading the numerical powers or radius of curvature at any analyzed point. The "score box" in the upper right hand corner provides the power, equivalent radius of curvature, and location of the cursor relative to the line of sight.

There is one confounding diagnosis in the determination of early keratoconus from analysis of corneal topography with this modern technology. It is a cone-appearing pattern in the color-coded contour map that results from warpage caused by contact lens wear. It is necessary to eliminate this possibility, particularly if the patient is a candidate for keratorefractive surgery. In a patient with a high-riding contact lens whose cornea also exhibits with-the-rule corneal astigmatism, the high-riding lens tends to flatten the superior segment of the cornea, mak-

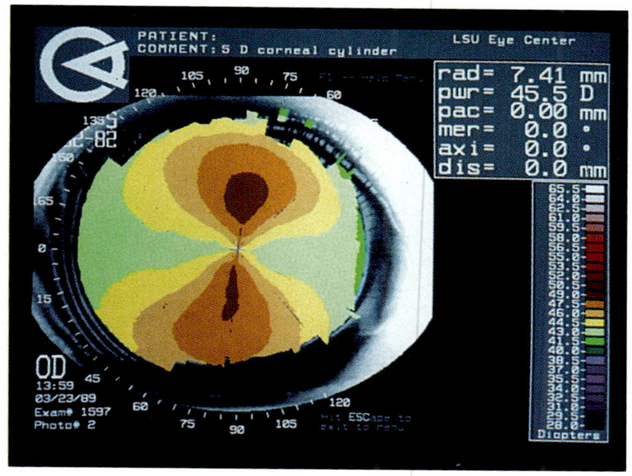

FIGURE 2.9. With-the-rule corneal cylinder, 5 D.

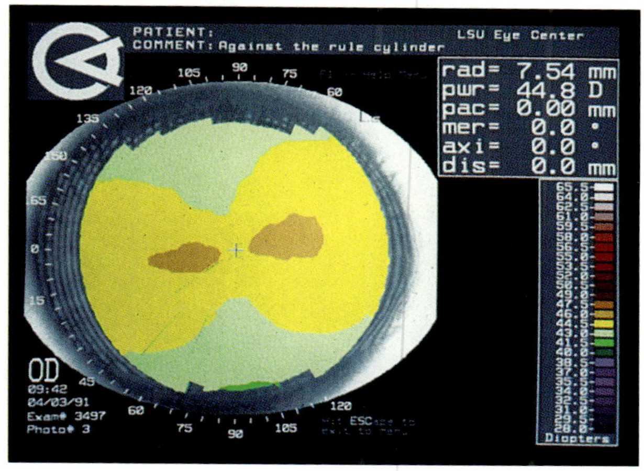

FIGURE 2.10. Against-the-rule corneal cylinder.

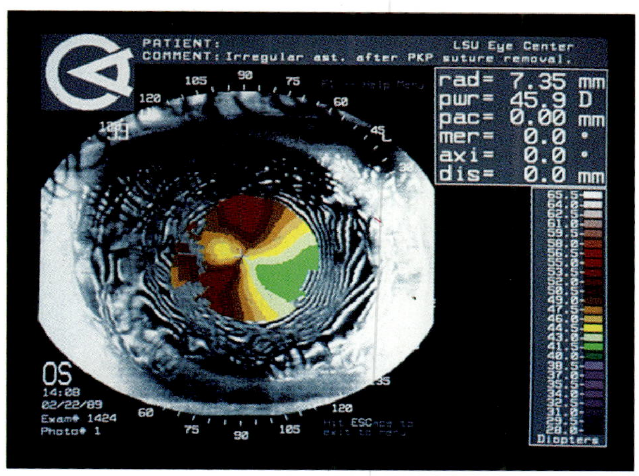

FIGURE 2.11. Irregular astigmatism after corneal transplantation.

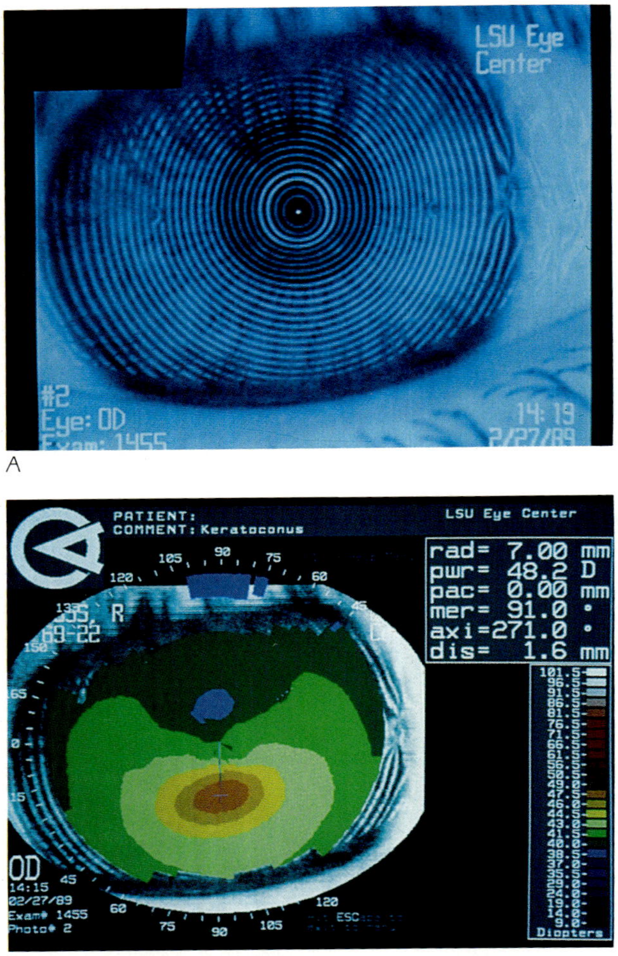

A

B

FIGURE 2.12. Early detection of keratoconus. (A) The presence of keratoconus is not obvious using the visual inspection method on this video image. (B) Analysis of the video image shows an obvious region of elevated power consistent with subclinical keratoconus. The K readings on this cornea were spherical.

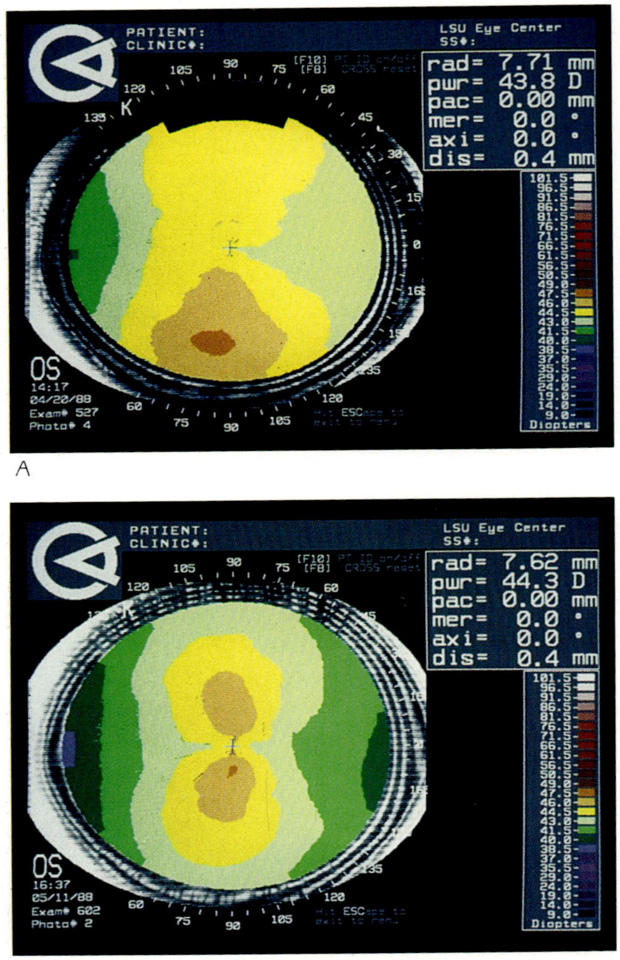

A

B

FIGURE 2.13. Keratoconus or contact lens warpage? (A) Keratoconus-like configuration in a contact lens–wearing patient. (B) Appearance of the same cornea after 3 weeks of not wearing the contact lens. Note the transition to a pattern of ordinary with-the-rule corneal astigmatism.

ing the upper half more spherical. This can leave an area of high power that resembles an incipient cone in the inferior portion of the cornea—the remnant of the preexisting corneal cylinder (Fig. 2.13).[30] Hence, the differential diagnosis between early keratoconus and contact lens warpage with the corneal topography technique is that if there is a history of contact lens use, contact lens wear should be discontinued to determine whether or not this pattern of apparent keratoconus is stable or whether it reverts to with-the-rule corneal cylinder. Contact lens wear may need to be discontinued for a period of months before corneal topography stabilizes, according to recent findings.[31]

Corneal topography analysis has been used productively in the development of specific refractive surgical procedures such as epikeratophakia.[32-35] Through the use of corneal topography analysis, it was found that the early myopic epikeratophakia lenticles had a smaller-than-expected optical zone and that positioning of the lenticle over the center of the pupil was not always optimal. As a result of these findings, the design of the peripheral area of the myopic epikeratophakia lenticle was modified to enlarge the diameter of the optical zone, and changes were made in the way the lenticle was surgically attached to the host cornea. With the information available from corneal topography analysis, these initial problems with this refractive surgical procedure were overcome to a large degree. These findings served to illustrate how powerful this diagnostic technique could be in the evolution of keratorefractive surgical technique.

Corneal topography analysis may be the only tool one can use to make certain evaluations when unexpected outcomes arise from keratorefractive surgery. For example, a patient who had undergone keratomileusis for myopia was referred to the LSU Eye Center. At 1 month postoperative, visual acuity was 20/400 uncorrected and 20/70 with +9.00 +0.25 × 85°. At 6 months there was little improvement and little change in the refraction. When first seen at the LSU Eye Center 9 months after surgery, the patient had an uncorrected visual acuity of 20/200 and a best spectacle-corrected visual acuity of 20/40 with −6.50 +4.50 × 155°. On analysis of this patient's corneal topography, it was clear why the best spectacle-corrected visual acuity was poor. The color-coded contour map showed a steady increase in corneal surface power from the center to the periphery (Fig. 2.14). No region of this cornea had a uniform corneal surface power. This patient refracted over a wide range of powers and achieved satisfactory vision (20/20) only with the use of a hard contact lens.[4] Multifocality can allow a patient to see clearly at near and far when the optics lead to two principal focal points, but in this case, a continuous range of powers present in the corneal surface seriously degraded contrast sensitivity.

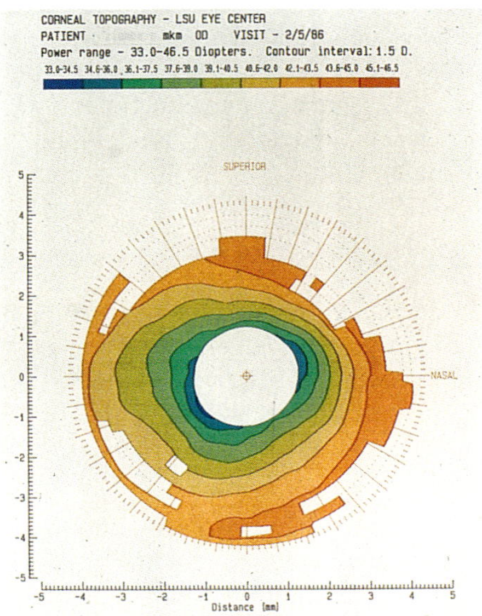

FIGURE 2.14. Original color-coded contour map from the LSU Research System[12,13] showing an analysis of a myopic keratomileusis procedure with poor visual result. (Reproduced with permission from Maguire LJ, Klyce SD, Sawelson H, et al: *Ophthalmic Surg* 18:352–356, 1987.[4])

Radial keratotomy has received worldwide attention in the keratorefractive community and is the most widely used and studied form of surgical correction for myopia. The PERK study[36] reports an 85% success rate in the predictability of outcome (eyes within 2 D of emmetropia) under the carefully controlled circumstances of the multicenter clinical trial. In general, the predictability of outcome is influenced by a number of variables—perhaps the greatest variable is the surgery itself. The micrometer precision of cut depth needed for reproducible results is not a talent that is easily transferred to all surgeons. A frustrating degree of variation can result even in the two eyes of the same patient. In the case illustrated in Figure 2.15, despite the fact that both eyes were operated on in close temporal proximity, by the same surgeon, with the same knife, at the same depth, with the same number of incisions, and with the same size spared optical zone, a disparity of 5 D resulted.

As with all keratorefractive procedures, success can also be limited by individual variations in the

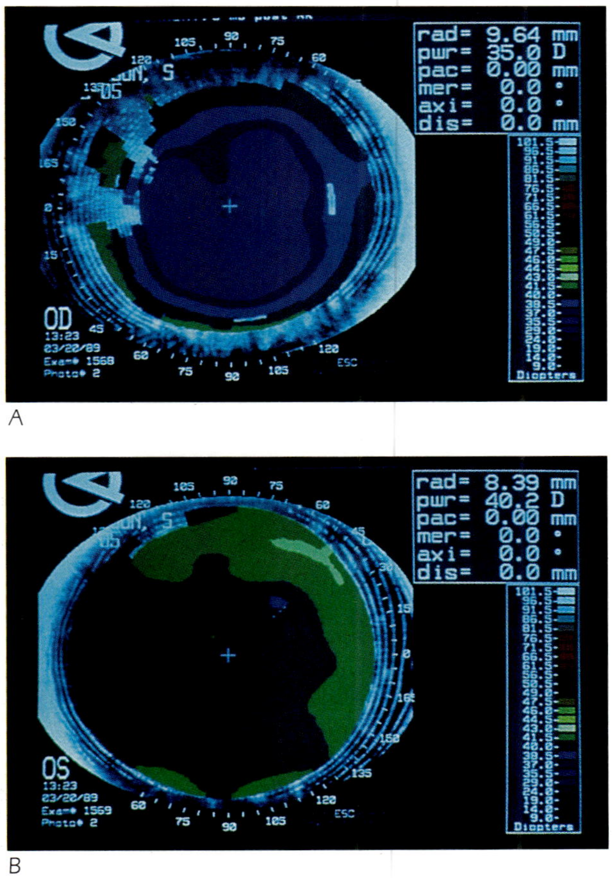

FIGURE 2.15. Corneal topography analysis of radial keratotomy patient. (A) Right eye, with a 7 D correction. (B) Left eye, with a 2 D correction.

biological wound-healing response. While surgical imprecision and biological wound-healing variations can trouble most keratorefractive procedures, it will be seen below that surgery with the excimer laser can largely overcome the precision limitation of both lathe and scalpel methods. The excimer laser removes corneal tissue at the rate of a quarter of a micrometer for each pulse, a level of precision that is far greater than has been achieved with other methods. This potential for accuracy can best be evaluated directly with corneal topographic analysis; color-coded maps and quantitative descriptors can be used to assess three features of the procedure: the optical quality (uniformity) of the treated zone, the predictability and stability of the procedure, and the accuracy of centration of the treated area over the entrance pupil. This information cannot be objectively and directly determined with any other measurement technique.

Parenthetically, for accurate evaluation of the topography of the ablation, it is critical that the excimer laser used to perform the keratorefractive surgery be carefully maintained, inspected, and calibrated prior to use. The extremely short wavelength light energy interacts to some extent with nearly all materials including the transmissive and reflective optical components of the excimer laser and associated delivery system. This interaction decreases the transmission of the beam and can alter the transverse spatial uniformity of the beam profile. The effect of this can seem to be merely a decrease in the apparent efficiency of the laser if the only check made is a measurement of lens power in a test block. However, a beam with a spatially nonuniform profile will produce a spatially nonuniform component to the altered curvature. In the example shown in Figure 2.16, the laser profile had less energy centrally, which inadvertently produced a pseudohyperopic correction. Use of an excimer laser without routine inspection of the beam profile, which can be done by measuring the lens power of a plano ablation in plastic, can impair predictability.

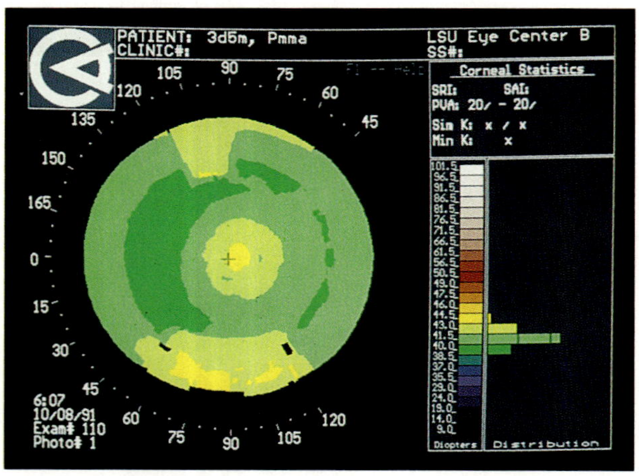

FIGURE 2.16. Plano excimer laser ablation of a 43 D PMMA surface using degraded laser optics. While the topography has the appearance of a hyperopic correction, in this case the nonuniform distribution of power was not intentional.

TOPOGRAPHIC ANALYSIS OF EXCIMER LASER PRK FOR MYOPIA

A number of clinical studies involving the use of the 193-nm excimer laser for the photoablative correction of myopia have been reported.[37-43] Some information in these clinical studies has appeared concerning the application of topographic analysis in the evaluation of the procedure.[44-46] The LSU study results will be described in some detail.

At the time that the data were collected for this review (8/1/91), a total of 98 human eyes had undergone PRK excimer treatment (Table 2.1). Only series III was still accepting new patients. All eyes in all series received preoperative and postoperative corneal topography exams with the TMS-1; postoperative examinations were scheduled at the 1-, 3-, 6-, and 12-month visits. All eyes were treated by the same physician (Dr. Marguerite B. McDonald). The laser used was the 193 nm excimer laser system prototype and later production version of the Twenty/Twenty™ Excimer Laser System (VISX, Sunnyvale, Cal.).

THE LSU BLIND EYE SERIES

As indicated in Table 2.1, nine eyes were included in the LSU blind eye study, which was initiated after extensive animal studies.[46,47] In this series, attempted corrections as high as −11 D were performed to examine the characteristics of the proce-

TABLE 2.1. LSU PRK series to August 1, 1991

Study	*Number of Eyes*
Blind eye	9
Partially sighted	10
Series IIA	19
Series IIB	19
Series III (in progress)	41

dure in humans. Parenthetically, it should be noted that good alignment of the cornea during the corneal topography analysis in these eyes was not possible; therefore, the results from these eyes could not be used to examine procedure centration characteristics. One of the first eyes treated is shown in Figure 2.17. The preoperative topography for this patient was normal, with a relatively spherical central area and flatter peripheral cornea. One month after treatment the power of the central cornea had been altered by −11.3 D. The apparent optical zone was close to the intended diameter of 5 mm, and the ablated area was uniform in its power distribution. Over the course of 1 year, there was a gradual loss of approximately 5 D of the correction, but the power in the treated area remained unchanged between the 6- and 12-month examinations.

A second result from the blind eye series is illustrated in Figure 2.18. This was also a −11 D intended correction, and the initial result at 1 week had the expected decrease in corneal surface power by topographic examination. At 9 weeks there was a pronounced reduction in the diameter of the apparent optical zone, and at 13 weeks essentially all evidence of the ablation had been eliminated. The transition was rapid enough to suggest that the power loss was primarily due to epithelial hyperplasia. With the patient's permission, the central cornea was deepithelialized and the eye patched with 1% atropine drops and gentamicin ointment. One month later (17 weeks postoperative) a final topographic examination gave the same appearance as seen at 13 weeks. During the deepithelialization process, it was noted that the anterior central corneal surface had a loose, gelatinous, and filamentous texture. It was concluded that the loss in cor-

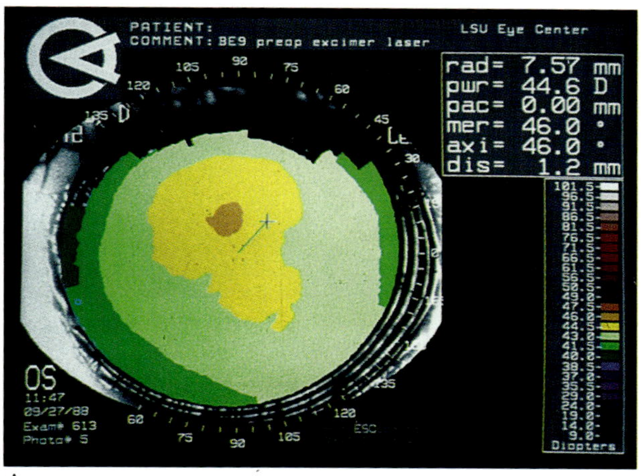

A

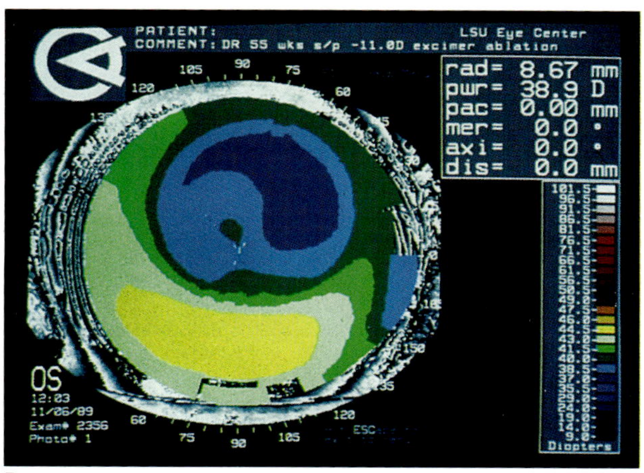

B

FIGURE 2.17. LSU PRK blind eye series. (A) Preoperative video keratograph. (B) One year after surgery.

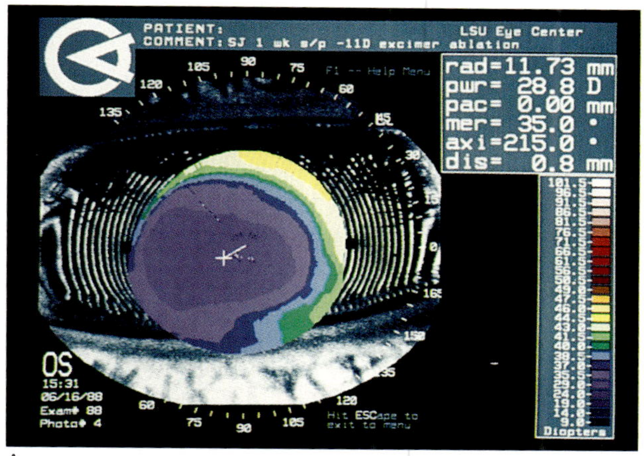

A

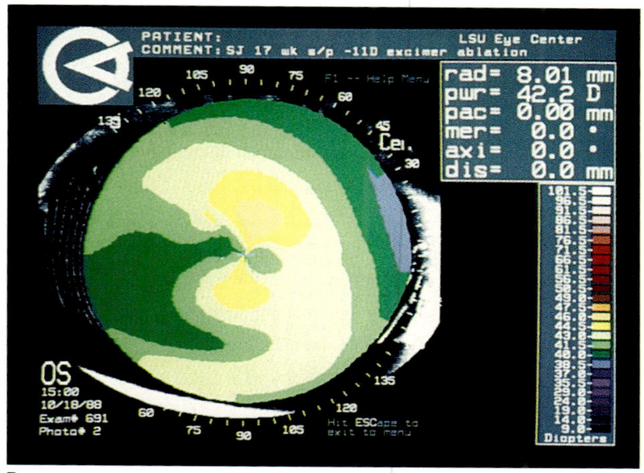

B

FIGURE 2.18. LSU PRK blind eye series: a case of complete regression. (A) One week postoperative. (B) Seventeen weeks postoperative after resurfacing following a deepithelialization.

neal surface power in this eye was due to stromal remodeling. While the pace with which the stroma is capable of remodeling seems on first reflection to be rapid, it should be considered that stromal keratocyes are extremely migratory and have an immense synthetic capacity when activated by an "adequate" stimulus. It is this characteristic that must be circumvented to maximize the successful application of excimer laser photoablation for myopia correction over a wide range of refractive errors. Recognition of this potential drawback, has been the focus of many research efforts; at LSU it renewed attention to the excimer topography studies, since only through such analysis could the specific nature of the "regression effect" be characterized.

THE INITIAL LSU SIGHTED EYE STUDIES: PHASES IIA AND IIB

In the LSU phase IIA series, 19 eyes were treated with attempted corrections ranging from 2.25 to 8.00 D. Seventeen of these eyes were available for follow-up with corneal topography analysis. In the analysis of these corneas, certain characteristics of the procedure became evident. The change in corneal topography generally underwent a transition during the postoperative period from an early (1–2 week) marked effect through a gradual diminution to stabilization at 6 months (Fig. 2.19). The temporal characteristics of the changes in corneal topography were assessed by recording and plotting the power of the ablation centers postoperatively; these are shown in Figure 2.20. Importantly, the mean change in corneal surface powers at the center of the ablations closely matched the cohort data based upon manifest refractions,[42] and in doing so provided independent, objective verification of a clinical data set with potentially confounding variables such as progressive increases in axial length.

THE CENTRATION ISSUE

The optimal keratorefractive surgical procedure is one that predictably alters the curvature of the entire cornea from limbus to limbus. Whereas radial keratotomy can provide a large optical zone of flattened corneal power, it does so only by encroaching on the scattering properties of the cornea by scarring the paracentral stroma, which produces the star-burst visual complaint. Neither is the excimer laser keratectomy procedure without drawbacks in terms of optical performance for two reasons: (1) Increasing the diameter of the treated zone raises the amount of laser energy needed by the square of

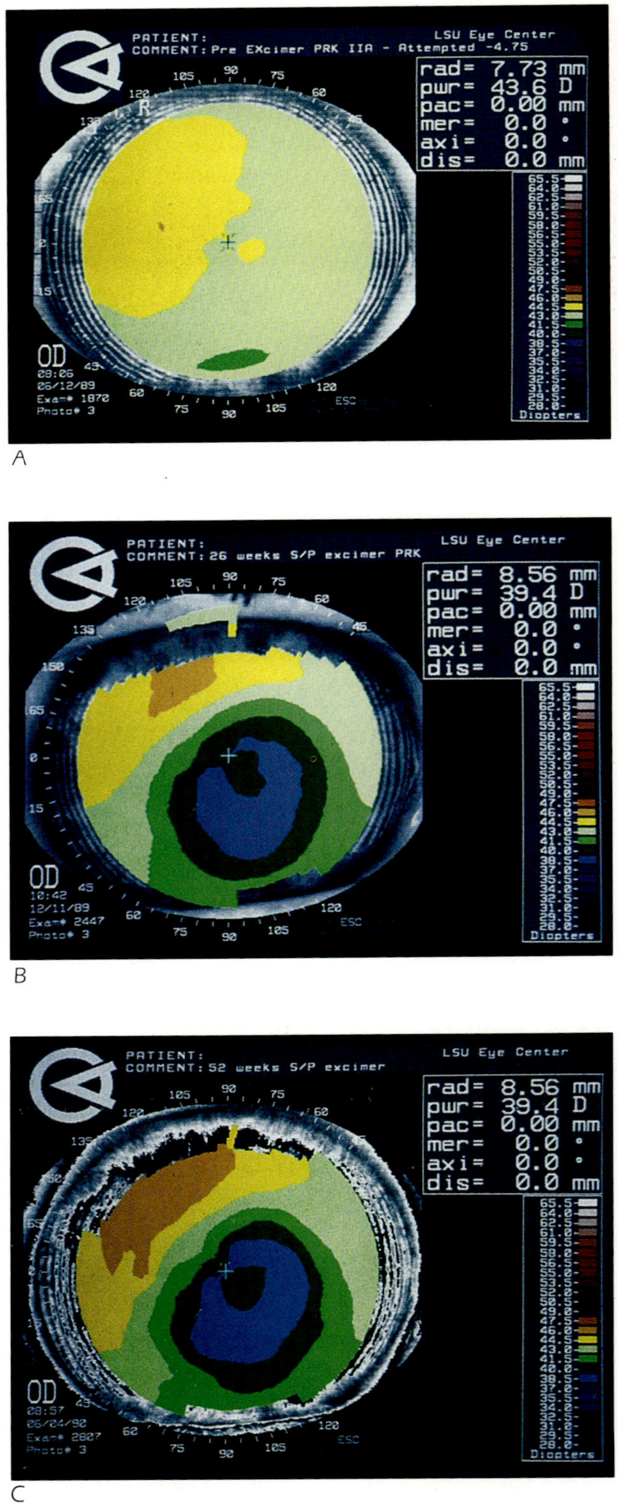

FIGURE 2.19. LSU PRK phase IIA example. (A) Preoperative. (B) Twenty-six weeks postoperative. (C) One year postoperative. Note the remarkable similarity in the ablation at 6 and 12 months. (Reprinted with permission from Wilson SE, Klyce SD, McDonald MB: *Ophthalmology* 98:1338–1347, 1991.[44])

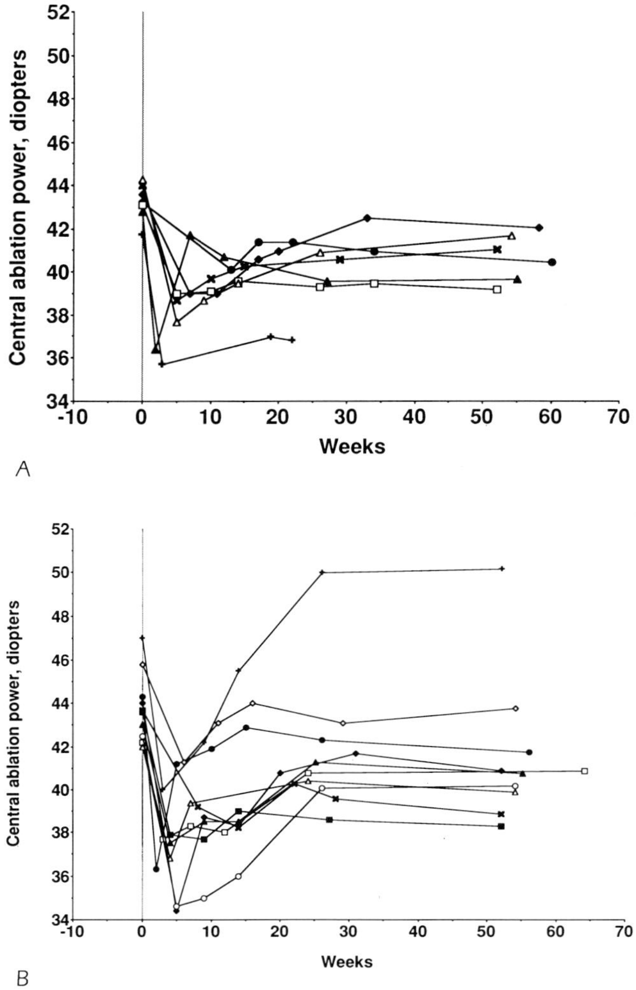

FIGURE 2.20. Change in central corneal power following PRK for myopia measured from video keratography: phase IIA. (A) Attempted corrections ≤ 5.0 D. (B) Attempted corrections > 5.0 D. Note the total regression of one eye in this series. (A and B reprinted with permission from Wilson SE, Klyce SD, McDonald MB: *Ophthalmology* 98:1338–1347, 1991.[44])

the radius, and in a keratorefractive tissue subtraction method, the diameter of the treated zone is limited by the desired correction; and (2) the higher the power change and the larger the desired optical zone, the greater the amount of stromal tissue that must be excised.

Among the findings in this LSU excimer laser series was an apparent problem with centration of the procedure over the intended corneal area. While it had been felt in the past that refractive surgical procedures should be centered on the line of sight, it is now generally accepted that the best visual performance results from a uniform alteration in corneal curvature centered on the entrance pupil.[48] Maloney[49] stresses the fact that keratorefractive surgical procedures should be centered on the pupil while the patient is fixating coaxially with the surgeon. He adds that a small or decentered optical zone may decrease visual acuity, reduce contrast sensitivity scores, and/or produce glare phenomena.

These predictions seem to be borne out by recent clinical results with the Summit Technology UV200 excimer laser, which has been used to produce ablations with 4 mm diameter optical zones.[50] Under ordinary daytime conditions, the adult human pupil will average 4 to 5 mm in diameter. It is to be expected that nonuniform powers within the entrance pupil will degrade optical performance,[27] and therefore it was not unexpected that results from this United Kingdom—Summit study found 78% of the patients reporting a halo effect at night. The halo effect is not a diffraction phenomenon as is Sattler's veil, which is caused by epithelial edema,[51] but is said to result from the refraction of light from untreated areas of the cornea that overlie the entrance pupil of the eye. This particular type of halo was thought to occur any time the ablation diameter is smaller than the active pupil and/or when marked decentration of the laser procedure exists. The halo complication was claimed to diminish with time; such a result could arise from a visual adaptation phenomenon or a change in data collection technique, since the ablation would not be expected to lessen the optical aberration by increasing in diameter. Corneal topographic assessment of this series was not provided; this sort of objective correlate would have been a powerful tool with which to support the authors' conclusions regarding the hypothetical basis for the psychometric findings.

The centration of a keratorefractive surgical procedure can be measured in a quasi-objective manner using the current capabilities of the TMS-1 corneal topography system.[44] In brief, every color-coded corneal topography map of every eye in each series at LSU was screened by measuring the displacement of the center of the ablation from the center of the pupil in order to evaluate the capabilities and qualities of methods used during surgery for centration over the pupil.

In LSU phase IIA, ablation decentration was found to average 0.88 ± 0.11 mm from the line of sight and 0.79 ± 0.11 mm from the center of the pupil (Fig. 2.21A). The conclusions drawn from these data were that (1) there were no systematic errors (consistently off-center in one direction or another), suggesting that the optics and alignment of the centering aids in the excimer laser were quite

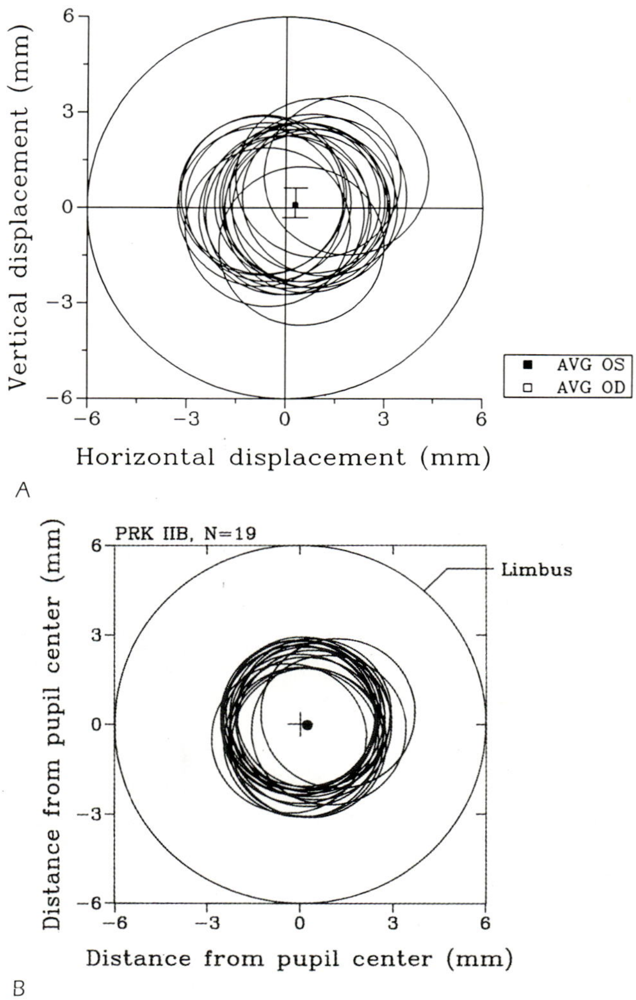

FIGURE 2.21. Measured centration of ablations from video keratography. (A) Phase IIA. (B) Marked improvement of centration in phase IIB. (A, reprinted with permission from Wilson SE, Klyce SD, McDonald MB: *Ophthalmology* 98:1338–1347, 1991.[44])

adequate, and (2) either the laser manufacturers or the users of these devices needed to develop methods or aids to improve the ability of the surgeon to lessen the error in centration.

In the phase IIA series we attempted to assess the visual consequence of the wide range of off-center ablations. The lack of a correlation between Snellen visual acuity and the amount of decentration for each eye is shown in Figure 2.22. The absence of an effect on acuity is encouraging; however, accurate contrast sensitivity measurements and well-designed psychometric tests should be done to fully evaluate the potential relationship be-

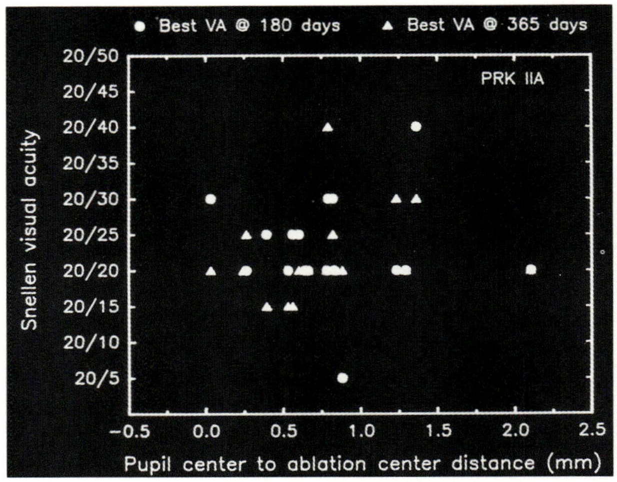

FIGURE 2.22. Lack of correlation between Snellen visual acuity and decentration in the PRK phase IIA study.

tween decentration and diminished visual performance.

A great deal of additional attention was subsequently given to alignment during the LSU series phase IIB (19 eyes were followed with topographic analysis) with an improvement in centration error (Fig. 2.21B). For the Phase IIB eyes, the average distance of the ablation centers was 0.47 ± 0.06 mm from the center of the pupil. An example of a well-centered and uniform ablation from the series is shown in Figure 2.23. In this series no corneas showed large amounts of regression and the predictability was excellent as indicated in Figure 2.24 (M. K. Smolek, S. D. Klyce, and M. B. McDonald,

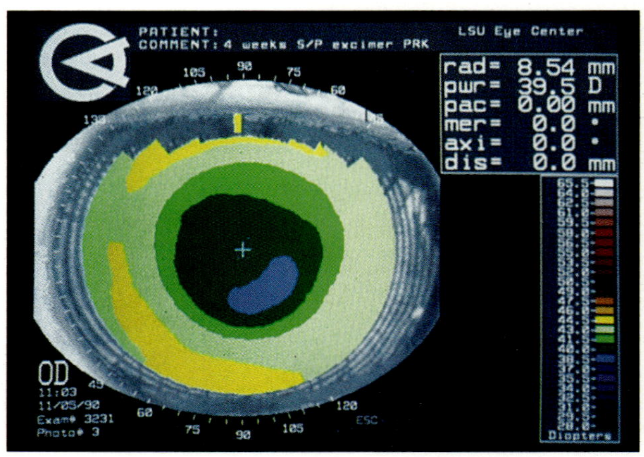

FIGURE 2.23. Example of uniform and well-centered ablation from the LSU PRK phase IIB series.

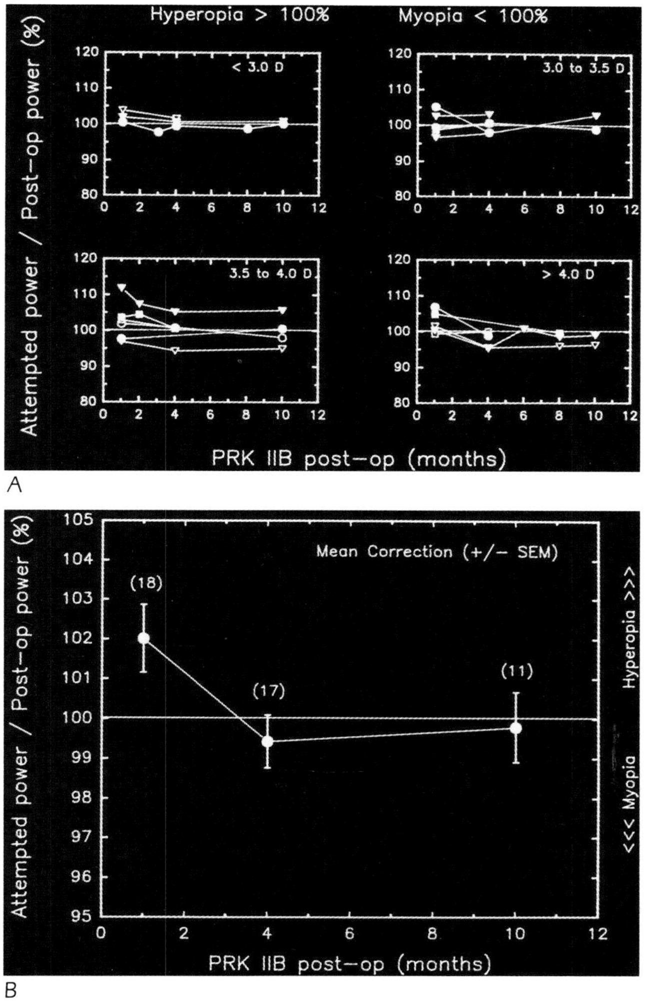

FIGURE 2.24. Predictability of LSU PRK phase IIB obtained from measuring the power of the central ablation for each of the eyes in the series. (A) Individual data. (B) Averages of the data.

unpublished data). Unfortunately, while improvement occurred, this success was achieved not with the addition of new insights or surgical alignment aids, but through careful attention by the surgeon and assistants to the centration detail. It remains a challenge for the future to develop procedural aid(s) to improve the ease with which this and other keratorefractive surgical procedures can be accurately placed over the center of the entrance pupil.

THE LSU SIGHTED EYE STUDY: PHASE III

In the LSU phase III series, 41 eyes had been treated at the time that data were collected for this chapter. Maximum follow-up was only 4 months. Nevertheless, the topographic data from this series are similar to the results presented above for LSU PRK phase IIB over the same postsurgical interval.

PREOPERATIVE SCREENING OF REFRACTIVE SURGICAL PATIENTS WITH TOPOGRAPHIC ANALYSIS

With the continuing expansion of refractive surgical modalities, careful screening for corneal shape anomalies with the most sensitive method available is not optional. It is a basic prediction from structural mechanics that the refractive surgical induction of an intended spherical change on a cornea that may progress to marked asphericity (keratoconus) will produce an unreliable effect. There is no question that the current generation of computerized corneal topography systems offer the most sensitive method available with which to diagnose keratoconus. No other clinical tool or diagnostic sign has the clear advantage afforded, in particular, by the color-coded contour map of corneal surface powers. With this technology, keratoconus appears as a regional area of surface power noticeably greater than its surround. Although there is a tendency for cones to emerge inferonasally,[52] this area of elevated power can be located anywhere on the corneal surface (including central and superior regions). Detection of keratoconus by means of video keratoscopy can occur before there are even mild symptoms such as spectacle blur. Finally, screening excimer laser refractive surgical candidates is particularly important since early keratoconus patients seem to choose contact lenses or keratorefractive surgery because their vision with spectacle correction is often suboptimal. Recently (M. B. McDonald and S. D. Klyce, unpublished observation) 8 of 22 eyes screened with topographic analysis for laser refractive surgery were found to have keratoconus, an incidence much higher than would normally be found in a random sample of the population. Finally, it is important to analyze the topography of both corneas of potential surgical candidates inasmuch as unilateral subclinical keratoconus may exist in the opposite cornea and could well be an early warning sign for the incipient development of a cone in the prospective surgical eye. In the preoperative topographic examinations for keratorefractive surgical candidates, a contact lens history should be mandatory. If a keratoconus-like pattern (as shown in Fig. 2.13A) is observed and the patient wears contact lenses, evaluation should be repeated every 2 weeks until the topography is stable, whereupon the keratoconus issue can be resolved.[30] A final point on the issue of contact lens wearers and excimer screening procedures is the fact that a fraction of lens wearers will have contact lens warpage that can alter their corneal power by 3 D or more. If contact lens wear is discontinued only 2 weeks prior to preoperative evaluation, the final refractive result may be unsuitable because the time for reestablishment of corneal stability after contact lens warpage may be as long as 5 (soft lenses) to 15 (PMMA lenses) weeks.[31]

PREDICTIONS FOR THE FUTURE AND CONCLUSIONS

From the perspective of corneal topography analysis, it is clear that excimer laser area ablation has enormous potential for becoming the standard keratorefractive surgical procedure for the correction of low-to-moderate amounts of myopia. One can forecast that controls for stromal remodeling and epithelial hyperplasia will be discovered, and even stable and predictable high-myopia correction will be achieved with the excimer. It is within the realm of modern cell biology to achieve this goal very shortly.

The ablation centration problem will likewise be solved either by application of real-time optical guidance or preferably by a clever (and inexpensive) optical alignment aid. Eventually, real-time corneal topographic analysis should find its way to the operating room to replace surgical keratometers[53] and to guide surgeons intraoperatively in reducing naturally occurring and induced astigmatism. With such a device for general anterior segment use, perhaps a special-purpose device for excimer laser guidance may not be necessary.

For the proper evaluation of excimer laser ablations, powerful algorithms will be implemented with corneal topography systems that will carefully translate preoperative and postoperative corneal topographies so that when they are in perfect registration, a subtraction method can be employed to examine the precise quality of the photoablative surgery. Quantitative descriptors of corneal optical performance will be strengthened by incorporation of pupil size considerations.[54] New fundamental aspects of visual function will be derived from the development of spatially resolved refractometry and comparison with corneal topography.[55,56] An advanced ray tracing approach[45] will be implemented on topography equipment so that patient vision can be simulated, which will be particularly valuable for diagnosis and evaluation when visual anomalies such as diplopia are experienced.

While corneal topography analysis has been essential for detailing the efficacy of the developing excimer laser procedure in the clinical research setting, it will become a routine and necessary tool for the corneal practitioner and will be used not only for diagnostic and surgical applications, but also for the rapid fitting of contact lenses using an onboard computer contact lens inventory, fitting guide, and clinical fluorescein simulation. This is the beginning of a new era, and the advantages to the patients will be numerous.

REFERENCES

1. Mandell RB: *Contact Lens Practice,* 3rd ed. Springfield, IL, Charles C Thomas, 1981, p 71.
2. Dingeldein SA, Klyce SD: The topography of normal corneas. *Arch Ophthalmol* 107:512–518, 1989.
3. Arffa RC, Klyce SD, Busin M: Keratometry in epikeratophakia. *J Refract Surg* 2:61–64, 1986.
4. Maguire LJ, Klyce SD, Sawelson H, McDonald MB, Kaufman HE: Visual distortion after myopic keratomileusis. Computer analysis of keratoscope photographs. *Ophthalmic Surg* 18:352–356, 1987.
5. Rowsey JJ: Ten caveats in keratorefractive surgery. *Ophthalmology* 90:148–155, 1983.
6. Waring GO: *Refractive Keratotomy for Myopia and Astigmatism.* St. Louis, Mosby-Year Book, 1992.
7. Dingeldein SA, Klyce SD: Imaging of the cornea. *Cornea* 7:170–182, 1988.
8. Wilson SE, Klyce SD: Advances in the analysis of corneal topography. *Surv Ophthalmol* 35:269–277, 1991.
9. McDonnell PJ: The corneal modeling system. In Schanzlin DJ, Robin JB (eds): *Corneal Topography: Measuring and Modifying the Cornea.* New York: Springer-Verlag, 1992, pp 145–164.
10. Arffa RC: Clinical uses of corneal topography analysis. *Curr Opinion Ophthalmol* 3:71–77, 1992.
11. Doss JD, Hutson RL, Rowsey JJ, Brown R: Method for the calculation of corneal profile and power distribution. *Arch Ophthalmol* 99:1261–1265, 1981.
12. Klyce SD: Computer-assisted corneal topography: High resolution graphical presentation and analysis of keratoscopy. *Invest Ophthalmol Vis Sci* 25: 1426–1435, 1984.
13. Maguire LJ, Singer DE, Klyce SD: Graphic presentation of computer-analyzed keratoscope photographs. *Arch Ophthalmol* 105:223–230, 1987.
14. Gormley DJ, Gersten M, Koplin RS, Lubkin V: Corneal modeling. *Cornea* 7:30–35, 1988.

15. Mammone RJ, Gersten M, Gormley DJ, Koplin RS, Lubkin VL: 3-D corneal modeling system. *IEEE Trans Biomed Engineer* 37:66–72, 1990.
16. Arffa RC, Warnicki JW, Rehkopf PG: Corneal topography using rasterstereography. *Refract Corneal Surg* 5:414–417, 1989.
17. Belin MW, Litoff D, Strods SJ, Winn SS, Smith RS: The PAR technology corneal topography system. *Refract Corneal Surg* 8:88–96, 1992.
18. El Hage SG: A computerized corneal topographer for use in refractive surgery. *Refract Corneal Surg* 5:418–423, 1989.
19. Koch DD, Foulks GN, Moran CT, Wakil JS: The Corneal EyeSys System: Accuracy analysis and reproducibility of first generation prototype. *Refract Corneal Surg* 5:424–429, 1989.
20. Wang JY, Rice DA, Klyce SD: A new reconstruction algorithm for improvement of corneal topographical analysis. *Refract Corneal Surg* 5:379–387, 1989.
21. Wilson SE, Wang J, Klyce SD: Quantification and mathematical analysis of photokeratoscopic images. In Schanzlin DJ, Robin JB (eds): *Corneal Topography: Measuring and Modifying the Cornea*. New York, Springer-Verlag, 1992, pp 1–9.
22. Hannush SB, Crawford SL, Waring GO, Gemmill MC, Lynn MJ, Nizam A: Accuracy and precision of keratometry, photokeratoscopy, and corneal modeling on calibrated steel balls. *Arch Ophthalmol* 107:1235–1239, 1989.
23. Wilson SE, Verity SM, Conger DL: Accuracy and precision of the corneal analysis system and the topographical analysis system. *Cornea* 11:28–35, 1992.
24. Wang J, Rice DA, Klyce SD: Analysis of the effects of astigmatism and misalignment on corneal surface reconstruction from photokeratoscopic data. *Refract Corneal Surg* 7:129–140, 1991.
25. Klyce SD, Wilson SE: Methods of analysis of corneal topography. *Refract Corneal Surg* 5:368–371, 1989.
26. Dingeldein SA, Klyce SD, Wilson SE: Quantitative descriptors of corneal shape derived from computer-assisted analysis of photokeratographs. *Refract Corneal Surg* 5:372–378, 1989.
27. Wilson SE, Klyce SD: Quantitative descriptors of corneal topography: A clinical study. *Arch Ophthalmol* 109:349–353, 1991.
28. Maguire L, Bourne W: Corneal topography of early keratoconus. *Am J Ophthalmol* 108:107–112, 1989.
29. Rabinowitz YS, McDonnell PJ: Computer-assisted corneal topography in keratoconus. *Refract Corneal Surg* 5:400–408, 1989.
30. Wilson SE, Lin DTC, Klyce SD, Reidy JJ, Insler MI: Rigid contact lens decentration—A risk factor for corneal warpage. *CLAO J* 16:177–182, 1990.
31. Wilson SE, Lin DTC, Klyce SD, Reidy JJ, Insler MI: Topographic changes in contact lens–induced corneal warpage. *Ophthalmology* 97:734–744, 1990.
32. Werblin TP, Klyce SD: Epikeratophakia: The surgical correction of myopia. I. Lathing of corneal tissue. *Curr Eye Res* 1:591–597, 1982.
33. McDonald MB, Klyce SD, Suarez H, Kandarakis A, Friedlander MH, Kaufman HE: Epikeratophakia for myopia correction. *Ophthalmology* 92:1417–1422, 1985.
34. Maguire LJ, Klyce SD, Singer DE, McDonald MB, Kaufman HE: Corneal topography in myopic patients undergoing epikeratophakia. *Am J Ophthalmol* 103:404–416, 1987.
35. Reidy JJ, McDonald MB, Klyce SD: Epikeratophakia: Corneal topography. *Refract Corneal Surg* 6:26–31, 1990.
36. Waring GO, Lynn MJ, Culbertson W, et al: Three year results of the prospective evaluation of radial keratotomy (PERK) study. *Ophthalmology* 94:1339–1354, 1987.
37. L'Esperance FA, Taylor DM, Warner JW: Human excimer laser lamellar keratectomy: short-term histopathology. *J Refract Surg* 4:118–124, 1988.
38. Taylor DM, L'Esperance FA, Del Pero RA, et al: Human excimer laser lamellar keratectomy: A clinical study. *Ophthalmology* 96:654–664, 1989.
39. McDonald MB, Frantz JM, Klyce SD, et al: Central photorefractive keratectomy for myopia. The blind eye study. *Arch Ophthalmol* 108:799–808, 1990.
40. Seiler T, Kahle G, Kriegerowski M: Excimer laser (193 nm) myopic keratomileusis in sighted and blind human eyes. *Refract Corneal Surg* 6:165–173, 1990.
41. Gartry DS, Muir MGK, Marshall J: Photorefractive keratectomy with an argon fluoride excimer laser: A clinical study. *Refract Corneal Surg* 7:420–435, 1991.
42. McDonald MB, Liu JC, Byrd TJ, et al: Central photorefractive keratectomy for myopia: Partially sighted and normally sighted eyes. *Ophthalmology* 98:1327–1337, 1991.
43. Zabel RW, Sher NA, Ostrov CS, Parker P, Lindstrom RL: Myopic excimer laser keratectomy: A preliminary report. *Refract Corneal Surg* 6:329–334, 1990.
44. Wilson SE, Klyce SD, McDonald MB, Liu JC, Kaufman HE: Changes in corneal topography after excimer laser photorefractive keratectomy for myopia. *Ophthalmology* 98:1338–1347, 1991.
45. Maguire LJ, Zabel RW, Parker P, Lindstrom RL: Topography and raytracing analysis of patients with excellent visual acuity 3 months after excimer laser photorefractive keratectomy for myopia. *Refract Corneal Surg* 7:122–128, 1991.
46. McDonald MB, Beuerman R, Falzoni W, Rivera L, Kaufman HE: Refractive surgery with the excimer laser. *Am J Ophthalmol* 103:469, 1987.
47. McDonald MB, Frantz JM, Klyce SD, et al.: One year refractive results of central photorefractive keratectomy for myopia in the nonhuman primate cornea. *Arch Ophthalmol* 108:40–47, 1990.
48. Uozato H, Guyton DL: Centering corneal surgical procedures. *Am J Ophthalmol* 103:264–275, 1987.
49. Maloney RK: Corneal topography and optical zone location in photorefractive keratectomy. *Refract Corneal Surg* 6:363–371, 1990.

50. Gartry DS, Muir MGK, Marshall J: Photorefractive keratectomy with an argon fluoride excimer laser: A clinical study. *Refract Corneal Surg* 7:420–435, 1991.
51. Lambert SR, Klyce SD: The origins of Sattler's veil. *Am J Ophthalmol* 91:51–56, 1981.
52. Wilson SE, Klyce SD: The corneal topography of keratoconus. *Cornea* 10:2–8, 1991.
53. Frantz JM, Reidy JJ, McDonald MB: A comparison of surgical keratometers. *Refract Corneal Surg* 5:409–413, 1989.
54. Applegate RA, Gansel KA: The importance of pupil size in optical quality measurements following radial keratotomy. *Refract Corneal Surg* 6:47–54, 1990.
55. Penney CM, Webb R, Thompson K: Representation of spatially resolved refraction data by a pseudo cornea. *Invest Ophthalmol Vis Sci* 32(*suppl*):922, 1991.
56. Webb R, Penney CM, Thompson KP: Measurement of ocular local wave front distortion with a spatially resolved refractometer. *Appl Optics* 31:3678–3686, 1992.

CHAPTER 3

Myopic Photorefractive Keratectomy: U.S. Experience

MARGUERITE B. McDONALD
DAVID H. LEACH

The use of the 193-nm argon fluoride excimer laser for treating myopia has evolved rapidly over the past decade. Early investigators used the excimer laser for ablation of various polymers and biological tissue.[1-4] In 1983, Trokel[5] noted the high degree of precision of excimer laser ablation, and the lack of thermal damage to adjacent corneal tissue. In this landmark paper, he proposed that the excimer laser could be used for surgery of the cornea.[5] Numerous other investigators followed with studies using the excimer laser for corneal surgery, exploring its therapeutic and refractive surgical potential.[6-12]

Early investigations centered on animal models used to determine the laser's usefulness for the correction of myopia.[13-21] There was much research interest in this concept, and at first, investigators attempted to perform radial keratotomy with the excimer laser. This effort failed, and researchers turned their attention to *wide-area ablation*—corneal sculpting, or photorefractive keratectomy (PRK) (Fig. 3.1). PRK was theoretically possible, since it had been demonstrated that submicron amounts of corneal tissue could be precisely removed with a relatively wide area of ablation. This resulted in a change in the corneal curvature and refractive properties of the eye (Fig. 3.2).[22]

Munnerlyn and coworkers[23] developed a computer-generated algorithm relating diameter and depth of the ablation to the required dioptric change. This algorithm was used in early investigations in an attempt to predict dioptric outcome of excimer laser surgery. Early investigations using nonhuman primate eyes showed stable change in the dioptric power of the cornea with a good healing response and long-term corneal clarity after PRK.[24-27] Beginning in 1987, the first human superficial keratectomies by excimer laser photoablation (PRKs) in the United States were performed on blind eyes or eyes destined for enucleation by L'Esperance and associates at Columbia University and McDonald at Louisiana State University (LSU) Eye Center.[28,29] Histopathologic examination showed the epithelium to be slightly hyperplastic, and there was no evidence of inflammation or other abnormal keratocyte activity.

The first excimer laser PRK for myopia on a "normally sighted" human eye was performed at the LSU Eye Center in July 1988 by McDonald and coworkers.[30] Under the direction of the Food and Drug Administration (FDA), VISX phase I of the (PRK) study had begun in that year (Fig. 3.3). First, McDonald performed central PRKs for myopia on

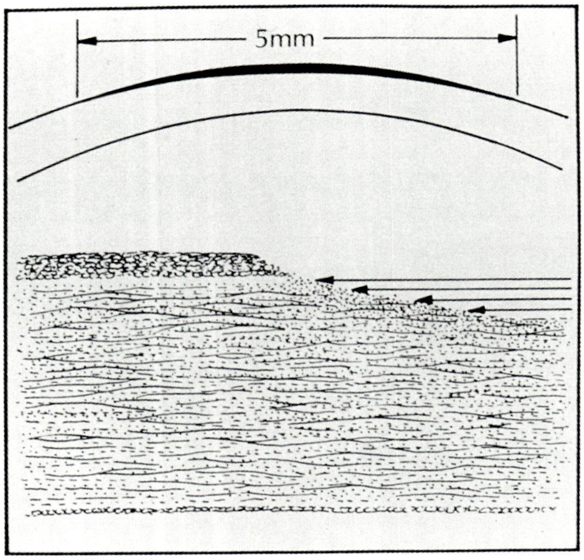

FIGURE 3.1. Photorefractive keratectomy (PRK), or *wide-area ablation,* involves stepwise removal of anterior corneal stromal tissue.

9 legally blind eyes. This was known as the "blind eye study."[29] Good results in this group led the FDA to allow PRK to be performed on 10 LSU patients who were "partially sighted" (20/50 or worse, best corrected), under the phase I protocol; these results also indicated that PRK had a good risk/benefit ratio.

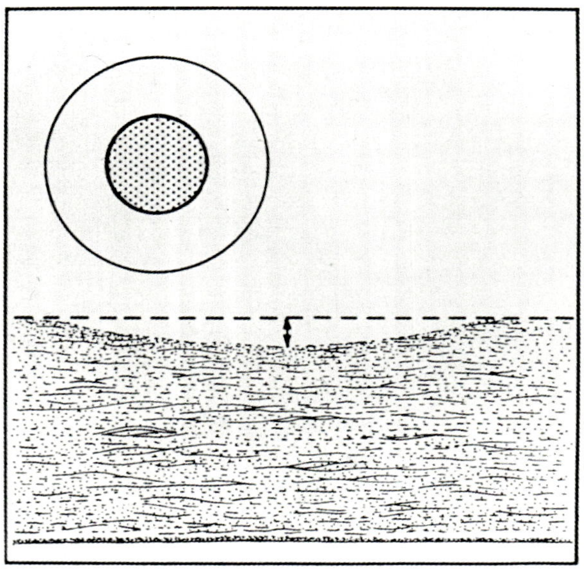

FIGURE 3.2. Following ablation of the central cornea (as shown), the anterior corneal surface is changed, resulting in new refractive properties of the eye.

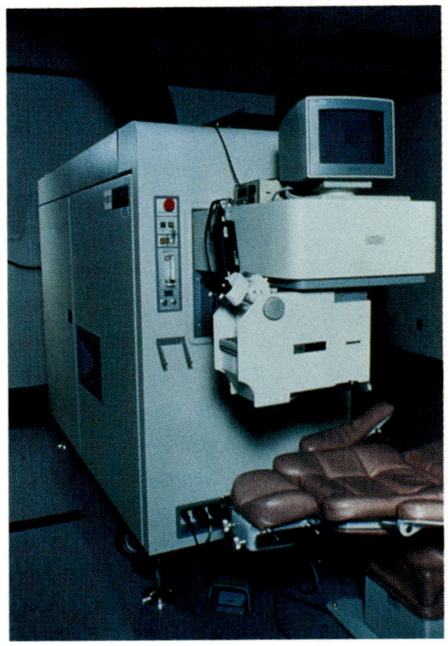

FIGURE 3.3. VISX Twenty/Twenty™ Excimer Laser System.

VISX phase IIA of the PRK study for the correction of myopia was begun on June 13, 1989, and included 40 patients who were considered "normally sighted" and were correctable to 20/50 or better. These studies were performed by McDonald at the LSU Eye Center and Michael R. Deitz and Larry W. Piebenga at the University of Missouri at Kansas City. VISX phase IIB of the clinical trial began in September 1990 and was expanded to include a total of five sites. Eighty fully sighted patients were treated in this series with very good results. Other studies were being done at this time to investigate the use of the excimer laser for removing corneal scars and corneal surface problems (phototherapeutic keratectomy, or PTK).[31-33]

The last phase of the FDA study, PRK III, was started in the spring of 1991 and was expanded to include three U.S. ophthalmic excimer laser manufacturers (Summit Technology, Watertown, Mass.; VISX, Sunnyvale, Calif.; and Taunton, Monroe, Conn.). VISX and Taunton are now currently merged as VISX in Sunnyvale, California. Phase III of the PRK study involves the enrollment of 700 patients at a maximum of 10 laser sites throughout the country for each of the three laser companies. A total of 2100 patients will be involved in the U.S. study. The follow-up examinations will extend through 2 years. This is the last phase of the study prior to FDA approval, which could conceivably occur in early 1994. The short-term results of the PRK phase III study are encouraging, with good uncorrected visual acuity, stability, and lack of significant complications. In the meantime, the excimer laser has been used extensively in countries outside the United States, and worldwide experience has accrued. The results abroad are also encouraging, although FDA-style multicenter studies have not yet begun outside the United States. However, various reports have indicated findings similar to the early phases of the PRK III study here in the United States. All these data will be helpful in determining the safety and efficacy of the excimer laser for the treatment of myopia.

PATIENT SELECTION

As in any ophthalmic refractive procedure, patient selection and education are important considerations. The patient should understand the preoperative evaluations and necessary tests, as well as all facets of the excimer laser procedure itself and postoperative evaluation. Initially, videotapes and printed information sheets are helpful in educating patients. At a later date, the patient should have an opportunity to discuss his or her concerns with the ophthalmologist and must be given an opportunity to ask questions.

It is important that the patient understand that early postoperative vision is often poor and should gradually improve over the ensuing weeks. Other important considerations include the problems of haze and glare, which are most marked at months 2, 3, and 4 but gradually resolve over time. The patient should also be aware of the risks of undercorrection, overcorrection, and regression. Early postoperative complications of corneal ulcers and later postoperative problems of steroid response leading to a rise in intraocular pressure should be mentioned as well.

It is essential that patients in their late thirties or early forties be instructed in detail about the excimer laser procedure as a correction for their distance vision only. They should understand that, depending on their degree of myopia, correcting their distance vision will make it more difficult for them to see near objects and will potentially require the use of reading glasses. They should also be given the option of full correction of one eye, with perhaps partial correction of the other eye, in order to achieve an "omnivision effect." This should be explained in detail beforehand, and a trial with contact lenses or trial lens set should be performed in order to allow the patients to decide which option is best for them. Invariably, some patients find these concepts difficult to understand. Simulating the end surgical result will allow them to make the best possible informed decision.

The patient's age, occupation, and hobbies should all be taken into consideration when planning the surgery. For the older patient, evaluation of possible incipient nuclear sclerosis should be taken into consideration.

Patients should be made aware that under present guidelines there will be a delay after treatment of the first eye before the second eye can be treated. Currently, according to the FDA protocol of PRK phase III, 6 months must elapse prior to treatment of the second eye. In the meantime, they may need to depend on a contact lens in the untreated eye, or allow for spectacle correction with a blank lens over the treated eye. It is important that patients understand the need for follow-up examination and be willing to return as scheduled so that a potential steroid regimen could be modified in the event of regression or steroid response. The fact that the procedure is investigational, and the necessity for FDA-required examinations should be explained. All these points and various options should be stressed to the patients before they undergo the excimer laser procedure.

The current inclusion criteria for the PRK phase III study include patients who are 18 years or older, with a mild to moderate degree of myopia, −1.00 to −6.00 D spherical equivalent at the corneal plane. It is necessary for the best corrected visual acuity to be 20/40 or better in both eyes. Phase III patients are limited to those with a cylindrical component of the manifest refraction of 1.00 D or less. The study requires that contact lens wearers remove their soft or hard gas-permeable contact lenses at least 2 weeks prior to baseline measurements. It has also been recommended that hard polymethyl methacrylate (PMMA) contact lenses be removed 3 weeks prior to measurements and that three central keratometry readings be performed, along with manifest refractions taken at approximately 1-week intervals. After the lens is removed it should be demonstrated that at least two of these measurements do not differ by more than 0.50 D in either meridian. It is also important that the mires be regular, without evidence of corneal warpage. These guidelines are probably a minimum, since corneal topographic changes have been noted in patients much longer after lens removal than had previously been described.[34] For non–contact lens wearers, the spherical or cylindrical portion of the manifest refraction should not change by an amount greater than 0.50 D from the date of the baseline exam.

Patients who have demonstrated contact lens intolerance, secondary to either marginal dry eye, allergies, or giant papillary conjunctivitis, are possibly good candidates for the excimer laser procedure. Other patients who might benefit from the procedure include those who need to have good uncorrected vision for occupational reasons. In this regard, compared with the radial keratotomy procedure, excimer laser surgery offers a theoretical advantage with no significant focal weakening of the cornea.

Certain criteria should be kept in mind to avoid performing the procedure on patients who might have a poor potential outcome. The PRK phase III exclusion criteria are potentially helpful guidelines for avoiding possible postoperative complications, or poor visual results.[35] First, it is best to perform this procedure on patients who are 18 years of age and older, since there is less likelihood of further refractive change. There is also greater likelihood that the patient understands what options are available and has had a trial of contact lens wear. Above all, it is important in a younger patient to show evidence of stability of refraction.

A patient demonstrating progressive myopia, with consecutive refractions showing increased myopic error, should be excluded until there is clear evidence of stabilization of the refraction. A progressive myopia might indicate pathologic myopia or perhaps early keratoconus. Keratoconus is an important consideration, and early signs should be looked for with retinoscopy, at slit lamp examination, and with corneal topography. Presently at the LSU Eye Center, we perform corneal topography on all patients prior to the excimer laser procedure to rule out subclinical cases of keratoconus, contact lens warpage, and other types of pathologic corneal conditions. Other contraindications for the excimer procedure include marked uveitis, severe lagophthalmos, advanced keratitis sicca, or severe blepharitis that has not been treated. Patients who are immunocompromised or taking systemic medications that would inhibit wound healing, such as corticosteroids or antimetabolites, are considered poor excimer laser candidates. Marked corneal neovascularization within 1 mm of the ablation zone would reduce the accuracy and evenness of the ablation zone in a patient having a myopic photoablation. Patients with systemic connective tissue diseases such as rheumatoid arthritis or lid abnormalities affecting epithelialization should be first evaluated and treated for their condition before PRK is attempted. Treatment of these patients should be avoided if the chance of reepithelialization remains uncertain after the medical condition has been treated.

PREOPERATIVE EVALUATION

The preoperative evaluation should be performed as near in time to the surgery as possible. Currently, the PRK phase III study requires the preoperative examination to be performed within 45 days of the surgery. Again, if the previously evaluated patient has reinserted his or her contact lenses, it should be stressed that contact lens wear must again be discontinued prior to surgery for at least 2 weeks in the case of soft or rigid gas-permeable lenses, and 3 weeks in the case of hard lenses. As stated previously, especially in the case of hard PMMA contact lenses, several keratometry readings and baseline refractions should be repeated prior to the procedure. This information is essential to make absolutely certain of stability and accuracy prior to planning the actual operation.

The preoperative evaluation should include a thorough and complete ocular examination of both eyes. Attention should be directed to any pertinent past ocular history, in particular contact lens wear. Uncorrected and best-corrected visual acuity measurements should be taken, along with both manifest and cycloplegic refractions. It is most important that keratometry be performed with accuracy. The cornea in particular should be examined for any signs of pathologic conditions.

The PRK III study currently requires other measurements, including pachymetry, glare testing, endothelial cell counts, and evaluation of visual fields and corneal sensitivity. These measurements will not necessarily be part of the normal preoperative and postoperative examinations once the study is completed and the FDA has approved excimer laser photoablation for patients with this degree of myopia. At the LSU Eye Center, we routinely obtain corneal topography measurements at baseline examinations as well as at the required follow-up visits.

As mentioned above, an important part of the preoperative evaluation is patient instruction and information. In addition to the previously mentioned points, patients should understand the potential need for correction at distance with either spectacle or contact lens in the event of overcorrection or undercorrection. In this regard, excimer PRK may have an advantage over radial keratotomy since it appears that the post–excimer laser ablation patient is easier to fit with a contact lens than the radial keratotomy patient. Patients should also be apprised of the haze that is most prominent during the 2 to 4 month interval, with possible glare and "doubling" of images. We find it useful to give the patient preprinted information about the excimer laser itself, preoperative evaluation, the procedure, and postoperative care. Videotapes are also useful. It should be remembered however, that, as in any ophthalmic refractive procedure, a good doctor–patient relationship established and fostered at the outset will provide for a much smoother procedure and more comfortable postoperative course for both patient and ophthalmologist.

On the day of the preoperative evaluation, the informed consent form can be given to the patient and discussed in detail as needed. We then routinely give patients their prescriptions for both pre- and postoperative medications. The informed consent form can be signed at this time, and a copy given to the patient. The patient is given an information sheet regarding the date and time of surgery, as well as the necessary preoperative preparation. We instruct the patient to have a very light meal on the day of the procedure, and to take one 5 mg tablet of diazepam (Valium®) prior to arrival in the laser suite. We recommend that patients be escorted by a friend or relative, since they will be medicated. If there was a poor refractive end point during the preoperative evaluation, or a disparity with a previous manifest refraction, the refraction can be repeated on the day of the surgery before the patient takes any sedatives or narcotics. This is the most important measurement taken prior to the excimer laser procedure. Therefore, it is essential that it be accurate.

SURGICAL TECHNIQUE

Once patients arrive at the LSU Eye Center, they are given a wrist band with their names and medical record numbers, with the operative eye indicated as a cross-check. This helps to prevent surgical mistakes, especially on a day when more than one patient is treated. Prior to the procedure, the patient is instructed in exactly what head and body positions are needed during the procedure, as well as the sights or sounds that may be perceived while in the laser room. This puts the patient at ease and makes for better cooperation. After this careful instruction, the patient is given two acetaminophen and codeine tablets (Tylenol® no. 3), as well as approximately 10 to 15 mg of diazepam. In certain instances, 25 to 50 mg of dimenhydrinate (Dramamine®) are given at least 30 minutes prior to surgery. The patient is supported and walked into the laser room and positioned in the chair.

Before the patient is positioned in the chair, much activity has taken place in the laser suite. The support staff, including, most importantly, the laser technician, has arrived, prepared the laser, and readied the instrumentation. There is a checklist that includes, most importantly, the laser energy reading and beam alignment, and a check on the uniformity and diameter of the beam. Before each procedure, one or more test ablations using PMMA are performed and read in a lensometer to be certain the amount of ablation is consistent with that desired for each patient (Fig. 3.4). The dioptrically proper ablation is, of course, predicated on a precise preoperative refraction. When the PMMA test lens is consistent with the desired correction, a calibration table supplied by the laser company (VISX) is consulted to be sure that the appropriate depth per pulse is used for computer entry. The TV monitor is checked to ensure that the ablation can be recorded. The patient's name and the date are recorded on a videocassette recorder. The eyepiece is adjusted to the proper pupillary distance, and the microscope is focused to the ophthalmologist's prescription unless the ophthalmologist is wearing his or her correction already.

The preoperative refraction and keratometry readings are then retransmitted from the computer to the laser, prior to the patient's entrance into the room. Once the patient is seated in the chair, a surgical head bonnet is used to prevent hair from impeding the laser ablation (Fig. 3.5). At this point the patient should be made as comfortable as possible, with armrests adjusted for maximum comfort. One drop of proparacaine is placed in each eye, and the nontreated eye is patched lightly but completely. This is to prevent the patient from cross-fixating during the procedure (Fig. 3.6). The patient is then lowered into position under the microscope until

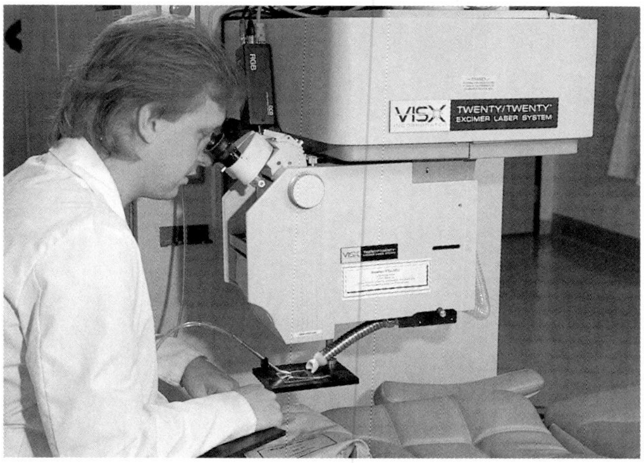

FIGURE 3.4. Test ablations are performed before each procedure to be certain the amount of ablation is consistent with that desired for each patient.

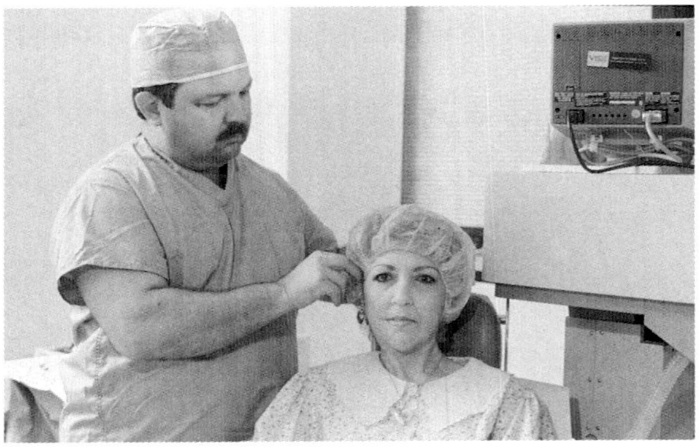

FIGURE 3.5. A surgical head bonnet is used to prevent hair from impeding the laser ablation.

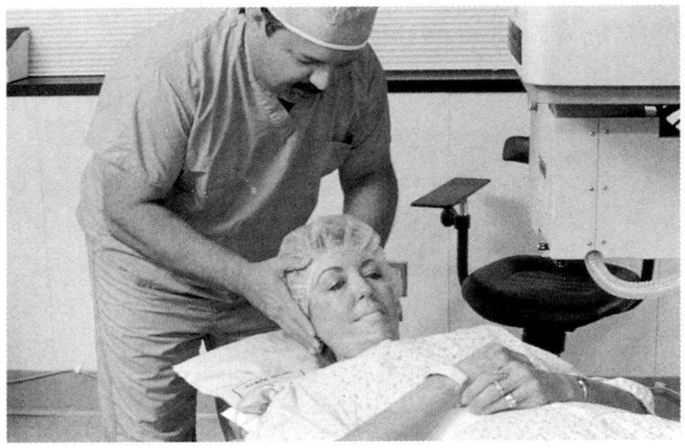

FIGURE 3.7. The patient is lowered into position under the microscope and maximum comfort is provided.

the eye to be treated is centered and in focus for the surgeon (Figs. 3.7 and 3.8). The patient's chin and head position should be adjusted and pressure applied to a "beanbag" headrest to prevent any head movement during the procedure. Next, a lid speculum is placed between the upper and lower lids, and an annular sponge soaked in topical anesthetic is placed on the eye (Fig. 3.9). The patient is asked to look directly at the blinking red fixation light, which is coaxial with the excimer beam, and a Sinskey hook is used to mark the center of the entrance pupil while the patient is looking at the red light (Fig. 3.10). This is done under three different levels of illumination in order to be certain that pupillary centration is exact. The importance of centration has been demonstrated in a previous study;[36] accurate centration makes a big difference with regard to dioptric accuracy, astigmatism, and quality of vision. Next, a circular radial keratotomy optical

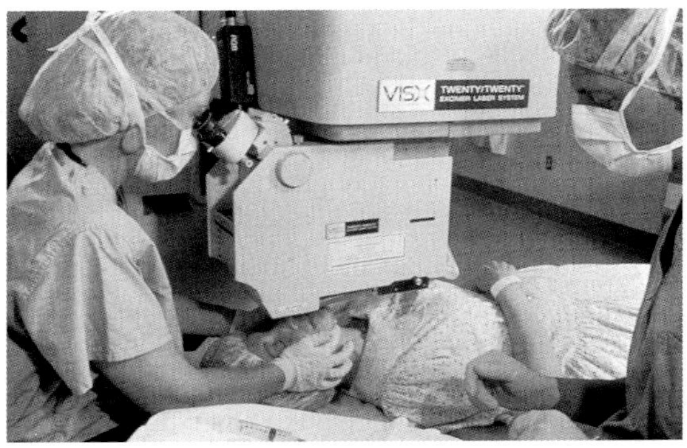

FIGURE 3.8. The head is properly positioned and the microscope adjusted until the eye to be treated is centered and in focus for the surgeon.

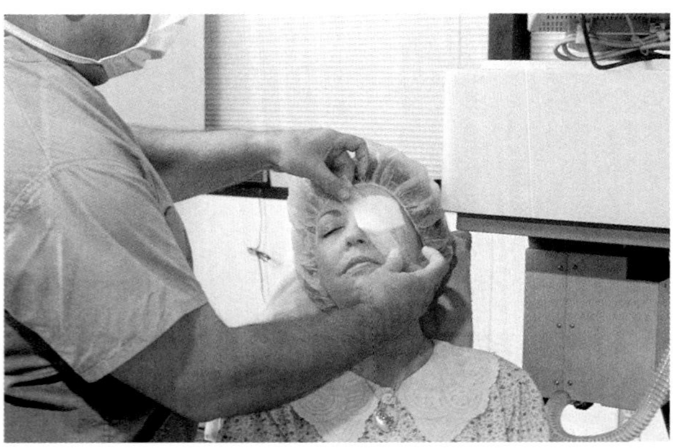

FIGURE 3.6. The opposite nontreated eye should be patched prior to the procedure to prevent cross-fixating.

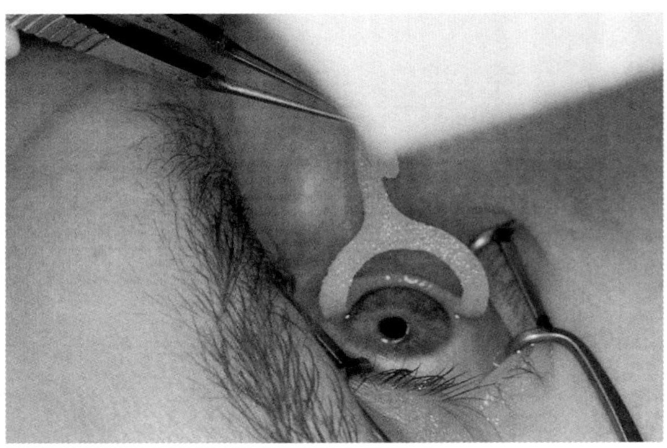

FIGURE 3.9. Annular sponge is placed on the eye following insertion of the lid speculum.

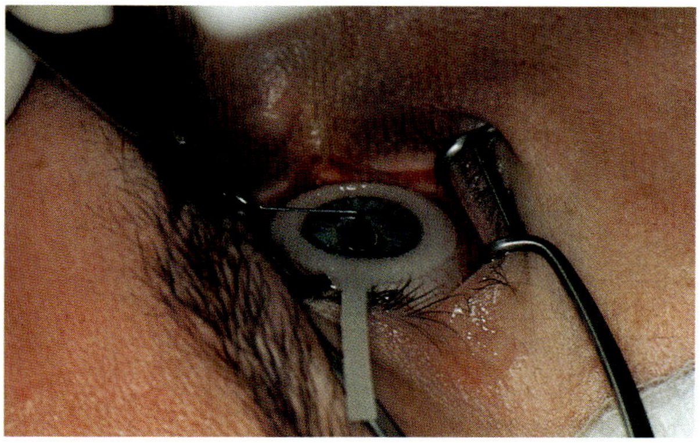

FIGURE 3.10. A Sinskey hook is used to mark the center of the entrance pupil.

zone marker 0.5 to 1 mm larger than the desired ablation zone is coated with methylene blue. At present, recommendations for the PRK phase III study (VISX) are that ablations up to 3.50 D use a 5.5 mm zone ablation, while ablations greater than 3.50 D use a 5.0 mm zone ablation. The cross hairs on the radial keratotomy optical zone marker are placed over the centration mark made on the cornea with the Sinskey hook (Figs. 3.11–3.14). After this, the central epithelium within the blue mark is carefully removed with the use of a Paton spatula (Figs. 3.15 and 3.16). The epithelium is pushed or moved to the side but saved, so that later it can be repositioned to facilitate reepithelialization.

It has been shown that the corneal surface is much smoother after ablation if corneal hydration is uniform just prior to ablation.[37] A tear substitute can be used to moisten the cornea during epithelial removal. Excess tear substitute should be gently wiped from the cornea with a moistened sponge prior to the treatment procedure, to ensure uniform surface hydration (Fig. 3.17). The VISX laser system has a surgeon handpiece that is used as an eye-fixation device. The surface has a soft sterilized sili-

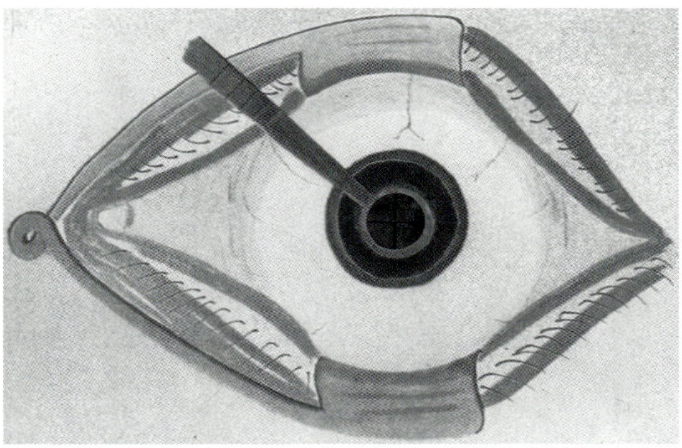

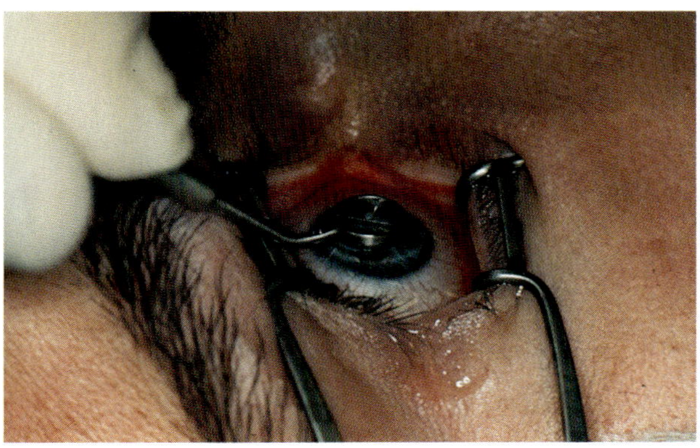

FIGURES 3.11 and 3.12. The cross hairs on the radial keratotomy optical zone marker are centered on the mark made on the cornea with the Sinskey hook.

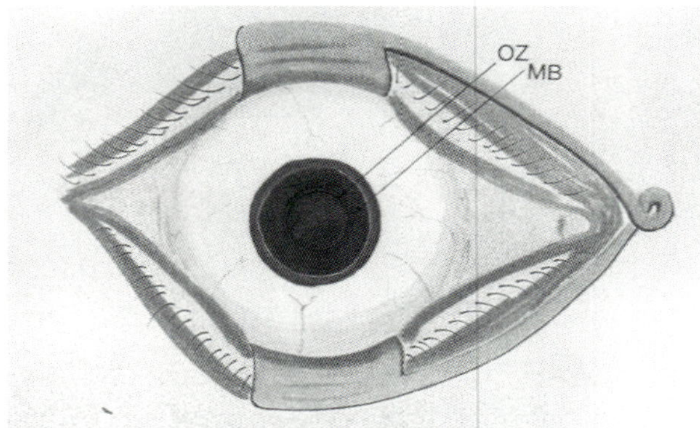

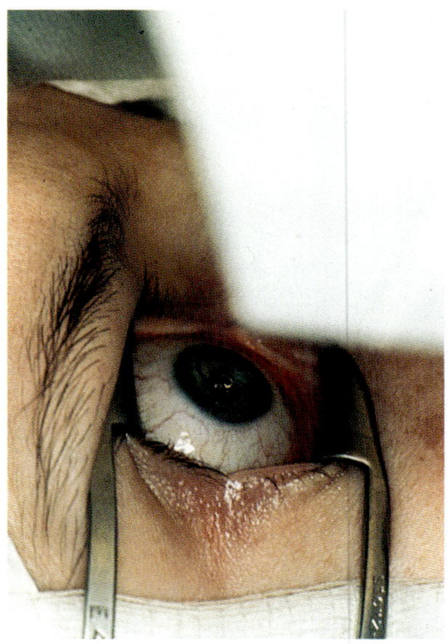

FIGURES 3.13 and 3.14. A methylene blue (MB) mark is made on the cornea surrounding the centered optical zone (OZ).

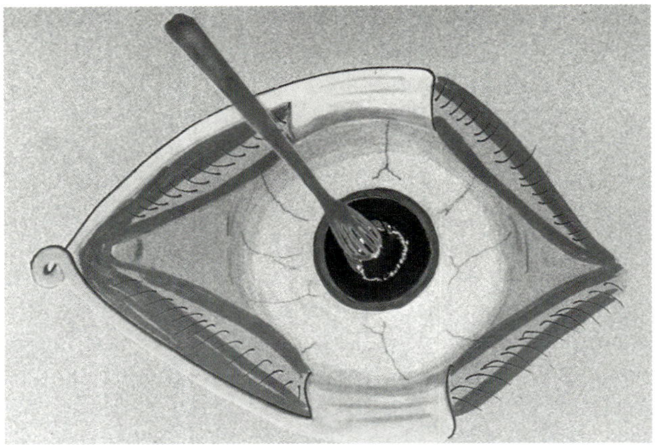

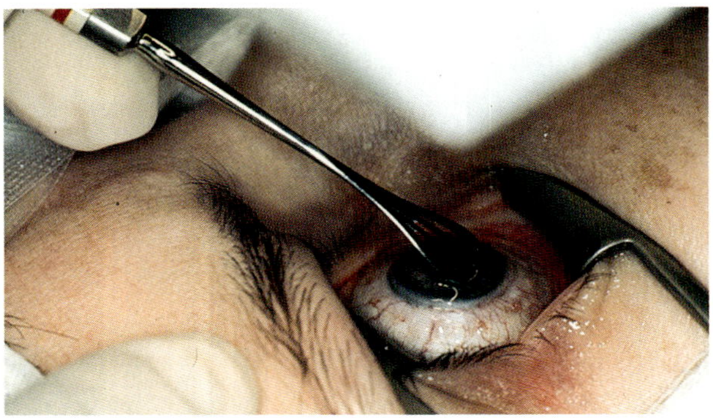

FIGURES 3.15 and 3.16. Central epithelium is carefully removed with the use of a Paton spatula.

cone ring with holes, hooked to a suction unit, as shown in Figure 3.18. The device effectively immobilizes the eye and allows the surgeon to control the position of the eye during the procedure (Figs. 3.19 and 3.20). However, this approach may be abandoned in the future as more surgeons choose to rely

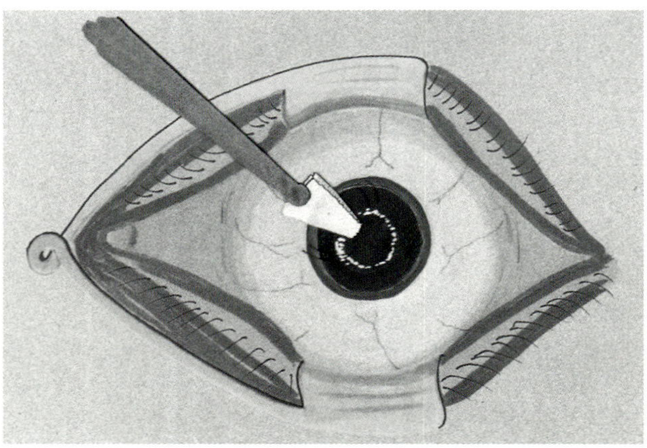

FIGURES 3.17. Excess tear substitute and debris are gently wiped from the cornea prior to the ablation procedure.

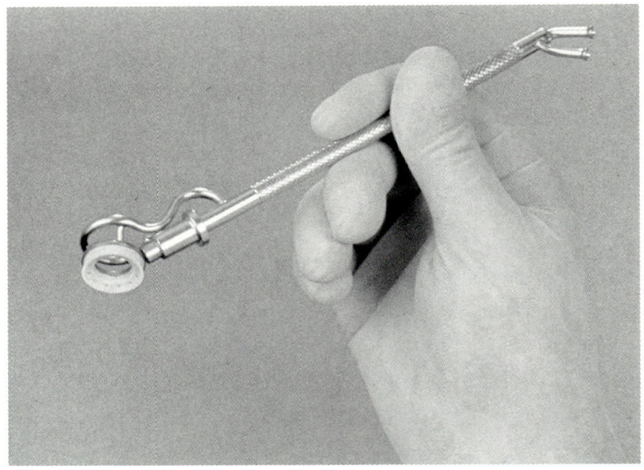

FIGURE 3.18. Surgeon handpiece has silicone ring with holes for suction.

on the patient's cooperation (i.e., voluntary fixation on the blinking red light). The handpiece may eventually be used only for PTK procedures if voluntary fixation is successful in large numbers of patients. Under a magnification setting of "12/14" on the operating microscope of the VISX system, the reti-

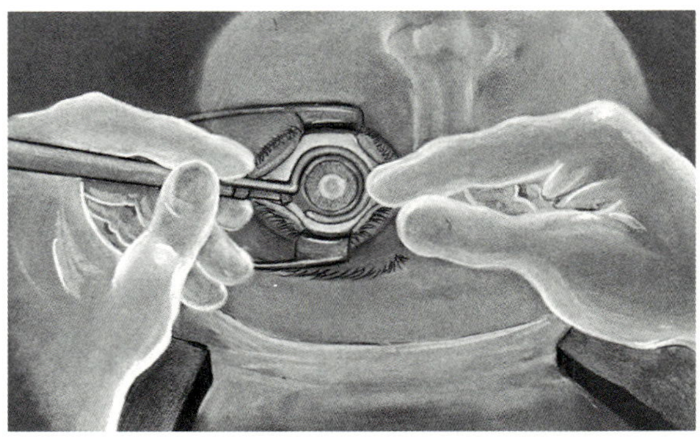

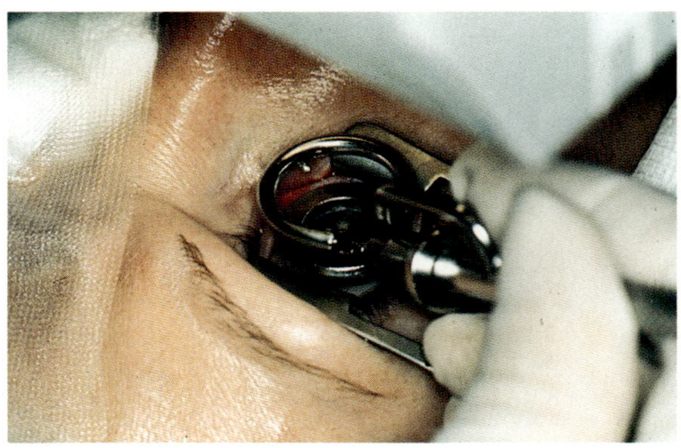

FIGURES 3.19 and 3.20. Surgeon handpiece effectively immobilizes the eye during the procedure.

cule of the eyepiece (in the right ocular of the microscope) is aligned with the methylene blue mark on the patient's cornea. For instance, if a 6.0 mm radial keratotomy marker was used to make the blue mark, the 6.0 mm ring of the reticule is aligned with it.

During this period of time, the debris aspirator should be moved into position as used in the Twenty/Twenty™ VISX Excimer Laser System. Current recommendations are to place the tip within 1.5 in. of the corneal plane and at a distance of 0.75 in. from the laser beam itself (Fig. 3.21). The importance of this has been demonstrated in previous studies.[38] Next, the position of the patient's iris plane is checked with respect to the floor; it should be parallel, that is, the patient's iris should be perpendicular to the laser beam's path. This position can be verified by the surgical assistant. The patient is then instructed to hold his or her head perfectly still prior to the procedure. If this appears to be a problem for the overly anxious patient and there is difficulty in getting cooperation, then intravenous meperidine (Demerol®) can be used to maintain sedation and augment the oral medication already given.

Next, the patient should be acclimated to the sound of the suction device, so that this noise will not cause alarm during the procedure, with resultant head movement. To start the ablation, the surgeon simply presses down on the foot pedal and holds it down until the ablation is completed. The ablation itself takes approximately 11 to 45 seconds for the treatment of myopia, depending upon the number of diopters to be corrected. It is most important that the ophthalmologist concentrate to maintain the position of the eye, so as to avoid a "drifting" ablation with resultant irregular astigmatism and unpredictable dioptric outcome.

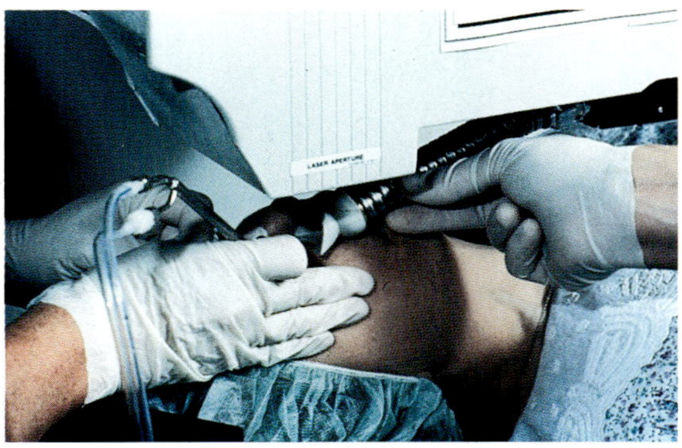

FIGURE 3.21. The debris aspirator is moved into position (as used in the VISX Twenty/Twenty™ Laser System).

Just as the ablation is completed, the assistant irrigates the eye. The epithelium that has been pushed or moved to the periphery of the ablation zone can be gently redistributed and patted into place. The patch on the opposite (untreated) eye is removed at this time. One drop of homatropine 5% is placed on the treated eye, as well as dexamethasone (Decadron®) and gentamicin (Garamycin®) ointments. A semipressure patch is applied to the eye. The patient can then be supported while leaving the room.

At the conclusion of the procedure, the VISX laser system generates a printout with all the laser parameters, including targeted ablation in diopters at the corneal plane, depth per pulse in the stroma, and number of shots at each of the different diameters of the diaphragm as it closes toward the center. Some machines, and in the future perhaps all machines, have diaphragms that open from a central, closed position *outward* to an open position.

The patient is instructed to remain in the recovery area of the laser suite, where he or she can be monitored for the next 30 to 45 minutes. A postoperative instruction sheet is given prior to the surgery, so the patient can be aware of what to expect following the surgery. However, these instructions should be reviewed with the patient and the friend or relative on hand.

POSTOPERATIVE EVALUATION

Follow-up examinations are generally scheduled at 24-hour intervals; the patch is removed and the same drops and ointment are applied until reepithelialization is complete. Reepithelialization usually takes from 3 to 5 days, after which the pressure patch is discontinued and the patient is placed on a topical steroid drop regimen. Currently, at the LSU Eye Center the patient receives one drop of fluorometholone (FML®) four times a day for the first month, three times a day for the second month, two times a day for the third month, once a day for the fourth month, and one drop every other day for the fifth month.

The patient experiences the greatest amount of pain during the first 24 to 28 hours. It is important to prepare the patient for this postoperative period and to prescribe adequate pain medications. A prescription for acetaminophen and codeine is written for postoperative discomfort, to be taken every 4 to 6 hours, 1 to 2 tablets, depending on the weight of the patient. We advise patients that if this is not adequate for pain control, meperidine-promethazine L (Mepergan Fortis®) tablets can be used instead for stronger pain control on a 6-hour basis.

During the first few days postoperatively the patient should be instructed to keep the patch on until the following day's visit. It should be noted that some ophthalmologists prefer not to patch the eye during the reepithelialization period. In either case, gentamicin and dexamethasone ointments are instilled after one drop of 5% homatropine for cycloplegia. After reepithelialization is complete (in approximately 3 to 5 days), the patient can be discharged from daily care. It should be explained to the patient that after patch removal his or her vision will be very blurry for the first week, and commonly is in the 20/200 range on the day the patch is removed. Following removal of the patch the patient can resume all normal physical activities and a normal work schedule.

Overcorrection is common in the first few weeks, so that vision, especially near vision for patients over 40 years of age, is noticeably decreased but often improves to approximately the 20/40 to 20/50 range over the ensuing 2 to 4 weeks. We tell patients that driving a car with good vision in the other eye is not a problem, whether it be corrected by contact lens or spectacle. If spectacles are worn, a blank lens can be placed over the operative eye. We advise patients that depth perception may be somewhat compromised in the early postoperative period, and this may require some adaptation. Presently the FDA mandates a 6-month interval before the excimer laser procedure is performed on the second eye. In addition, per the PRK III protocol, patients are instructed to return at 1 month, 3 months, 6 months, and 1 year. Since they are on a topical steroid regimen, we feel it is important to obtain an intraocular pressure check two months after surgery. At that time, we adjust the steroids as required, or add timolol maleate (Timoptic®) if necessary to control the intraocular pressure. The patients are instructed that if a marked change in vision should occur, they should report sooner for an evaluation, so the steroid regimen can be modified if dioptric regression is diagnosed. The efficacy of this, however, has not been conclusively proved, and experience is limited.

RESULTS OF PRK STUDIES

At this time, investigations are still continuing regarding the refractive efficacy of the excimer laser. The first clinical human application of the excimer laser—creating T-cuts for the correction of astigmatism—was performed by Theo Seiler and associates in Germany in April 1985, as described by Trokel.[39] These studies continued through 1987 and included both blind human eyes and normally sighted eyes.[40]

As stated earlier, researchers then began to direct their attention to wide-area ablation, or PRK. McDonald and associates at LSU performed the first successful PRK on a normally sighted myopic eye in June 1988.[30] They recently demonstrated stability throughout 4 years of follow-up examinations on this particular patient with approximately 5.5 D of correction, and 20/20 uncorrected vision. In addition, in this case, it was demonstrated that the subepithelial haze seen in the early postoperative period was almost completely resolved by 4 months, and the cornea was completely clear at the 5-month visit (Fig. 3.22). At LSU, nine patients underwent PRK for myopia with attempted corrections as high as 11 D, as part of the blind eye study beginning in July 1988.[29] Significant flattening of the cornea occurred as expected. There was no significant increase in refractive or keratometric astigmatism, but there was some regression of initial effect at 6 months. It was also noted at this time that the amount of regression appeared to be greater when higher dioptric corrections were attempted.

Long-term follow-up with these patients has shown clear corneas with stability of keratometric and retinoscopic findings. This study was followed at LSU by treatment of 10 partially sighted eyes as part of the PRK phase I study, and 19 normally sighted eyes as part of the PRK phase IIA study.[41] In both the partially sighted eyes and normally sighted eyes, corneas receiving greater than 5.00 D of correction at the corneal plane were more likely to experience undercorrection than corneas receiv-

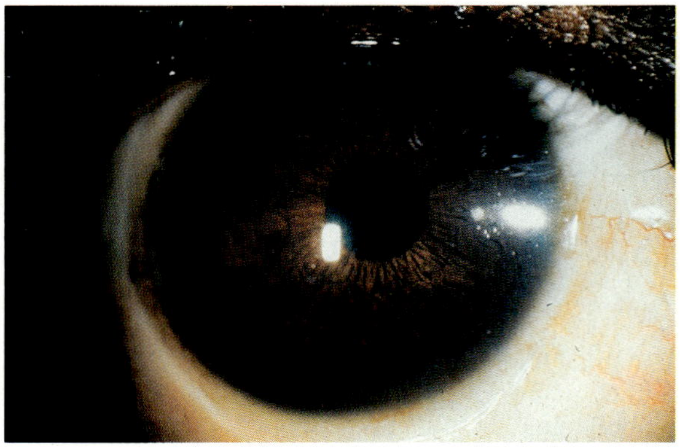

FIGURE 3.22. First normally sighted myopic patient in the United States to undergo PRK, 30 months postoperative. No significant corneal haze is detectable.

ing attempted corrections of 5.00 D or less. For the normally sighted eyes, uncorrected visual acuity improved by two or more Snellen lines, compared with preoperative values in 15 of 18 patients in the phase IIA study. One patient was lost to followup. Overall, 8 of the 18 eyes (44%) achieved uncorrected visual acuities of 20/40 or better. This result was achieved in 6 of 7 eyes (86%) with attempted corrections of 5 D or less and 2 of the 11 eyes (18%) with attempted corrections greater than 5 D. Best-corrected visual acuity in the normally sighted eyes averaged approximately 20/20 from before laser surgery to the end of the study. Corneal clarity was maintained. There appeared to be no relation between haze and depth of ablation, as had been previously discussed in the blind eye study. In this group of patients, there were no medical complications—no recurrent erosions, nonhealing epithelial defects, or corneal ulcers. The eyes tended to be overcorrected at 1 month with a regression toward myopia by 6 months, after which the refractions appeared to be stable. It was theorized that stromal remodeling was a possible mechanism of regression. Therefore, deeper stromal ablations could possibly incite a greater wound-healing response. Similar results were found by Seiler and coworkers, using the Summit laser to treat 10 blind and 13 sighted eyes; they found a difference in dioptric accuracy between higher and lower degrees of attempted correction (higher attempted corrections usually resulted in undercorrections).[42,43]

A multicenter study of PRK in sighted eyes phase IIA, was performed by Sher and coworkers[44] with the Taunton laser. In this study the excimer laser was used to perform PRKs on 31 sighted myopic eyes. The preoperative refractive errors ranged from −3.75 D sphere to −12.00 D sphere. These patients were divided into a moderate-myopia group with a spherical equivalent between −3.12 D and −6.00 D, and a high-myopia group with a spherical equivalent preoperatively of −6.12 to −12.00 D. At 6 months, 67% of the moderate-myopia group had a postoperative spherical equivalent refraction of plano to −1.00 D. This was in contrast to the high-myopia group, in which only 16% had a spherical equivalent refraction of plano to −1.00 D, and 26% had a refraction of −1.12 to −2.00 D. In this study, as in previous studies, subepithelial haze in a reticular pattern was noted. This haze peaked at 3 weeks and diminished over the ensuing 3 to 4 months. The authors concluded that this was not visually significant. There was no significant change in astigmatism, contrast sensitivity, corneal sensation, or endothelial cell counts. The authors also discussed PRK in relation to the 1-year follow-up results of the Prospective Evaluation of Radial Keratotomy (PERK) study. The 1-year follow-up examination showed that these two surgical methods of correcting myopic refractive error were comparable. The PERK study demonstrated that 30% of eyes with a baseline refraction of −4.50 to −8.00 D achieved corrections within ± 1.00 D of emmetropia. In the study by Sher et al,[44] 41% of patients achieved this result. The authors also reported no evidence of diurnal shifts, progressive myopia, or hyperopia after the 3-month interval. It was noted that there were no significant glare problems in this group of excimer patients, in contrast to the results of the PERK study, and there was virtually no chance of perforation. None of the eyes in this PRK study had symptoms of recurrent erosions. The study highlighted one patient with significant regression, which was associated with a marked amount of haze. The patient's epithelium was mechanically removed, and significant epithelial hyperplasia was noted on histologic examination. This hyperplasia was thought to be the cause, or one of the causes, of dioptric regression and variability in the intended postoperative refractive results in this group of patients.

A retrospective study with analysis of clinical correlations of the excimer PRK for myopia was performed by Liu and coworkers at LSU,[45] looking for significant clinical correlations that could predict clinical outcome. The study included the previously mentioned blind, partially sighted, and normally sighted eyes. This analysis found that larger attempted corrections resulted in less accurate postoperative refractions and poorer uncorrected visual acuity. It also found that the relationship between the amount of attempted correction or depth of ablation and corneal clarity was weak and not statistically significant. Again, in this study it was determined that corneal haze was not statistically significant in disturbing visual acuity (Figs. 3.23 and 3.24). The study mentioned that older patients tended to have better postoperative results than younger patients, regardless of the amount of attempted correction or depth of ablation. A more recent clinical impression is that older patients tend to be more hyperopic or overcorrected postoperatively, and the rate of regression is slower toward myopia. However, this needs to be statistically analyzed, as more excimer ablations are performed on older patients.

Other issues that were evaluated in phase II patients following excimer laser PRK included contrast sensitivity, long-term stability of correction, and corneal topography with degree of centration. Hogan, McDonald, and coworkers at the LSU Eye

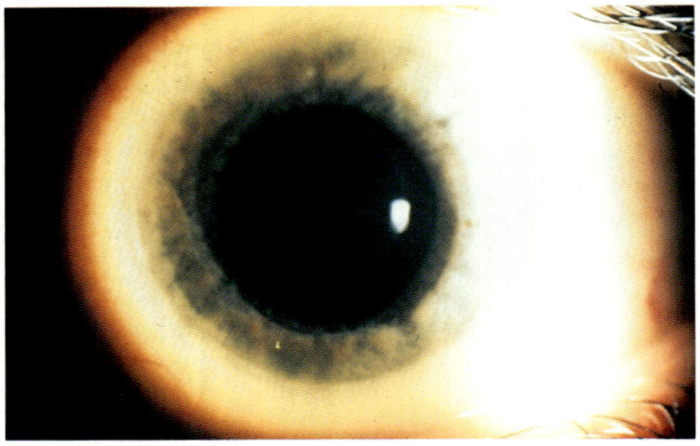

FIGURE 3.23. Patient (PRK phase IIB) 4 months following excimer laser ablation. Central haze is visible in the area of ablation.

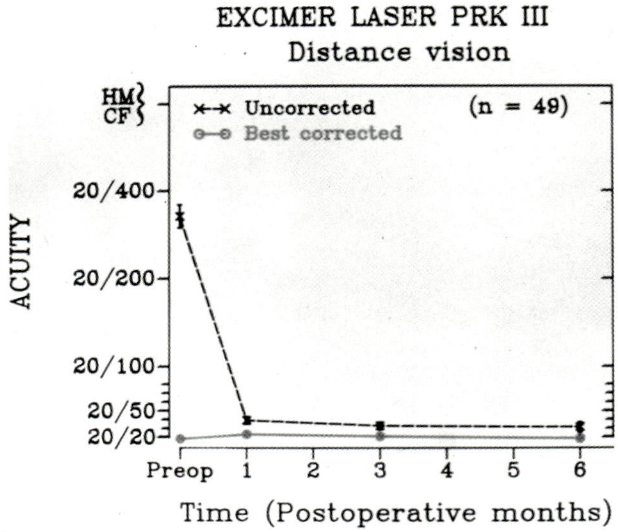

FIGURE 3.25. Recent data from the PRK phase III study (VISX) showing stability of uncorrected and corrected visual acuity at 6 months.

Center[46] evaluated contrast sensitivity in a group of 17 excimer PRK patients from phases IIA and IIB using the Vistech MCT 8000. The results showed that contrast sensitivity of eyes undergoing PRK for myopia was temporarily depressed 6 months postoperatively. By 12 months after surgery, however, the eyes had recovered and there was no significant difference from preoperative values.

An issue as important as dioptric accuracy is that of the dioptric stability of the correction after the procedure. Stability must be evaluated over many years on a very large group of patients, but it has been demonstrated in short-term studies that dioptric stability occurs 6 months postoperatively (Fig. 3.25).[29,36]

Parker and coworkers[47] evaluated six patients with preoperative myopia between −5.00 and −8.25 D who were followed for 1 year. These patients were also evaluated for any possible diurnal variations by performing manifest refractions and keratometry measurements at two time periods in the same day. There was minimal regression in this group from the third week to the 1-year follow-up visit. In addition, no diurnal fluctuation of visual acuity or refraction was noted during the study.

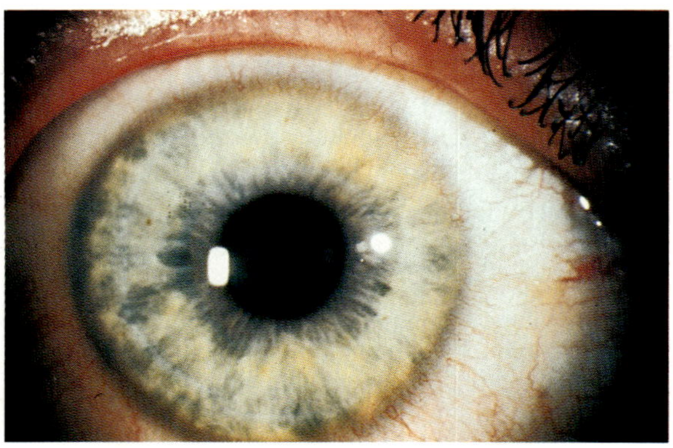

FIGURE 3.24. Same patient as in Figure 3.23, showing almost complete resolution of corneal haze at 10 months postoperative.

Corneal topography has been used postoperatively to evaluate eyes following excimer laser ablation. Wilson and coworkers[36] noted some cases of decentration in a series of 17 normally sighted phase IIA patients 1 year following excimer laser PRK for myopia. In an evaluation of 17 normally sighted eyes, the majority (10) showed decentration of 0.5 to 1.0 mm. Three eyes were decentered 1 to 1.5 mm, and one eye was decentered 2.1 mm. Decentration of this degree could conceivably result in a multifocal lens effect and significant astigmatism. (These and other considerations are the subjects of a corneal topography chapter, chapter 2, in this book.) The authors mentioned that improved methods to align the ablation zone with the center of the entrance pupil are needed to avoid this effect.

More recently, PRK phase III laser surgery has been completed. For the VISX investigators, the phase III study involves treating 700 patients with moderate degrees of myopia, divided among 10 treatment centers. These patients will be followed for 2 years postoperatively prior to FDA approval. Some early results are available, and recently data analysis was expanded to include all low to moderately myopic eyes ($\leq$5.00 D) treated at the LSU Eye Center, beginning with the PRK phase II study. Though the patients in these three series had three different postoperative steroid regimens, and the surgical team added many technique refinements along the way, the postoperative results were remarkably similar. In this analysis, 41 of 48 (85%) of eyes were within 1.00 D of emmetropia at 6 months. Twenty of 24 eyes (83%) were within 1.00 D of emmetropia at 10 to 12 months. Uncorrected visual acuity was 20/40 or better in 44 of 48 eyes (92%) at 6 months, and in 22 of 24 eyes (92%) at 10 to 12 months. Manifest refractions averaged -3.45 ± 0.20 D before treatment, $+0.91 \pm 0.12$ D at 1 month, $+0.28 \pm 0.13$ D at 3 months, -0.26 ± 0.13 D at 6 months, and -0.50 ± 0.09 D at 10 to 12 months after PRK. Best-corrected visual acuity of 20/20 or better was 93% (43 of 46 eyes) at 6 months and 96% (23 of 24 eyes) at 10 to 12 months. No astigmatism was induced following these excimer laser ablations. Evaluation of the corneas revealed on average trace haze or less after treatment, never exceeding 1+ (scale: 0 = clear; 5+ = opaque) in any eye. This pooled data analysis once again demonstrated the safety and effectiveness of excimer laser PRK in the treatment of low-to-moderate myopia in humans.

COMPLICATIONS

In comparing various refractive procedures for the correction of myopia, it is important to have information regarding the severity of possible complications and the rate of frequency of these complications. In the United States, the rate of medical complications related to the excimer laser procedure has been exceedingly low. At the LSU Eye Center, of the 38 eyes that had undergone the procedure as part of the Blind Eye Study, phases I, IIA, and IIB, only one medical complication occurred. A *Staphylococcal epidermidis* corneal ulcer occurred outside the zone of ablation. This was presumably the result of removal of epithelium prior to the excimer laser procedure itself.[29] The multicenter phase IIA study by Sher and associates, which included 31 sighted eyes, made no mention of medical complications associated with the excimer laser procedure.[44]

Postoperatively, some patients demonstrated a temporary increase in intraocular pressure referred to as the steroid response. An evaluation of a more intensive steroid regimen following excimer laser photoablation versus a less intensive one during the phase II study demonstrated no significant difference between the two groups with regard to postoperative visual results, regression, or corneal haze (Marguerite B. McDonald, Michael R. Deitz, and Larry W. Piebenga, unpublished data). The only difference between the two groups was the percentage of people demonstrating a steroid response. However, the role of steroids following the excimer laser ablation needs much more study and further evaluation.

The most common complications in these earlier phase I and II studies[29,41,44] and in the phase III study of excimer laser photokeratectomy for myopia were optical, not medical—either undercorrection or overcorrection. More recently, at LSU, the pooled data from the phase I, II, and III studies have been compiled and showed a slight overcorrection in 9 of 48 eyes (19%) at 6 months. Forty-one of these 48 eyes (85%) were within 1 D of emmetropia at 6 months.

The most common optical (or refractive) complication of PRK for myopia is undercorrection. As previously mentioned, early work by McDonald and coworkers has shown that those corneas receiving attempted corrections greater than 5.00 D were more likely to experience undercorrection and regression compared with corneas receiving attempted corrections of 5.00 D or less.[41] It was noted that a few corneas lost 70% or more of the attempted correction.[41] The problem of regression with higher dioptric correction is also illustrated by the LSU Blind Eye Study.[29] For example, one 11.00 D correction showed an initial overcorrection, but at 6 months the net dioptric change was approximately only 32% of the attempted correction. In the Taunton multicenter study for myopic photorefractive keratectomy in sighted eyes (phase II) by Sher and coworkers, the question of regression is complicated by problems with calibration on several patients.[44] One patient demonstrated almost complete regression that was thought to be due, in large part, to epithelial hyperplasia. The authors, however, thought that there was marked stability after 3 months with no further significant regression toward myopia or drift toward hyperopia.

During the early years of excimer laser PRK, there was significant concern about superficial subepithelial and anterior stromal haze. This was felt to be a factor that might limit the acceptance of the excimer laser procedure compared with radial keratotomy, since excimer PRK for myopia involves the central cornea, over the visual axis. In the past, there have been a few instances of haze causing a somewhat reduced visual acuity for extended periods of time. One patient in the normally sighted PRK phase II study at LSU had a loss of two lines of best-corrected visual acuity at the 12-month visit. This was thought to be secondary to a reticulated haze.[41] This patient had a 6.50 D attempted correction. In addition, one other patient with an attempted correction of 7.00 D lost one line of best-corrected visual acuity at the 12-month visit as a result of reticulated haze. Both were highly myopic patients treated early in our experience, and both recovered their best-corrected acuity by 18 months with no medications of any kind. The multicenter phase IIA study by Sher and coworkers[44] for myopic photorefractive keratectomy in sighted eyes found that corneal haze was not a significant problem. The haze was found to be transient and disappeared over time. It was not felt to be visually significant. The haze in this group of patients tended to peak at 3 weeks and diminished over the ensuing 3 to 4 months. Contrast sensitivity testing in both this study and at the LSU Eye Center[46] has shown contrast sensitivity to be depressed at 6 months compared with the unoperated eye, but almost the same at 12 months. These changes seem to concur with corneal haze assessments. Long-term follow-up of the blind-eye patients at 42 months has shown no evidence of corneal haze on slit-lamp examination, with barely detectable or undetectable zones of ablation in most cases.

There is speculation that this postoperative haze may be a result of fibroblastic keratocytes in the subepithelial zone. Experts debate whether or not topical corticosteroids affect postoperative haze and/or prevent the loss of refractive effect. It is not clear whether normal healing will occur as soon as steroid drops are stopped, or if therapeutic intervention with steroids is needed at all. Some leaders in the field think no steroids should be used at any time. Others feel that low doses should be used for 5 months or more. Prospective randomized trials are now underway to address this issue more thoroughly.

No other significant complications have been demonstrated in these two major myopic photoablation studies. Endothelial cell counts and corneal sensitivity have been found to be unchanged. No reports of cataract formation or perforations of the eye have been reported in any myopic PRK patients in the United States. To date, the photorefractive keratectomy procedure for myopia appears to be a safe procedure with good results for the low to moderately myopic group. The PRK phase III study will provide more information about the safety and efficacy of PRK for myopia prior to FDA approval, which is estimated to occur in 1994.

REFERENCES

1. Taboada J, Archibald CJ: An extreme sensitivity in the corneal epithelium to far UV ArF excimer laser pulses. *Proc Sci Prog Aerospace Med Assoc* 1981.
2. Taboada J, Mikesell GW Jr, Reed RD: Response of the corneal epithelium to KrF excimer laser pulses. *Health Phys* 40:677–683, 1981.
3. Srinivasan R: Action of far-ultraviolet light on organic polymer films: Applications to semiconductor technology. *J Radiation Curing* Oct 12–15, 1983.
4. Srinivasan R: Kinetics of the ablative photodecomposition of organic polymers in the far ultraviolet (193 nm). *J Vac Sci Technol B* 1(4):923–926, 1983.
5. Trokel SL, Srinivasan R, Braren B: Excimer laser surgery of the cornea. *Am J Ophthalmol* 96:710–715, 1983.
6. Puliafito CA, Steinert RF, Deutsch TF, Hillenkamp F, Dehm EJ, Adler CM: Excimer laser ablation of the cornea and lens: Experimental studies. *Ophthalmology* 92:741–748, 1985.
7. Serdarevic O, Darrell RW, Krueger RR, Trokel SL: Excimer laser therapy for experimental *Candida* keratitis. *Am J Ophthalmol* 99:534–538, 1985.
8. Krauss JE, Puliafito CA, Steinert RF: Laser interactions with the cornea. *Surv Ophthalmol* 31:37–53, 1986.
9. Marshall J, Trokel SL, Rothery S, Krueger RR: A comparative study of corneal incisions induced by diamond and steel knives and two ultraviolet radiations from an excimer laser. *Br J Ophthalmol* 70:482–501, 1986.
10. Seiler T, Wollensak J: In vivo experiments with the excimer laser—Technical parameters and healing processes. *Ophthalmologica* 192:65–70, 1986.
11. Seiler T, Marshall J, Rothery S, Wollensak J: The potential of an infrared hydrogen fluoride (HF) laser (3.0 μm) for corneal surgery. *Lasers Ophthalmol* 1(1):49–60, 1986.
12. Bath PE, Mueller G, Apple DJ, Brems R: Excimer laser lens ablation. *Arch Ophthalmol* 105:1164–1165, 1987.
13. Dehm EJ, Puliafito CA, Adler CM, Steinert RF: Corneal endothelial injury in rabbits following excimer laser ablation at 193 and 248 nm. *Arch Ophthalmol* 104:1364–1368, 1986.
14. McDonald MB, Beuerman R, Falzoni W, Rivera L, Kaufman HE: Refractive surgery with the excimer laser. *Am J Ophthalmol* 103(3, part II):469, 1987.
15. Tuft S, Marshall J, Rothery S: Stromal remodelling following photorefractive keratectomy. *Lasers Ophthalmol* 1:177–185, 1987 (cited in Marshall J et al: *Ophthalmology* 95:1411–1421, 1988).
16. Berns, MW, Liaw LH, Oliva A, Andrews JJ, Rasmussen RE, Kimel S: An acute light and electron microscopic study of ultraviolet 193-nm excimer laser corneal incisions. *Ophthalmology* 95:1422–1433, 1988.
17. Marshall J, Trokel SL, Rothery S, Krueger RR:

Long-term healing of the central cornea after photorefractive keratectomy using an excimer laser. *Ophthalmology* 95:1411–1421, 1988.
18. Del Pero RA, Gigstad JE, Roberts AD, et al: A refractive and histopathologic study of excimer laser keratectomy in primates. *Am J Ophthalmol* 109:419–429, 1990.
19. Malley D, Dobi E, Steinert R, Puliafito CA, Stern D: Immunohistochemical analysis of primate corneal wound healing following excimer laser large area ablation. *Invest Ophthalmol Vis Sci* 29(suppl):310, 1988.
20. Thompson KP, Barraquer E, Loerscher H: New collagen production and wound morphology following corneal laser excisions. *Invest Ophthalmol Vis Sci* 29(suppl):310, 1988.
21. Tuft S, Zabel R, Marshall J: Corneal remodelling following anterior keratectomy. *Invest Ophthalmol Vis Sci* 29(suppl):310, 1988.
22. Marshall J, Trokel SL, Rothery S, and Krueger RR: Photoablative reprofiling of the cornea using an excimer laser: Photorefractive keratectomy. *Lasers Ophthalmol* 1(1):21–48, 1986.
23. Munnerlyn CR, Koons SJ, Marshall J: Photorefractive keratectomy: A technique for laser refractive surgery. *J Cataract Refract Surg* 14:46–52, 1988.
24. Marshall J, Trokel SL, Rothery S, Krueger RR: Long-term healing of the central cornea after photorefractive keratectomy using an excimer laser. *Ophthalmology* 95:1411–1421, 1988.
25. McDonald M, Frantz J, Santana E, et al: Excimer laser surface shaping of the primate cornea for the correction of myopia (ARVO abstract). *Invest Ophthalmol Vis Sci* 29(suppl):310, 1988.
26. Fantes F, Hanna KD, Waring G III, Thompson K, Savoldelli M, Pouliquen Y: Myopic laser keratomileusis on monkeys: Clinical, microscopic and ultrastructural observations (ARVO abstract). *Invest Ophthalmol Vis Sci* 29(suppl):217, 1989.
27. Shofner RS, McDonald MB, Beuerman RW, et al: Serial histological studies of monkey corneas after central photorefractive keratectomy (PRK) with the 193 nm excimer laser. *Invest Ophthalmol Vis Sci* 30(suppl):216, 1989.
28. L'Esperance FA Jr, Taylor DM, Warner JW: Human excimer laser keratectomy: Short-term histopathology. *J Refract Surg* 4:118–124, 1988.
29. McDonald MB, Frantz JM, Klyce SD, et al: Central photorefractive keratectomy for myopia: The blind eye study. *Arch Ophthalmol* 108:799–808, 1990.
30. McDonald MB, Kaufman HE, Frantz JM, Shofner S, Salmeron B, Klyce SD: Excimer laser ablation in a human eye. *Arch Ophthalmol* 107:641–642, 1989.
31. Stark WJ, Gilbert ML, Gottsch JD, Munnerlyn C: Optical pachometry in the measurement of anterior corneal disease: An evaluative tool for phototherapeutic keratectomy (letter to the editor). *Arch Ophthalmol* 108:12–13, 1990.
32. Sher NA, Bowers RA, Zabel RW, et al: Clinical use of the 193-nm excimer laser in the treatment of corneal scars. *Arch Ophthalmol* 109:491–498, 1991.
33. Stark WJ, Goodman GL, Gilbert ML, Gottsch JD, Kamp MT, Enger C: 193-nm excimer laser phototherapeutic keratectomy (ARVO abstract 271). *Invest Ophthalmol Vis Sci* 32(suppl):720, 1991.
34. Wilson SE, Lin DT, Klyce SD, Reidy JJ, Insler MS: Topographic changes in contact lens–induced corneal warpage. *Ophthalmology* 97:734–744, 1990.
35. *Protocol: VISX Twenty/Twenty Excimer Laser System Photorefractive Keratectomy (PRK) Phase III*, VISX, Sunnyvale, CA, 1991, p 3.
36. Wilson SE, Klyce SD, McDonald MB, Liu JC, Kaufman HE: Changes in corneal topography after excimer laser photorefractive keratectomy for myopia. *Ophthalmology* 98:1338–1347, 1991.
37. McDonald MB, Frantz JM, Klyce D, et al: One-year refractive results of central photorefractive keratectomy for myopia in the nonhuman primate cornea. *Arch Ophthalmol* 108:40–47, 1990.
38. Puliafito CA, Stern D, Krueger RR, Mandel ER: High-speed photography of excimer laser ablation of the cornea. *Arch Ophthalmol* 105:1255–1259, 1987.
39. Trokel SL: Evolution of excimer laser corneal surgery. *J Cataract Refract Surg* 15:373–383, 1989.
40. Seiler T, Bende T, Wollensak J, Trokel S: Excimer laser keratectomy for correction of astigmatism. *Am J Ophthalmol* 105(2):117–124, 1988.
41. McDonald MB, Liu JC, Byrd TJ, et al: Central photorefractive keratectomy for myopia: Partially sighted and normally sighted eyes. *Ophthalmology* 98:1327–1337, 1991.
42. Seiler T, Kahle G, Kriegerowski M: Excimer laser (193 nm) myopic keratomileusis in sighted and blind human eyes. *Refract Corneal Surg* 6:165–173, 1990.
43. Wilson SE: Excimer laser (193 nm) myopic keratomileusis in sighted and blind human eyes. (Letter to the Editor.) *Refract Corneal Surg* 6:383–385, 1990.
44. Sher NA, Chen V, Bowers RA, et al: The use of the 193 nm excimer laser for myopic photorefractive keratectomy in sighted eyes. *Arch Ophthalmol* 109:1525–1530, 1991.
45. Liu JC, McDonald MB, Varnell R, Andrade HA: Myopic excimer laser photorefractive keratectomy: An analysis of clinical correlations. *Refract Corneal Surg* 6:321–328, 1990.
46. Hogan C, McDonald M, Byrd T, Andrade A, Varnell R, Ginsberg A: Effect of excimer laser photorefractive keratectomy on contrast sensitivity (ARVO abstract 277). *Invest Ophthalmol Vis Sci* 32(Suppl):721, 1991.
47. Parker P, Chen V, Lindstrom RL, et al: Stability of correction after excimer photorefractive keratectomy (ARVO abstract 276). *Invest Ophthalmol Vis Sci* 32(Suppl):721, 1991.

CHAPTER 4

Photorefractive Keratectomy: European Experience

THEO SEILER

HISTORICAL ASPECTS

At about the same time that Stephen Trokel published his results with the first keratectomies performed with the excimer laser, J. Wollensak and myself visited Lambda Physik (Göttingen, Germany), a producer of technical excimer lasers, in order to perform some in vivo experiments in rabbits. After the investigation of the histologic sections, we ordered our first excimer laser in early 1984 and developed a preliminary delivery system that allowed us to perform in vitro slitlike keratectomies. In early 1985 a cooperation venture with Meditec, of Heroldsberg, Germany, was initiated, resulting in a delivery system that coupled our excimer laser to a slit lamp capable of performing linear cuts of variable width and orientation. We realized that excimer laser surgery has to be performed on patients who are in a supine position and by means of a wide beam, but for various reasons Meditec and our group established different approaches: Whereas Meditec started the project to create a large-area ablation by the scanning slit technique, we continued our work by establishing wide-field ablation by optically homogenizing a high-energy excimer laser beam and coupling it to a surgical microscope. This new delivery system was used in 1985 to correct astigmatism by linear and arcuate keratectomies in blind eyes and since January 1986 in sighted eyes.[1] In addition, we performed the first phototherapeutic keratectomies (PTKs) in 1986 in cases of Salzmann's degeneration (Fig. 4.1) and for smoothing of the cornea after pterygium operations by means of an immersion technique (with methycellulose 0.5%). These first results, presented at the Laser Congresses in Interlaken 1986 and Crans-Montana 1987, were interesting enough to draw the interest of Summit Technology to our work, and in 1987 we commenced a cooperative program with this company. In 1988 we started a program of photorefractive keratectomy (PRK) for myopic corrections in blind eyes and in 1989 in sighted eyes.

Since then, in Europe we have had two different approaches to PRK:

- The scanning slit technique
- The large-area technique

Whereas the scanning slit technique has been further developed by Meditec-Aesculap, in Heroldsberg, Germany, the large-area concept has been continued independently by different companies: Summit Technology in Waltham, Massachusetts; VISX in Sunnyvale, California; Schwindt in Aschaffenburg, Germany; and Impro in Hamburg,

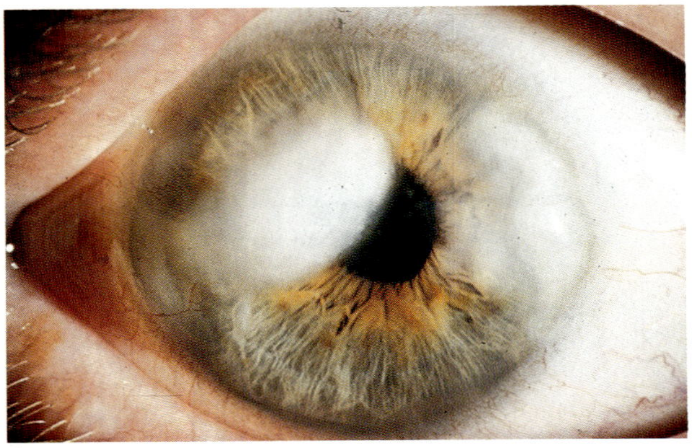

A

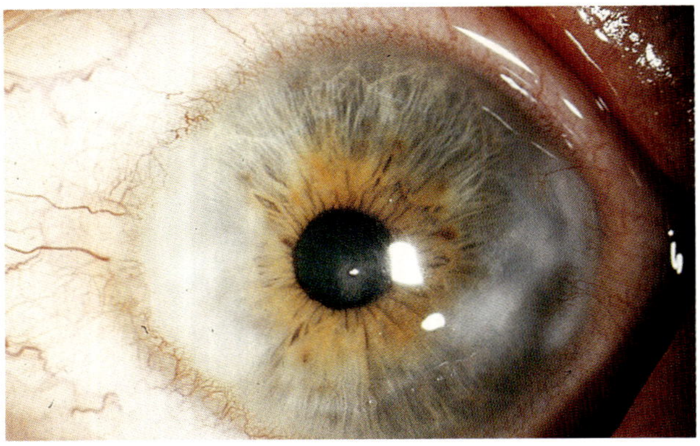

B

FIGURE 4.1. Probably the first PTK in the world, (A) preoperative and (B) 1 year postoperative. This patient was treated with the excimer laser and immersion technique in 1986 because of Salzmann's nodular degeneration. The preoperative best-corrected visual acuity was 20/200. One year after surgery, his visual acuity was 20/40 (+2). There was a hyperopic shift of about 4 D, which has remained stable since 1987.

Germany. Today (early 1992) in Europe more than 150 excimer lasers are in clinical use:

Summit Technology	78 units
Meditec-Aesculap	65 units
VISX	5 units
Impro	5 units
Schwindt	2 units

Publications on clinical European experience are available only on the trials with the Summit and the Meditec systems.

SCANNING SLIT TECHNIQUE

TECHNICAL DETAILS

In contrast to all other excimer laser systems used, the Meditec device MEL 60 creates a large-area photoablation by scanning a slitlike exposure area of 7 × 1 mm^2. The laser works at a repetition rate of 25 Hz and an average fluence of 250 mJ/cm^2. Usually a field of 7 × 10 mm^2 is scanned with a sweep time of 2 seconds. A PRK procedure takes several minutes. Repetition frequency and scan time are adjusted in such a way that with each one sweep 1 μm of corneal tissue will be ablated.[2]

The photoablation pattern for myopic or hyperopic corrections is achieved by masks mounted on suction rings that have to be adjusted and fixed on the patient's eye. For myopic corrections it consists of a standard iris diaphragm driven by a stepper motor, whereas hyperopia is corrected by means of a rotating diaphragm with spirallike perforations. The aperture has to be rotated by a fixed angle between subsequent laser exposures.

The patient is located on the bed, and the articulated arm is connected to a surgical microscope to swing over the patient's head (Fig. 4.2). The patient is asked to fixate a target mounted inside the articulated arm, and the mask is positioned onto the eye.

CLINICAL RESULTS

Unfortunately there are no scientific peer-reviewed reports on really prospective studies presenting refractive and visual results and complications. So far, to my best knowledge, I could find only two publications of results of PRK performed with the Meditec system, one of them already published[2] and another one in press.[3]

In a retrospective study, the 6-month results of myopic PRK in 134 sighted eyes of 106 patients were presented.[2] However, the dropout rate of patients who have not been followed was not reported. The postoperative medical treatment con-

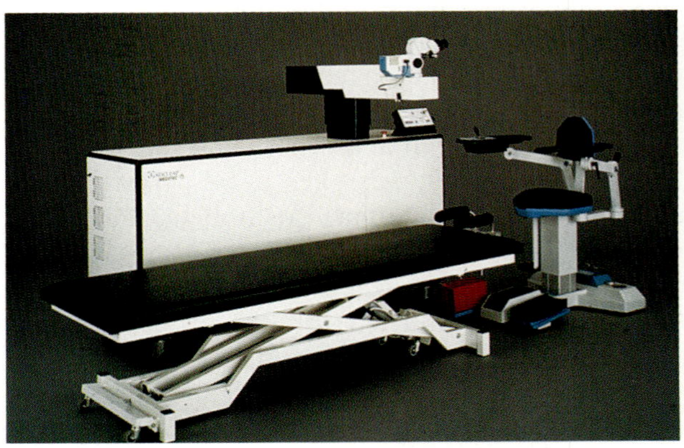

FIGURE 4.2. Medical excimer laser system using the scanning slit technique (MEL 60, Meditec-Aesculap, Heroldsberg, Germany).

TABLE 4.1. Refractive results of myopic PRK 6 months after surgery performed with scanning slit technique*

Preoperative Refraction (D)	*Number of Patients*	*Achieved Corrections (D)*
−3.0 to −6.0	36	88% within ± 1.0
−6.1 to −10.0	12	72% within ± 1.0
−10.1 to −20.0	60	Average 10.6
>20.0	16	Average 13.4

*SOURCE: Ref 2.

sisted of dexamethasone drops five times a day for 1 month with reduction of the dosage during months 2 and 3. The attempted correction ranged from −3.0 to −15.0 D. The refractive results are listed in Table 4.1. From the published data one can extrapolate that regression continues after 6 months.

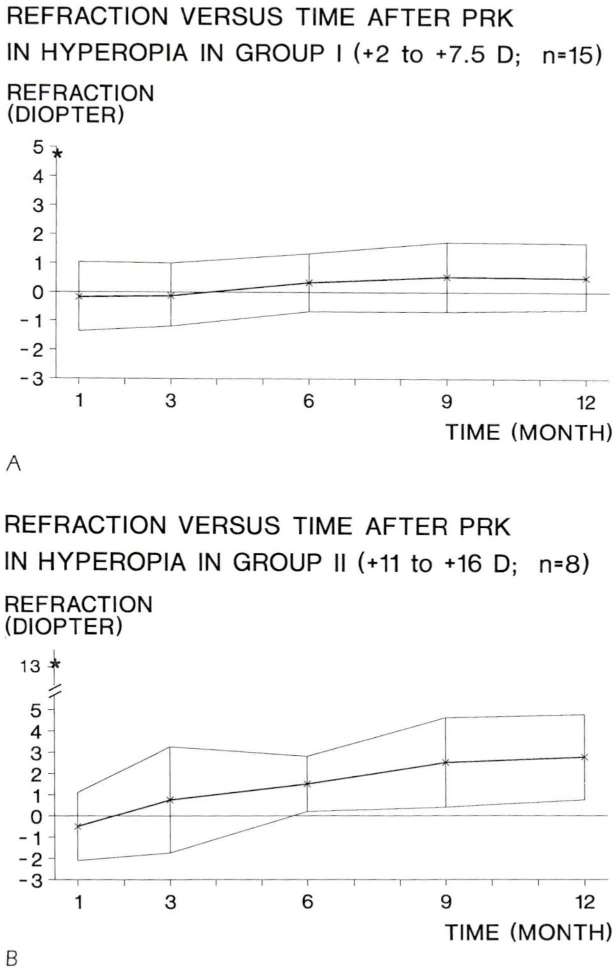

FIGURE 4.3. Temporal evolution of refraction after hyperopic PRK using the scanning slit technique. (A) Only a minimal regression takes place after hyperopic corrections up to +7.5 D. (B) The results of corrections of aphakic eyes. The regression is much higher. (From D. Dausch, Amberg, Germany.)

Only 3 eyes (2.2%) had a reduction of visual acuity due to scar formation. The complications were minimal: 2 patients (1.5%) had recurrent erosions without consequences; 6 patients (4.5%) had a steroid-induced increase of intraocular pressure; most patients complained about glare, which disappeared within 3 to 4 months; and 10 patients (8%) showed marked subepithelial haze without interference with visual acuity. No astigmatism was induced. Obviously, the results are remarkably good.

The same authors reported on results of hyperopic PRK in 23 patients treated unilaterally with a follow-up of 1 year.[3] Fifteen eyes were hyperopic (range +2.0 to +7.5 D), and eight eyes were aphakic (range +11.0 to +16.0 D). Full correction was attempted in all cases. The postoperative care included soft contact lenses for 3 months. The temporal evolution of the postoperative refraction is shown in Fig. 4.3A and 4.3B. None of the patients had an increase in astigmatism of more than 0.5 D. Two eyes lost more than one line in visual acuity. Halos were not a problem in the low-correction group, but all eight aphakic patients complained about glare and halos even 12 months after surgery. A ring-shaped haze was seen in all treated corneas; however, it was minimal in eyes of the lower-correction group and marked in the aphakic group. All eyes showed a central steepening detected by corneal topography (Fig. 4.4).

Again, the results of this first-in-the-world cohort of patients treated by hyperopic PRK seem to be very good for corrections up to +7.5 D.

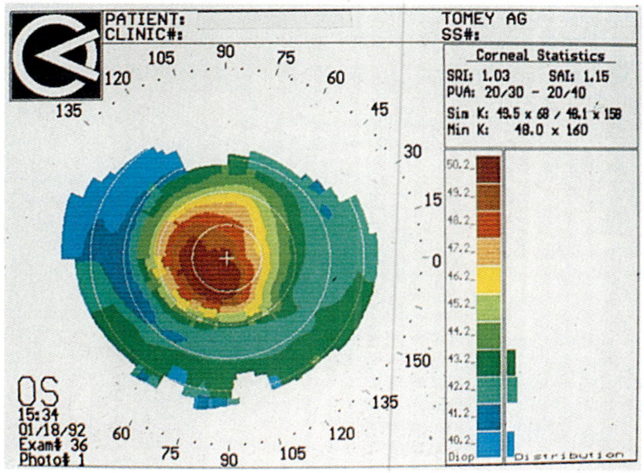

FIGURE 4.4. Corneal topography 12 months after surgery for hyperopic correction. The attempted correction was +3.5 D. Pre- and postoperative best spectacle-corrected visual acuity was 20/20. One year after surgery the refraction was −0.5 D. (From D. Dausch, Amberg, Germany.)

LARGE-AREA TECHNIQUE

TECHNICAL DETAILS

As most European reports are based on the Summit system, this device is described briefly. The laser beam has an energy density (fluence) of about 180 mJ/cm^2 per pulse within a circular area of a diameter of 5 mm. The laser runs at a repetition rate of 10 Hz. The average fluence is controlled internally, and an external control of the homogeneity of the beam has to be performed by means of ablation patterns in polymethyl methacrylate (PMMA) discs weekly. A daily control of homogeneity and fluence has to be performed by the surgeon prior to surgery by means of calibrated gelatin filters (Wratten gelatin filter no. 96, Kodak, Rochester, N.Y.). The myopic correction pattern is obtained by an iris diaphragm mounted inside the laser. The iris diameter increases in small increments with each subsequent laser pulse from 0.5 to 5.0 mm on the eye. The operation plane is defined by two crossed helium-neon pilot beams merging on the center of the ablative zone at the outer surface of the cornea.

The patient is positioned supine on a chair (Fig. 4.5) and is asked to fixate a target (green light–emitting diode) mounted in the center of the beam. A 5 D correction is completed within 20 seconds. Therefore, in most cases an additional mechanical fixation of the patient's eye (Thornton ring, suction ring) is not necessary.[4] In order to accommodate the patient to the procedure and the environment, prior to the final operation some training procedures are performed on topically applied methylcellulose and on the epithelium. The epithelium is removed manually prior to surgery. No gas flow is directed

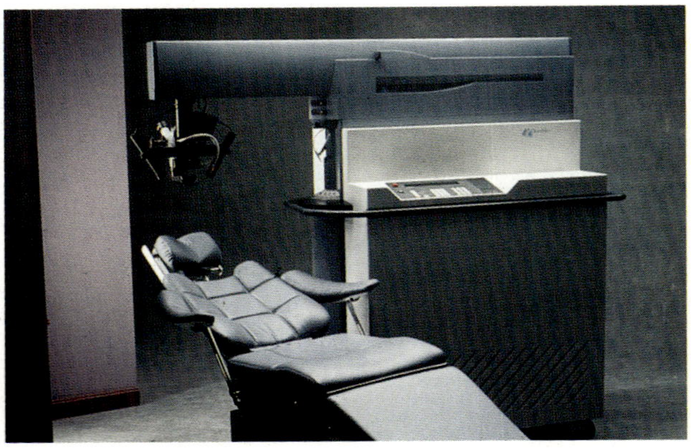

FIGURE 4.5. Medical excimer laser using large-area technique (Summit Technology, Waltham, Mass.). The laser system is capable of performing standard PRK using a non-touch technique and erodible mask procedures.

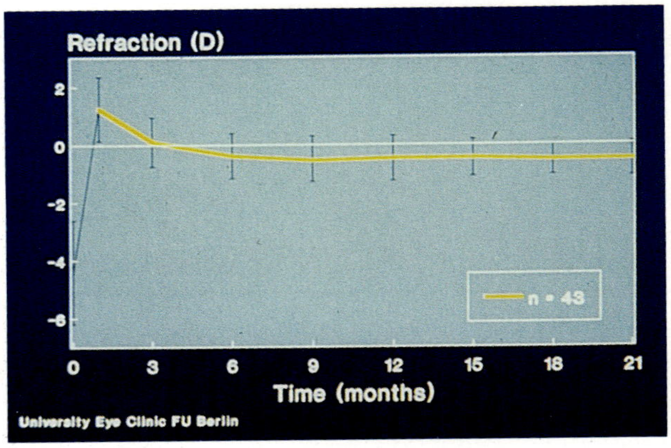

FIGURE 4.6. Temporal evolution of refraction in 43 treated eyes (range −1.5 to −6.0 D). After an initial overcorrection, stabilization of the refraction takes place between 3 and 6 months.

onto the cornea to remove ablated products or to create a defined atmosphere in the operation field.

CLINICAL RESULTS

Two European groups have published clinical experiences in peer-reviewed journals: the London group[5] and our group in Berlin.[6] Both groups used the same type of laser but different microcomputer software, different laser parameters, and different postoperative medical treatment regimens. Therefore, it is not surprising that the results (mainly regarding refractive outcome) are somewhat contradictory.

Refraction

After a period of overcorrection of about 1 month, the refraction tended to stabilize between 3 and 6 months after surgery, and only minimal change in mean refraction took place up to 2 years (Fig. 4.6). However, in our series this was true in eyes with corrections up to 6.0 D, whereas the London group found this pattern of evolution of refractive error in corrections up to 5.0 D only. Eyes with greater corrections showed continued regression of the refractive effect [Fig. 4.7]. In most of the high corrections we saw an epithelium much thicker in the center than in the periphery of the cornea, indicating that the regression is at least partly related to changes in epithelial thickness.

The success rate for refractive correction, defined as the percentage of treated eyes in the range of ±1.0 D from the intended final refraction after 1 year, is about 90% for corrections up to 6.5 D (Ber-

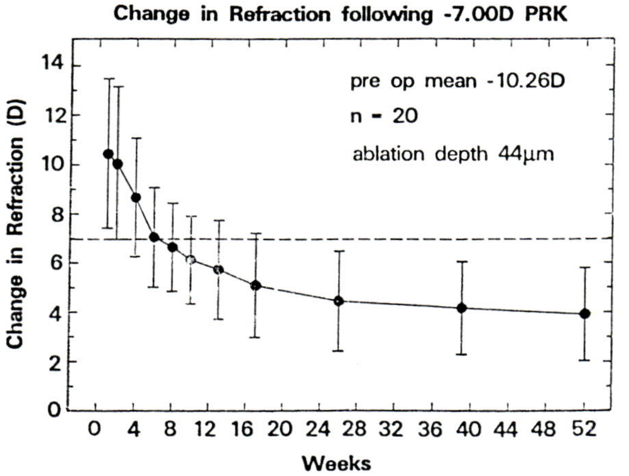

FIGURE 4.7. Regression of refractive effect in high-myopia corrections. The English study ($n = 20$) did not attempt emmetropia. The baseline refraction ranged from −6.25 D to −17.5 D.

lin data). At 6 months, the London colleagues found fewer patients within ±1.0 D of expected postoperative refraction: 90% in eyes with a −2.0 D correction, 75% in the 3.0 D correction group, and 50% in eyes with a −4.0 D correction, further decreasing in higher corrections. This discrepancy may be explained in part by different software: In Berlin we used a different nominal ablation rate and a different algorithm. The postoperative medical treatment included a different steroid protocol. Also, the baseline myopia was much more heterogeneous in the London patients.

Based on results in 281 eyes treated with myopic PRK, the incidence of undercorrection (more than −1.0 D) 12 months after surgery is clearly dependent on attempted correction (Table 4.2). In contrast, overcorrection occurs independently of intended refractive change in about 5 to 6% of the operated eyes.

Visual Acuity

Best-corrected visual acuity was equal or better than preoperative in 93% of the English patients.

TABLE 4.2. Incidence of undercorrection of more than 1 D 12 months after surgery (Berlin data)

Attempted Correction (D)	*Number of Treated Eyes*	*Incidence of Undercorrection (%)*
Up to −6.0	202	2.7
−6.25 to −10.0	65	36.9
More than −10.0	14	42.8

Three patients (2.5%) lost two lines of Snellen acuity; all of them had undergone −6.0 D or −7.0 D procedures. Unfortunately, the authors did not offer an explanation for this visual loss. Based on 281 treated eyes with a minimal follow-up of 3 months, we found 8 eyes lost two lines or more of best-corrected visual acuity due to scarring (4 of them had corrections of more than −7.0 D) and 1 eye due to a grossly eccentric ablation zone. Our overall percentage of patients with visual loss is therefore 3.2 including high corrections and 2.2 in patients with corrections of 6.0 D and less.

Consistent results were received in London and Berlin regarding uncorrected visual acuity. About 50% of eyes had an unaided visual acuity of 20/20 or better when considering corrections of 5.0 D or less in London (6 months postoperative) or 7.0 D or less in Berlin (12 months postoperative).

"Haze" and Scarring

In virtually all patients a change in corneal clarity can be detected. In most of the patients a faint diffuse subepithelial haze appears after about 1 month, increasing in intensity during the next 2 to 3 months. This haze is maximal at about 3 to 6 months after surgery, and then decreases gradually. After 18 months most corneas are clear except for a central brownish spot representing an epithelial iron line (Fig. 4.8). The subepithelial haze at its greatest shows substantial variety in severity (Figs. 4.9–4.13). Although it is clear that the histologic correlate to this haze is scar tissue,[7] only haze of grade 2+ and more interferes with best-corrected visual acuity and is therefore called manifest corneal scar. Again, the incidence of these manifest

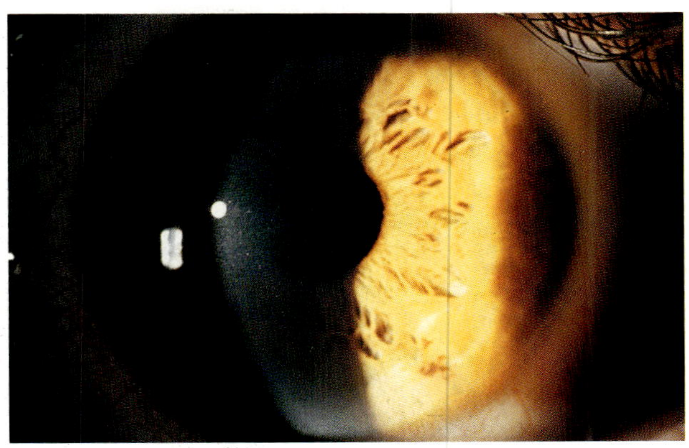

FIGURE 4.8. Clear cornea 12 months after PRK (5.0 D correction, 4.5 mm optical zone). Note the brownish iron spot in the center.

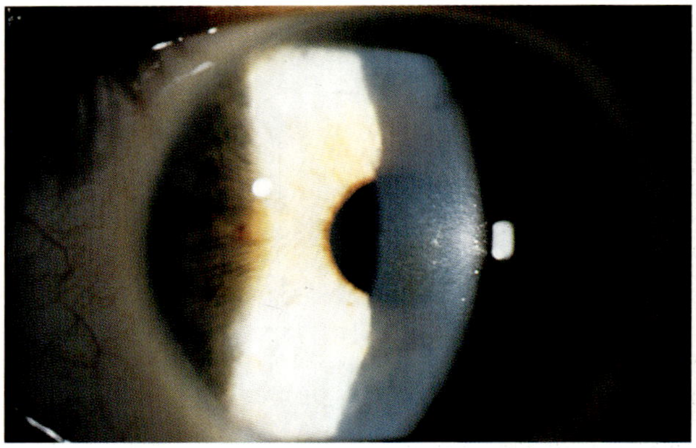

FIGURE 4.9.

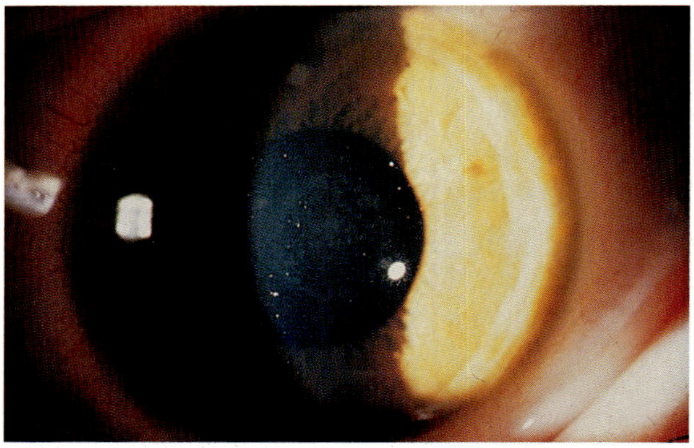

FIGURE 4.10.

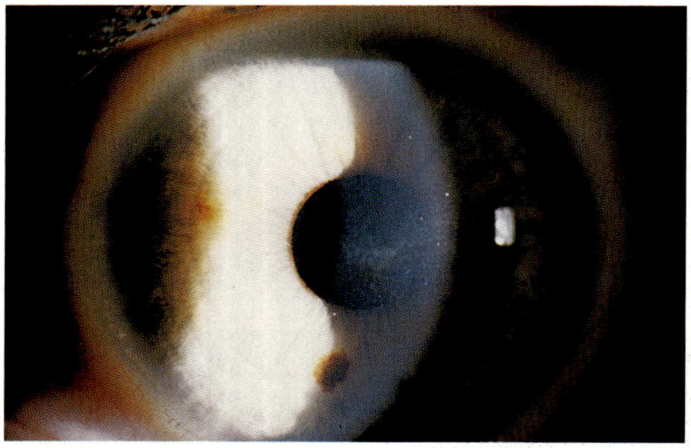

FIGURE 4.11.

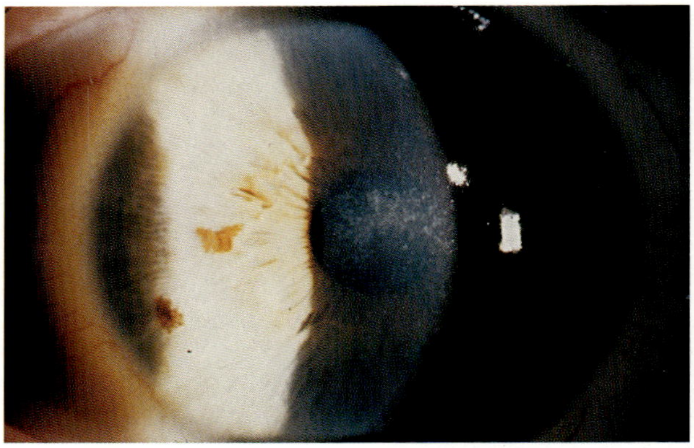

FIGURE 4.12.

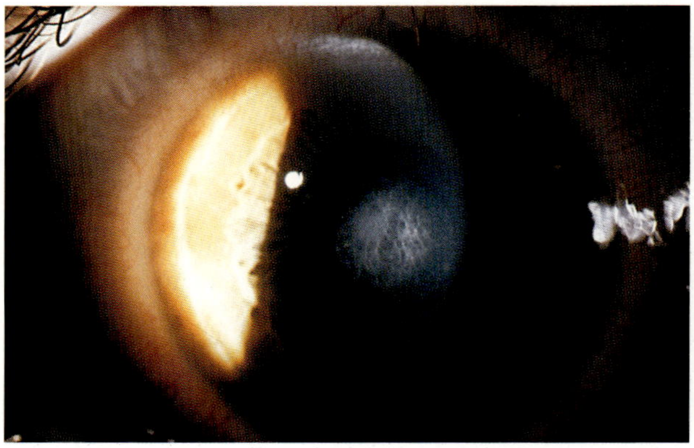

FIGURE 4.13.

FIGURE 4.9–4.13. Postoperative haze at its maximal expression (3–6 months). The photographs were taken by a standard technique to make even small changes of corneal clarity visible. Fig. 4.9. Trace haze. Fig. 4.10. Haze grade 1+. Fig. 4.11. Haze grade 1.5+. Fig. 4.12. Haze grade 2+. Fig. 4.13. Haze grade 4+.

scars is clearly related to the attempted correction (Table 4.3). Although any change in postoperative transparency of the cornea is of concern, mild and moderate haze seems to interfere neither with best-corrected visual acuity[5,6] nor with low-contrast visual acuity.[8] In addition, manifest scars may be removed by a reoperation using the excimer laser and a different PTK-technique (Fig. 4.14). Only 1 of 11 such retreated eyes showed repeated mild scar formation within 6 months after reoperation.[9]

TABLE 4.3. Incidence of manifest corneal scars (grade 2+ and more; Berlin data)

Attempted Correction (D)	*Number of Treated Eyes*	*Incidence of Manifest Scars (%)*
Up to −6.0	202	0.5(n = 1)
−6.25 to −10.0	65	9.2(n = 6)
More than −10.0	14	7.1(n = 1)

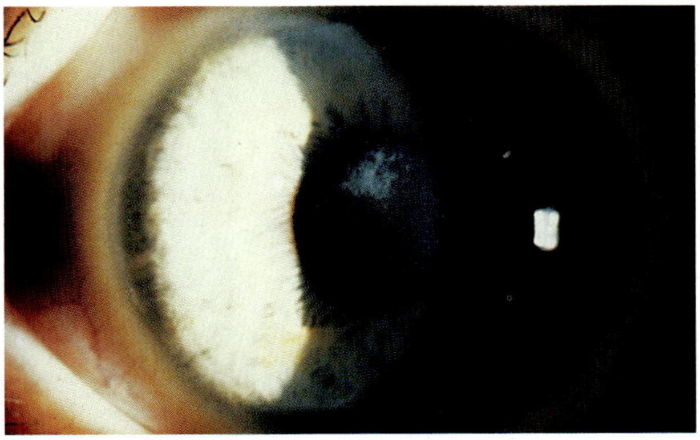

A

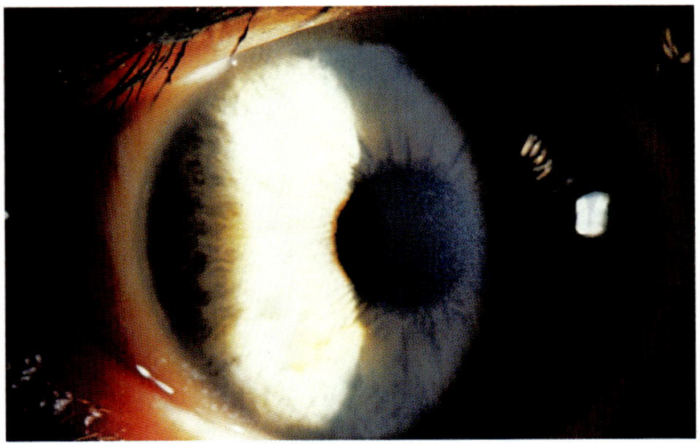

B

FIGURE 4.14. (A) Eccentric scar 12 months after initial PRK. (B) Six months after reablation the cornea shows a trace haze.

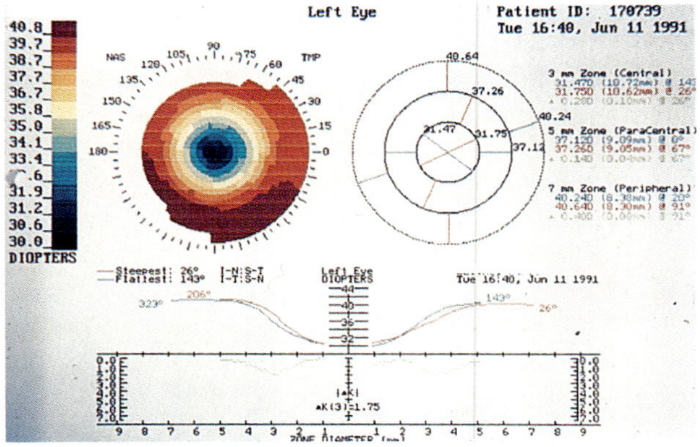

A

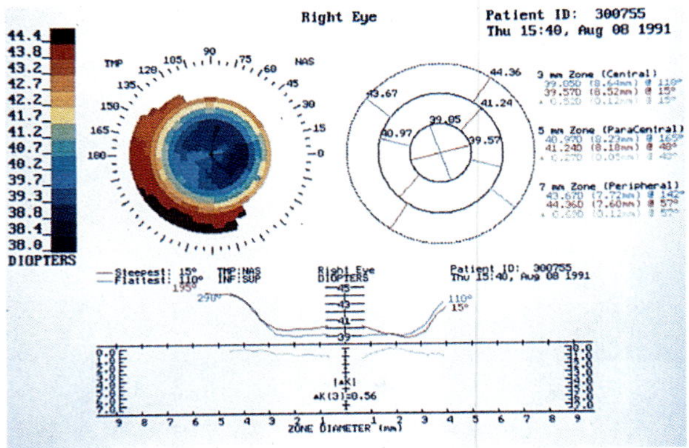

B

FIGURE 4.15. Topographies of corneas 6 months after PRK (5.0 D corrections, 5 mm ablative zone). (A) A standard spherical correction was performed. (B) An aspheric correction was performed. Clearly, the effective optical zone is greater in the aspherically corrected eye.

Subjective Symptoms

The pain arising from the erosion created during surgery has been managed by different approaches. Usually antibiotic ointment such as gentamycin (known to be toxic to the epithelium) or oflaxocin (of very low toxicity) is instilled combined with systemic pain medication. Also, bandage lenses have been tried (B. Tengroth, personal communication). Another medical approach is to use a topical anesthetic such as oxybuprocain 0.4% (diluted 1:10), which has only minor epitheliotoxic properties (D. Maurice, personal communication).

Halos around bright sources of light occur mainly under night lighting conditions. On direct questioning in the early postoperative period, 70 to 80% of the patients report observing these halos. The intensity of the halos diminishes with time; only 34% of the patients report seeing halos after 9 months. The halo effect may be interpreted as a consequence of the spherical aberration of the cornea being increased by any keratorefractive surgery. This concept also explains the dependence of the halos on pupil diameter.[10] Greater ablation zones would probably solve the halo problem, but greater ablation zones would require deeper keratectomies,[11] and, there is some clinical evidence that deeper excisions result in a higher incidence of scar formation and regression. Alternatively, aspheric corrections including a peripheral overcorrection can be performed to create greater effective optical zones (Fig. 4.15A and 4.15B) and minimize the halo effects. The incidence of halos is as small as 10% in eyes with aspheric corrections using 5 mm ablative zones.

Other Complications and Side Effects

We saw in a few patients, postoperative mild blepharoptosis, lasting for up to 3 months. Anisocoria with mydriasis in the operated eye occurred in about 5% of the patients and was detectable for up to 12 months after surgery. Both side effects were not bothersome to the patients.

About 30% of the patients showed an intraocular pressure increase of more than 5 mm Hg after 1 month. Reduction of the steroid dose and application of β blockers returned the intraocular pressure to normal within 2 weeks. The incidence of corticosteroid-induced increase in intraocular pressure was significantly reduced since we changed the postoperative medical treatment to fluorometholone (FML®) four times a day for 2 months. It is worth mentioning that about 60% of the overcorrected eyes showed corticosteroid-induced pressure elevation. There might be a correlation between the increased corticosteroid response of corneal wound healing and the increase in corticosteroid response of intraocular pressure. It would be advantageous if such steroid treatment could be avoided. Double-blind studies are underway in London and Stockholm to clarify this issue but, so far, have been leading to absolute contradictory results (J. Marshall and B. Tengroth, personal communications).

Epithelial disorders persisting longer than 1 week after surgery are fortunately rare. In 1 case out of more than 600 of ours, the patient reported symptoms comparable to an attack of a recurrent erosion within the first postoperative month. In addition, in 20% of their patients Gartry and coworkers[5] reported various symptoms of minimal discomfort, including mild foreign body sensation on waking or tenderness on eye rubbing. All these symptoms resolved within a 6- to 9-month period.

Grossly decentered ablation zones may occur during the learning curve of the surgeon. Gartry and coworkers[5] reported one case in which the patient moved bodily during the operation. The resultant ablation was located approximately 1.0 mm above the desired position, resulting in induction of minimal astigmatism and asymmetric halos. In our study group including 281 cases we found two ablation zones eccentric by 1.0 and 1.5 mm (−6.5 and −7.5 D corrections).[12] Increased experience of the surgeon should help to avoid these eccentricities since the surgeon controls the position of the eye relative to the laser beam and can interrupt the photoablation at any time, continuing as soon as the patient fixates the target again.

Of a total of more than 600 patients we had one vision-threatening complication. A 62 year-old woman showed an extraordinary delay in healing of the epithelium defect, which required 10 days to close. After the defect healed, standard steroid therapy was begun. The patient returned at postoperative day 32 with a perforated painless sterile corneal ulcer (Fig. 4.16). A penetrating keratoplasty was performed, and reepithelization of the graft required more than 8 weeks. In retrospect, we discovered the patient suffered from undiagnosed occasional rheumatic attacks, which had occurred over a period of more than 10 years. Results of rheumatologic evaluation eventually led to a diagnosis of systemic lupus erythematosus in this patient. At the present time, therefore, we consider autoimmune and connective tissue diseases known to be associated with corneal ulcers as absolute contraindications for PRK.

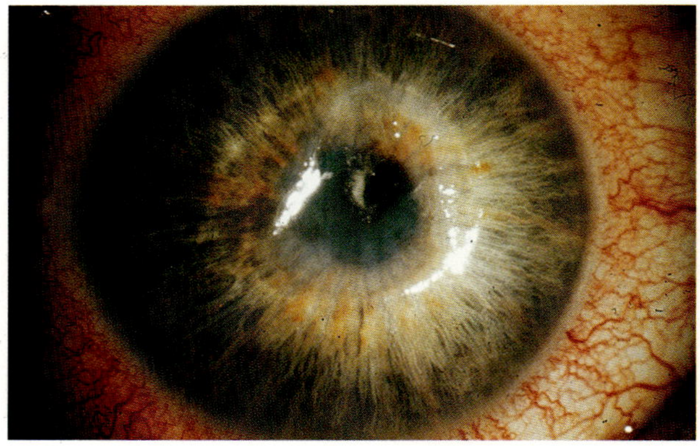

FIGURE 4.16. This noninfectious perforated corneal ulcer occurred 30 days after PRK. The patient suffered from systemic lupus erythematosus.

ERODIBLE MASK TECHNIQUE

The concept of using an erodible mask to perform PRK was suggested by Muller.[13] The mask consists of a precisely shaped plastic button that exhibits an ablation rate strictly related to that of corneal tissue (Fig. 4.17). The mask is held a short distance above the eye on a thin quartz substrate that is transparent at 193 nm. The laser beam is designed to illuminate the entire mask. During the first few pulses the radiation is totally absorbed by the mask material. As the mask material is photoablated from the thinner portions (for myopia correction in the center, for hyperopia correction in the periphery of the mask), laser light eventually penetrates this region and reaches the surface of the eye, removing corneal tissue. With subsequent pulses, the area of removed mask material increases, leading to ever-increasing areas of photoablation on the cornea. When the mask material is totally removed, the shape of the corneal ablation approximates inversely, to the first order, the original shape of the mask.

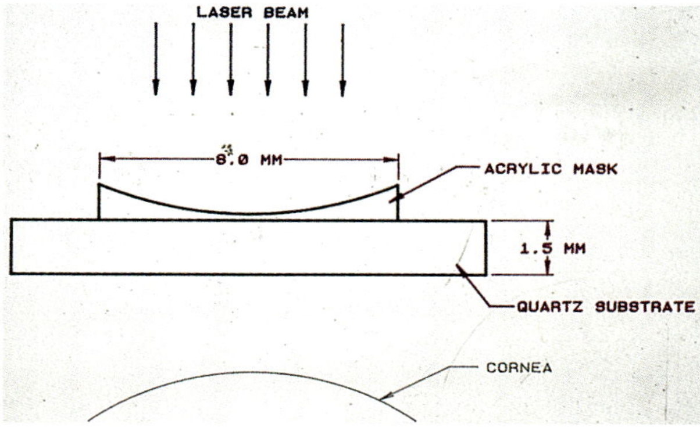

FIGURE 4.17. Principle of the erodible mask technique. The plastic button (erodible) is adherent to a quartz substrate (transparent for 193 nm radiation). The shape of the mask is transferred by the laser beam as a negative shape onto the cornea positioned underneath the mask.

In order to align the mask on the eye, a special eye cup has been developed that includes internal illumination and a humidified air flow to prevent corneal ablation by-products from condensing underneath the mask, where they could affect the transmission of 193 nm radiation.

In principle, almost any shape can be transferred which can be numerically described. The concept has been realized for correction of myopic astigmatism and hyperopia. Future applications also include irregular astigmatism, for which the masks will have to be produced individually as negative duplicates of the irregularities to be removed.

No clinial trials have been published hitherto. However, we have some experience in hyperopic PRKs and corrections of myopic astigmatism.

In Figure 4.18 a cornea 1 year after hyperopia correction (approximately 5 D) is shown with an ablation zone 4.5 mm in diameter. The ringlike haze developed during the first 6 months after surgery with a slight tendency to fade during the following months. The refraction change 1 month after surgery was about +5 D but showed a regression of 3.75 D within the first year. Currently we are testing new mask designs with larger transition zones at the edges of the optical zone, which we hope will minimize the disappointing regression.

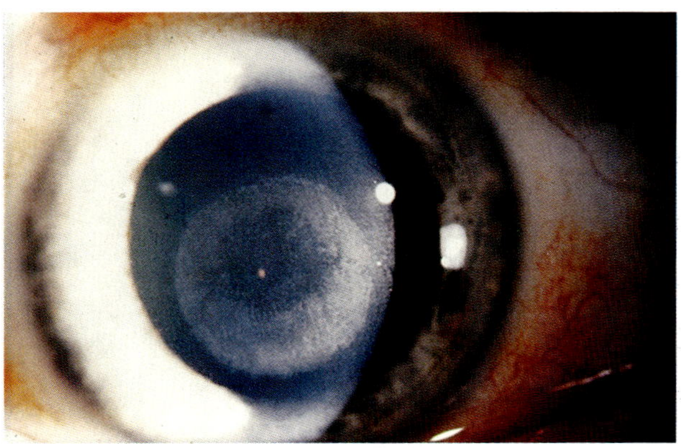

FIGURE 4.18. Slit lamp photograph of a cornea with a +5.0 D hyperopic correction. The ring-shaped haze is easily visible. The scar formation is accompanied by substantial regression.

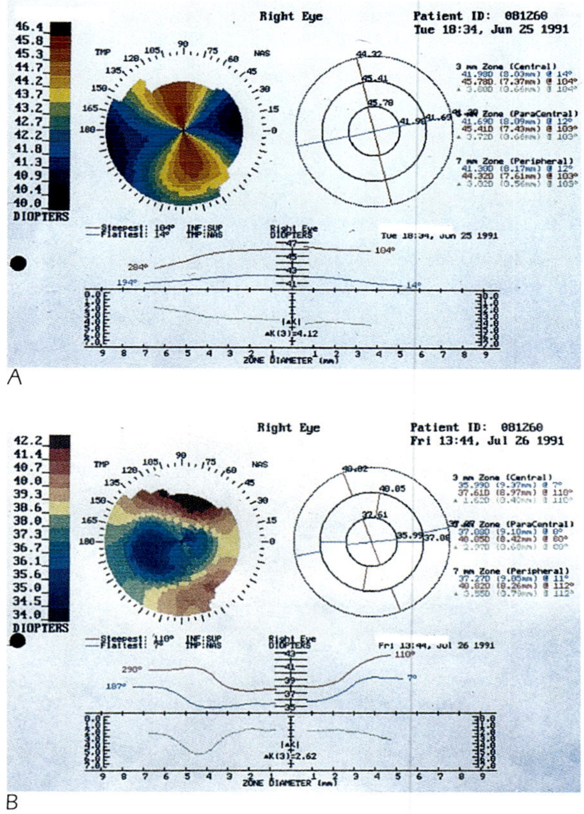

FIGURE 4.19. (A) Pre- and (B) postoperative corneal topographies of an eye with a correction of myopic astigmatism using the erodible mask technique (attempted correction: −5.0 cyl −2.5/10°). The ablative zone is eccentric.

Much better results were obtained with corrections of myopic astigmatism. Myopia as well as astigmatism could be reduced significantly in more than 20 eyes. Figure 4.19 compares the preoperative corneal topography to the map of the cornea 1 month postoperatively in a typical example. Because of the reduced visual acuity (20/100) of the treated eye, fixation and centration of the mask were difficult.

The erodible mask technique is a promising approach to corrections of other than myopic refractive errors. With further improvement of alignment techniques, large-area beams (6 mm diameter and more are available), and mask designs, it will be a true alternative to incision techniques.

CONCLUSION

In the hand of an experienced surgeon, PRK is capable of correcting myopia reliably within a refraction range up to about −6.0 D. Although the present data show stability of the refraction within the second postoperative year, long-term stability is still a concern. Vision-threatening complications seem to be extremely rare. Currently we consider PRK a clinically acceptable procedure for the correction of myopia, ranked clearly behind spectacles and contact lenses.

REFERENCES

1. Seiler T, Bende T, Wollensak J, Trokel S: Excimer laser keratectomy for correction of astigmatism. *Am J Ophthalmol* 105:117–124, 1988.
2. Dausch D, Klein R, Schröder E: Photoablative refractive keratectomie (PRK) zur Behandlung der Myopie. Eine Fallstudie an 134 myopen Augen mit sechsmonatiger Nachbeobachtungszeit. *Fortschr Ophthalmol* 88:770–776, 1991.
3. Dausch J, Klein R, Schröder E: Excimer laser photorefractive keratectomy for hyperopia. *Refract Corneal Surg* 1992, in press.
4. Seiler T, Kahle G, Kriegerowski M: Excimer laser (193 nm) myopic keratomileusis in sighted and blind human eyes. *Refract Corneal Surg* 6:165–173, 1990.
5. Gartry D, Kerr Muir M, Marshall J: Photorefractive keratectomy with an argon fluoride excimer laser: A clinical study. *Refract Corneal Surg* 7:420–435, 1991.
6. Seiler T, Wollensak J: Myopic photorefractive keratectomy with an excimer laser—one year follow-up. *Ophthalmology* 98:1156–1163, 1991.
7. Fantes F, Hanna K, Waring G III, et al: Wound healing after excimer laser keratomileusis (PRK) in monkeys. *Arch Ophthalmol* 108:665–675, 1990.
8. Lohmann C, Gartry D, Kerr Muir M, Timerlake G, Fitzke F, Marshall J: Corneal haze after excimer laser refractive surgery: Objective measurements and functional results. *Eur J Ophthalmol* 1:173–180, 1991.
9. Seiler T, Derse M, Pham T: Repeated excimer laser treatment after photorefractive keratectomy. *Arch Ophthalmol* 1992, in press.
10. Seiler T, Reckmann W, Maloney R: Longitudinal spherical aberration of the cornea as a quantitative descriptor in corneal topography. Unpublished data.
11. Munnerlyn C, Koons S, Marshall J: Photorefractive keratectomy: A technique for laser refractive surgery. *J Cataract Refract Surg* 14:46–52, 1988.
12. Seiler T, Wollensak J: Komplikationen der Laserkeratomileusis mit dem Excimer laser (193 nm). *Klin Mbl Augenheilkunde,* in press.
13. Muller D: Laser reprofiling system and methods. U.S. Patent Number 4, 856, 513.

CHAPTER 5

Radial Keratotomy Versus Photorefractive Keratectomy

JAMES J. SALZ

BACKGROUND INFORMATION ABOUT THE AUTHOR

My interest in refractive surgery techniques began in 1979 when my good friend Dr. Richard Villasenor convinced me to spend some of my free time studying and practicing the Barraquer techniques of keratomileusis and keratophakia on eye bank eyes at the Doheny Eye Institute in Los Angeles. We also participated in several studies of radial keratotomy (RK) in cadaver and primate eyes which were instrumental in reducing the number of RK incisions from the 16 originally recommended by Fyodorov to the current 4 and 8 incision approaches favored by most surgeons. I have performed RK for over 10 years, and I was the principal surgeon at the University of Southern California during the PERK study.

My interest in the excimer laser began with a trip to Germany to attend the first excimer laser symposium sponsored by Meditech in July of 1987. Dr. Alf Tenner and Dr. Thomas Neuhann had performed excimer laser radial "excisions" on a small number of blind eyes of human volunteers. Although the Meditech delivery system was most impressive, it was unclear whether a more elegant method of creating RK incisions would really improve the results. We studied biopsies of some of these incisions at the Doheny Eye Institute and were concerned by the large epithelial plugs that remained up to 1 year following the surgery.[1] These epithelial plugs were much larger than those observed following incisional RK, and we felt that stromal healing might never occur, thus leading to a markedly weakened cornea and an unstable result.

It was only after attending the first VISX excimer laser symposium at Louisiana State University under the direction of Drs. Herbert Kaufman and Marguerite McDonald that I became convinced precise reshaping of the cornea could become a viable alternative to RK. After examining and questioning several photorefractive keratectomy (PRK) patients, with follow-ups of a few weeks to 1 year, our group of Cedars Sinai in Los Angeles decided to apply to become one of the VISX investigational sites for the FDA-sponsored clinical trials of PRK. Dr. Anthony Nesburn is the principal investigator for the phototherapeutic study, and I am the principal investigator for the photorefractive study at Cedars Sinai. Our coinvestigators are Drs. Michael Berlin, John Hofbauer, Jonathan Macy, and Ezra Maguen. We performed our first procedure in October of 1990, and as of this writing we have completed approximately 100 procedures.

The comparison of RK and PRK in this chapter will include the following topics: mechanism of action, patient selection, patient experiences at surgery and postoperatively, results, safety and side effects, PRK after RK, financial considerations, and conclusions.

MECHANISM OF ACTION

RADIAL KERATOTOMY

How does RK change the refractive power of the eye? Basically the deep radial incisions cause a weakening of the peripheral cornea and flattening of the central cornea. The mechanism of action is succinctly described by Holladay and Waring:[2]

> The partial thickness (80 to 90% depth) incisions in the paracentral and peripheral cornea create wounds that gape open under the force of the intraocular pressure. This gaping is sustained as the wounds are filled acutely with edema, then with an epithelial plug, and finally with scar tissue. The gaping wounds increase the corneal surface area and weaken the cornea so that the paracentral and peripheral areas are displaced anteriorly and steepened, creating a compensatory central posterior displacement and flattening.

A number of factors influence the results of RK, but the principal ones are the number of incisions, the size of the optical clear zone, and the age of the patient. Smaller clear zones (usually no less than 3.0 mm), more incisions (usually no more than 16 total), and older patients combine to produce larger corrections. Even though these general principles are now well understood, precisely predicting the effect of RK in a given patient can be quite frustrating, and herein lies one of the major disadvantages of RK.

For example, I have personally observed as little as 3 D and as much as 10 D of effect from an 8-incision, 3.0 mm clear zone RK and as little as 2 D and as much as 6 D of effect from 4-incision, 3.0 mm clear zone RK in similarly aged patients. It is this individual patient variability in the response to RK that is primarily responsible for the significant number of over and undercorrections in reported series on the results of RK. This will be discussed in more detail in the results section of this chapter. Unfortunately this "patient response factor" has remained elusive, and significant numbers of over and undercorrections following RK will continue.

A major advantage of the mechanism of action of RK is that the central cornea, hopefully including the patient's visual axis, is untouched by the incisions. Thus when RK is properly performed, significant visual loss is extremely unlikely.

PHOTOREFRACTIVE KERATECTOMY

How does PRK change the refractive power of the cornea? The excimer laser reshapes, or sculpts, the anterior corneal surface by precisely removing Bowman's membrane and the anterior corneal stroma centrally with virtually no thermal damage. The laser physics and details of the laser delivery systems have been covered by Dr. L'Esperance in Chapter 1. Three aspects of the mechanism of action of PRK deserve special emphasis.

The first is that in contrast to RK, PRK works on the central cornea, exactly over the patient's visual axis. If there are problems with the laser–cornea interaction, such as increased haze or an irregular corneal surface, they will definitely have an effect on the quality of the patient's vision.

The second aspect involves the removal of Bowman's membrane in the area of the ablation. Questions about the significance of the absence of Bowman's membrane, such as the quality of the resultant optical surface and the adherence of the epithelial cells to the underlying stromal surface, have been answered in the short term. The vast majority of patients have recovered their preoperative best-corrected visual acuity, and recurrent corneal erosions have not been a problem thus far.

The final important aspect of the PRK procedure is the relationship between the diameter and depth of the ablation zone and the diopters of correction. Larger-diameter optical zones require deeper ablations per diopter of attempted corrections. For example, for an attempted correction of −6 D, a 4.0 mm optical zone requires a depth of only 30 μm, while a 6.0 mm zone would require a depth of 80 μm. This relationship may limit the amount of myopia that can be safely and accurately corrected. To correct −10 D with a 6.0 mm optical zone requires an ablation depth of 130 μm, while the same correction could be accomplished with a 4.0 mm zone by removing only 50 μm of stromal tissue. Seiler and Wollensak[3] reported that PRK utilizing 3.5 mm optical zones in a small series resulted in frequent patient complaints of excessive glare and halos, and most investigators are now performing PRK with 5.0 to 6.0 mm diameter ablation zones.

Whether the deeper ablation zones required for higher amounts of myopia with larger ablation zone diameters will produce an increased incidence of corneal haze and loss of effect has not yet been established. The preliminary reports by Seiler and Wollensak[3] and McDonald and coworkers[4] have already shown that PRK is less accurate for corrections over 6 D. Current investigations utilizing multiple ablations with different optical zones at the same time for higher amounts of myopia (for example, a −10 D patient might have a 4 D ablation with a 6.0 mm zone followed immediately by a 6 D ablation with a 5.0 mm zone) should help determine the upward limit of accurate, safe PRK.

Although the excimer laser is capable of removing corneal tissue with an unprecedented degree of accuracy, it is already apparent that this will not ensure uniformly excellent results in all cases. The reader should not find this surprising since ablating corneal tissue is not like ablating plastic. There are bound to be biological differences in the cornea's response to the laser. The amount and quality of the new collagen deposited, the degree of corneal haze, and the extent of epithelial hyperplasia will undoubtedly vary from patient to patient and will combine with other yet-unknown factors to produce under- and overcorrections as well as occasional decreases in best-corrected visual acuity. Only time will tell whether the incredible accuracy of the excimer laser will minimize the effects of biological variability and allow PRK to become the preferred refractive surgery technique for most myopic patients.

PATIENT SELECTION AND INFORMED CONSENT

RK PATIENT SELECTION

The most satisfying results in terms of uncorrected visual acuity following RK have been in patients with between −1 and −6 D of myopia and less than 1 D of astigmatism. Within this range of myopia the age of the patient is important only in determining the surgical plan. For patients with more than −6 D, especially younger patients, a complete correction of their myopia is far less likely.

A useful formula for estimating the amount of correction possible from an 8-incision, 3.0 mm optical zone RK is 2.5 + 0.1 (patient age). Thus a 25 year-old patient could expect 5 D of correction, while a 50 year-old might obtain 7.5 D. Most young prepresbyopic patients are not satisfied unless they can essentially eliminate their need for glasses, and therefore it is unwise to attempt corrections greater than 6 D in this group. Presbyopic patients, however, are often quite pleased with an undercorrection of 1 to 2 D, allowing them to read without glasses and wear much lighter spectacles. Because these older patients obtain more effect from RK, satisfactory results can be obtained in 50 year-olds with up to 10 D of myopia.

RK INFORMED CONSENT

In addition to discussing the possibility of over- and undercorrections and demonstrating various possible outcomes with trial lenses, the RK informed consent should include a thorough discussion of "star bursting" around lights at night, morning to evening fluctuations in vision, the possibility of progressive hyperopic shift with time, and the permanent structural weakening of the cornea.

Some of the normal side effects of RK can be important factors in a patient's decision to go ahead with the surgery. For example, a patient with large pupils who drives a truck at night will be more concerned about star bursting than a patient with small pupils who rarely drives at night. Although many patients undergo RK to qualify for positions in law enforcement or fire fighting, some occupations such as certain commercial airlines and the military specifically exclude candidates who have had RK. The weakened cornea can at times be an important consideration. I recently counseled a karate instructor not to have an RK because of the increased risk of corneal rupture in the event of ocular trauma. He elected to have a PRK.

PRK PATIENT SELECTION

At the present time, patient selection for PRK is determined by the FDA protocols. The protocol for myopic PRK is limited to patients with 1 to 6 D of myopia and no more than 1 D of astigmatism. The astigmatism protocol is limited to patients with 1 to 6 D of myopia and 0.75 to 4.50 D of astigmatism and the high-myopia protocol is for patients with −10 to −20 D. VISX has also recently submitted a protocol for myopic patients with refraction between −6 and −8 D.

PRK INFORMED CONSENT

In all the FDA PRK trials, the experimental nature of the procedure must be emphasized, and an extensive written informed consent must be read and signed. The informed consent at our hospital is 10 pages long and was approved after extensive revisions by our human subjects committee. This committee requires periodic reports on the results and complications of PRK.

In discussing PRK with potential patients, several differences between the ablation technique and the incisional procedures should be emphasized.

PRK causes considerably more pain, and recovery of useful vision is much slower than with RK. The fact that PRK is performed on the central cornea with the inherent risk of loss of best-corrected visual acuity can be extremely important to a patient who requires correctable vision of 20/20. I have already observed loss of best-corrected visual acuity to 20/50 and 20/40 following PRK due to excessive corneal haze in our small series of PRK patients (details later), and I have not encountered this degree of visual loss in 10 years of performing RK.

This potential for loss of best-corrected vision must be emphasized during the informed consent process. I recently discussed PRK versus RK with a 38 year-old commercial airline pilot with 5 D of myopia. If his uncorrected visual acuity could be improved to 20/70 or better, he would be able to obtain a superior position as a pilot, but only if his correctable vision remained 20/20. If his corrected vision fell below 20/20, he would be in danger of losing his present job. Although I felt that he had an excellent chance of obtaining uncorrected vision of 20/70 or better with either procedure, I felt that PRK was more likely than RK to cause a decrease of one line or more in his best-corrected visual acuity. After extensive discussions, we decided to perform 4-incision RK on his nondominant eye. At 6 weeks postoperatively his vision was 20/30 uncorrected and 20/20 with a −0.5 D sphere. Four weeks after a similar procedure in his other eye, he has 20/20 uncorrected visual acuity in that eye, and he is obviously pleased with the results of his surgery.

In contrast to the pilot, the −2 D karate instructor discussed earlier chose PRK for both eyes, and he now has 20/20 uncorrected visual acuity in both eyes. At the present state of our knowledge about both procedures, either one may at times be preferable for a given patient, and the complete refractive surgeon should be capable of performing either as soon as FDA approval for PRK is obtained.

PATIENT EXPERIENCES

RK AT SURGERY

RK is typically performed with topical anesthesia in an outpatient operating room or, more commonly, in a minor procedure room in the surgeon's office. The patient experiences minimal pain during the surgery, usually only a slight pinching sensation during fixation of the globe and little or no discomfort from the incisions. The entire procedure is usually completed in less than 15 minutes, and the eye is patched. Most patients remove the patch in less than 2 hours and have only mild-to-moderate discomfort, usually described as a burning or scratchy sensation requiring only mild analgesics such as hydrocodone and acetaminophen (Vicodin®) or acetaminophen with codeine (Tylenol®).

RK POSTOPERATIVELY

The RK patient usually obtains a good night's sleep and arrives at the office the next day with the eye open, mild photophobia, and usually excellent functional visual acuity. A mild overcorrection of 1 to 2 D usually improves within the first 2 weeks, and a near-final result is present at 4 weeks. If an additional procedure is required, such as adding 4 additional incisions, it can be performed in 4 to 6 weeks.

The quality of the patient's vision with an overcorrection is usually excellent from day 1, and a decrease in best-corrected visual acuity is rare. Although most patients are aware of the star bursting phenomenon around lights, it is rarely bothersome to them and improves during the first 3 months. The fact that most RK patients elect to have the surgery on their second eye certainly indicates a high level of satisfaction.

PRK AT SURGERY

Compared with an office RK, the patient experience with PRK can be somewhat more intimidating because of the presence of a high-tech laser in a dedicated room. The surgery is again performed with topical anesthesia. Because of the sounds created by the laser pulses and additional noises from suction pumps and the nitrogen flow in the VISX system, most surgeons perform some type of preliminary training to familiarize the patient with the experience. With the Summit system, which depends solely on the patient's own fixation, the training consists of applying a few pulses to the patient's epithelium prior to its mechanical removal. With the VISX, we have the patient present in the laser room during the ablation of the calibration plastic so that they can hear the various sounds and see the laser beam. Despite this training session, I have had a few patients experience a brief startle reaction with the initial laser pulses.

The most time-consuming aspect of PRK is the mechanical epithelial removal on the central 6 mm of the cornea, which can be quite variable. At times the epithelium can be easily removed as a sheet with a blunt spatula, but it can also be very adherent to the underlying Bowman's, requiring more tedious removal with sharper instruments. Although the entire procedure is painless, the epithelial removal is usually the part the patients most vividly remember. One patient described it as "tap dancing on my cornea."

PRK POSTOPERATIVELY

The eye is patched after application of a steroid antibiotic ointment and a cycloplegic drop. In contrast to RK, PRK patients experience moderate to severe pain requiring strong analgesics, such as deoxycortisone acetate (Percoset®) or meperidine (Demerol®), which are relatively ineffective. The pain is most severe for the first 8 to 10 hours and then gradually eases so that most patients are able to sleep on the night of surgery, and they are reasonably comfortable by the next morning.

On the first postoperative day the patients have a significant central corneal abrasion causing tearing, photophobia, blurred vision, and mild-to-moderate discomfort. The epithelium usually covers the defect in 2 to 4 days, and although patching is optional during this phase, most patients seem more comfortable unpatched.

Patients usually begin to have reasonable vision after about 1 week. The low-myopia patients may have near- 20/20 vision by this time, but the higher-myopia patients are usually about 20/50. All patients are usually hyperopic during the first 3 months, approximately 1 to 3 D, so the quality of their uncorrected vision depends on their amplitude of accommodation. Although the corneal reticular haze is obvious on slit lamp examination, especially during the first 3 months, it causes surprisingly few complaints of glare or foggy vision. The majority of patients are unaware of the corneal haze. The final visual result is generally obtained at about 3 months but with progressive clearing of the corneal haze and continued improvement in hyperopia, especially in older patients.

RK VERSUS PRK COMPARISON BY ONE PATIENT

In order to give the reader a true patient perspective about the similarities and differences between RK and PRK, I have asked one of our patients who had an RK in one eye and a PRK in the other to describe his experience at surgery and postoperatively with special emphasis on the quality of his vision. The patient, R. S., is a 33 year-old man who was not satisfied with contacts or spectacles for the correction of his vision. His preoperative refraction was: OD -2.00 $-1.25 \times 05°$; OS -2.25 $-0.50 \times 165°$. Because he had too much astigmatism to qualify for PRK in his right eye, he elected to have an RK in this eye followed by a PRK in the other.

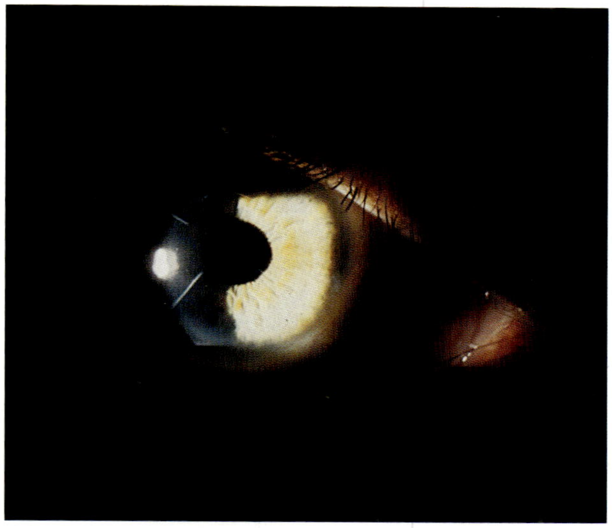

FIGURE 5.1. Slit lamp photograph of patient R. S. at 3 months postoperative RK in right eye.

He underwent 4-incision RK, 4.0 mm clear zone plus 1 superior arcuate incision in the vertical meridian at a 6-mm optical zone to the right eye and had a PRK, 5.5-mm optical zone, to the left eye. Six months postoperatively he has an uncorrected visual acuity in each eye of 20/20, and his refraction is plano $-0.25 \times 85°$ OD and plano $-0.50 \times 160°$ OS. Because he has obtained such an excellent result in each eye from each procedure, he is particularly well suited to contrast the two techniques. Figures 5.1 and 5.2 are slit lamp views of each eye at 3 months, and Figures 5.3 and 5.4 are computerized corneal maps of each eye at 6 months. The following is R. S.'s description of his experience:

> During the summer of 1990 several of my fellow swimmers on the West Hollywood Aquatics team mentioned that they had undergone eye surgery to correct their nearsightedness. They had the RK procedure and were thrilled with the results, and now they no longer had to wear contacts when they swam. I was interested but not quite sure I was willing to "go under the knife."
>
> In the spring of 1991 I read an article in Cedars-Sinai Medical Center's internal newsletter, *Currentlines,* about a new experimental eye surgery utilizing a laser to correct the shape of the cornea. Now I was interested. The article said that doctors here at Cedars were looking for people to volunteer to have this experimental eye surgery, PRK, done on them. I felt that this might be my chance to finally stop wear-

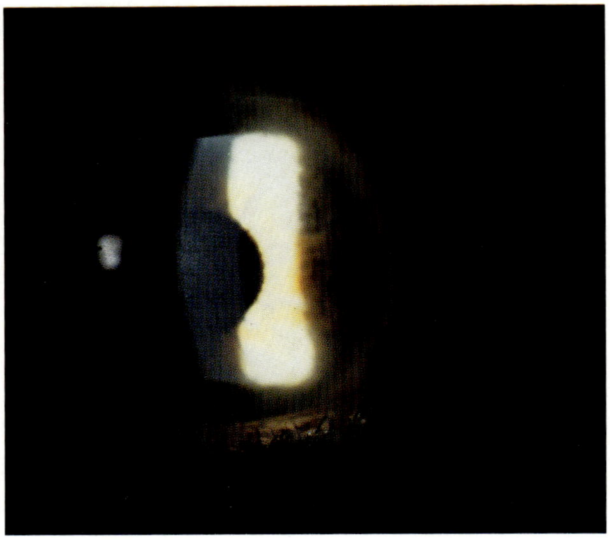

FIGURE 5.2. Slit lamp photograph of patient R. S. at 3 months postoperative PRK in left eye.

ing contacts and glasses, so I arranged an appointment to be interviewed as a possible candidate.

I was prescreened over the phone, and after meeting the criteria, I went to meet Dr. Salz's technician. She showed me video interviews with patients who had this new procedure, and these patients seemed very confident and pleased with their results. I was given a long informed consent form explaining the possible risks involved, and I was told to read it at home

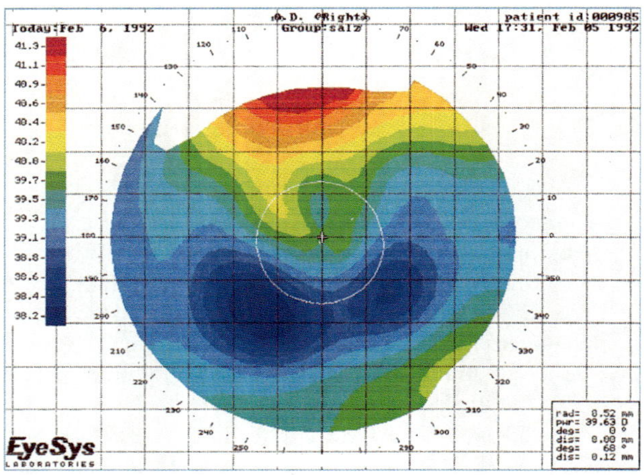

FIGURE 5.3. Computerized corneal map of patients R. S. at 6 months postoperative RK in right eye. The white circle represents the pupil. The blue inferior area is 1 D flatter than the central optical zone and probably represents excessive flattening over the two inferior RK incisions.

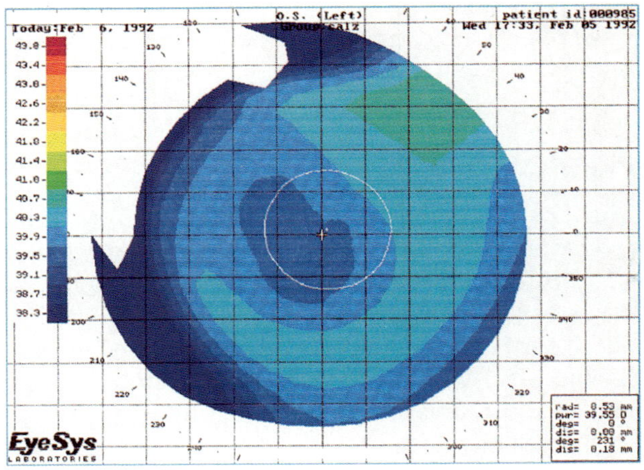

FIGURE 5.4. Computerized corneal map of patient R. S. at 6 months postoperative PRK in left eye. The central blue zone represents the area of the ablation. The white circle represents the pupil.

and let them know if I wanted to schedule the surgery. I immediately knew I would go ahead with this surgery, so I scheduled my initial examination.

When Dr. Salz examined my eyes he concluded that my right eye had too much astigmatism to qualify for the PRK study, so we decided to perform the PRK on my left eye. He explained that I could have the RK procedure on my right eye and later the PRK on my left eye. This would also eliminate the need to wait 6 months between eyes as would be necessary if PRK was performed on both eyes. After hearing about the risks of RK and the differences between the two procedures, I agreed to have the RK on my right eye.

The RK procedure was supposed to be less painful than the PRK, so I thought it was going to be a piece of cake. The procedure took about 15 minutes, and Dr. Salz was assisted by a technician and Dr. Le. Dr Salz's procedural style includes the education of his patients (which really did help my anxiety). He talked me through the entire procedure and made me feel very comfortable. The procedure itself was somewhat uncomfortable; I had to make sure my eye would stay open (even though they had opened my eye with a speculum). I would look up and Dr. Salz would apply pressure to my eye and tell me to hold steady. I would see the light above me fade out and move about my vision. Dr. Salz made several incisions and seemed very confident afterwards. They bandaged my eye, gave me some Tylenol® with codeine, and sent me on my way until the following day.

When I returned home my eye started to hurt even though I had taken some of the Tylenol®. The pain was almost unbelievable. It would come in waves and get real bad and then somehow ease. (I assume it was the buildup and release of endorphins.) After about 3 hours I could not stand it any longer, so I took off the bandage and lifted my eyelid off my eye. This seemed to ease the irritation of my eyelid rubbing against my cornea. After another hour and a half I felt much better and I was able to get to sleep.

The next day I went in to see Dr. Salz and had my RK eye tested. It was somewhat watery, but my vision had already improved to 20/30. Dr. Salz was quite excited about the improvement although he did expect this type of reaction. We then scheduled my PRK surgery for 1 month later. During that time I had to wear a contact in my left eye. I was only allowed to do this for 2 weeks as I was not allowed to wear the contact lens for 2 weeks prior to the PRK.

My vision in my RK eye was sensitive to light, and I would have problems with night driving due to the star bursting effect around lights. I thought if this was what the RK results were, I would not recommend RK to anyone because of the reduction in my night vision. Dr. Salz informed me that this was normal and would fade away in the next couple of months. I also noticed for the next couple of weeks that my eye would really sting when I touched my cornea or eyelid.

I was scheduled for the PRK on June 12, 1991. Before my PRK I had talked with a person who works here at Cedars who had the PRK procedure several months earlier. I had some concern about the amount of pain I would have to endure, since Dr. Salz warned me that the PRK was going to be much more painful than the RK. This other patient told me she did not have much pain because she got prescriptions for Valium® and Percoset®, so I requested the same prescriptions.

The morning of the surgery, I of course was anxious. Dr. Salz arrived and showed me with a sample piece of plastic how the laser reshapes the eye. The assistants in the Ellis Eye Center set me up in the chair, and Dr. Salz again talked me through the procedure. However, this time there was no pressure applied to my eye. The only thing Dr. Salz told me to do was to continue to look at the red light above me and try not to blink. During the procedure, I lost sight of the red light and all I could see was a white color. I did not feel any discomfort during this procedure, and when the laser was finished they rinsed my eye and patched me up. I was given my prescriptions and driven home by a friend. I honestly do not remember experiencing any pain (the Valium® really did the trick!).

The next day I went in to see Dr. Salz and he removed the patch. I could see much better now that at least one eye wasn't completely blind. It seemed to balance my vision out (one of the chief drawbacks was not being able to see out of one eye for 2 weeks). I rested for 2 days and watched some TV. I was told that I should probably remain quiet for a few days so I did.

After the PRK surgery, my eye did not hurt when I touched it (unlike the RK eye). I could rub it and nothing irritated it. Another subtle difference was when I walked outside, I would automatically close the RK eye. It seemed to be more sensitive to the light. My night vision in the RK eye gradually got better, and I was not seeing as much star bursting. The PRK eye had a different type of night vision. I don't notice it much, but I see a haze around lights. The haze was similar to the haze that I would see if my contacts have been on all day long. I only notice this at night. Also, in my PRK eye when I travel at night and look up at the freeway signs, the lettering has a slight double image. Nothing serious, but if I have to scrutinize my vision, I must mention that.

It's been roughly 6 months since both procedures. I almost can't remember what it was like to have to deal with my contacts. My eyes seem to be the same every day. I don't notice any fluctuation in my vision, and I don't double-check my night vision abilities. I feel very strongly that the PRK seems to be the better procedure overall in the amount of pain and irritation involved. I also feel that the fact I don't have the star bursting is an added benefit.

RESULTS

RADIAL KERATOTOMY

Table 5.1 summarizes the 1-year results of RK from the PERK,[5] Deitz,[6] and Salz[7] studies for low, medium, and high myopia. The PERK study utilized 8-incision RK with three different optical zones, ignoring patient age, and is based on only one operation. The Deitz series included 8- and 16-incision RK with multiple optical zones, considered patient age, and is again based on only one operation. The Salz series included both 4- and 8-incision RK with multiple optical zones, considered patient age, and included additional incisions in 15% of the eyes. All three studies employed micrometer diamond knives, ultrasonic pachymetry, and an incision direction from optical zone to limbus without redeepening.

The results of RK in all three series were excellent for low-myopia patients, with over 90% of the patients achieving an uncorrected visual acuity of 20/40 or better, but the PERK and Deitz studies resulted in overcorrections greater than 1 D in 11 and 13%, respectively. Since we now know that 20 to 30% of patients experience a progressive hyperopic shift greater than 1 D after the first year, this represents a major disadvantage of RK. The overcorrection rate in the Salz series was only 3%, primarily because all the patients received a 4-incision RK.

In the group with medium myopia, the results were not as satisfactory, with 74 to 88% of the eyes achieving uncorrected visual acuity of 20/40 or better. Again a major problem of the PERK and Deitz studies was an overcorrection rate more than 1 D

TABLE 5.1. Comparison of RK studies—Results at one year

*Study**	*Low (≤ −3.0 D)*	*Medium (3.1 to 5.9 D)*	*High (6.0 to 12.0 D)*
PERK			
20/40 sc (%)	92	76	48†
+1 to −1 D SE (%)	84	55	24
>+1 D SE (%)	11	11	4
Deitz			
20/40 sc (%)	95	88	77
+1 to −1 D SE (%)	90	76	53
>+1 D SE (%)	13	13	16
Salz			
20/40 sc (%)	100	74	47
+1 to −1 D (SE (%)	96	80	45
>+1 D SE (%)	3	3	4

*SE = spherical equivalent; sc = without correction.
†PERK −6 to −8 D.

in 11 and 13%. This was again only 3% in the Salz study, in which many of the patients received an initial 4-incision RK.

Only 47 to 77% of the eyes with more than 6 D of myopia achieved an uncorrected visual acuity of 20/40 or better. Correcting high myopia with RK is very age-dependent. With proper patient selection in high myopia, even patients who are not corrected to 20/40 may be quite satisfied with a significant reduction in their myopia, allowing them to read comfortably without glasses.

A major problem with RK is the progressive hyperopic shift first described by Deitz. It is certainly frustrating to see a patient with a near-emmetropic result at 1 year become progressively more hyperopic with time. The incidence of a progressive hyperopic shift of more than 1 D has been reported as 22% by PERK,[8] 31% by Deitz and coworkers,[9] and 13% by Salz and coworkers.[7] The magnitude of the shift can at times be quite alarming. Damiano and Forstot[10] recently reported on two patients who were near-emmetropic at 1 year and now have spherical equivalent refractions of +6.25 and +8 D, 5 and 10 years after their original surgery. In those patients who are experiencing this shift, it is uncertain if and when it will stop.

PHOTOREFRACTIVE KERATECTOMY

Since PRK is a relatively new procedure, 1-year results are just now beginning to appear. Because of differences in the method of reporting, it is not possible to summarize the results in tabular form as was done with RK, so studies by McDonald et al.,[4] Seiler and Wollensak,[3] Sher et al.,[11] and Gartry et al.[12] will be discussed separately.

McDonald and coworkers reported on a 1-year follow-up on 18 normally sighted eyes that had a PRK with the VISX system. Eight eyes (44%) achieved an uncorrected visual acuity of 20/40 or better. In eyes with −5 D of myopia or less, 6 of 7 (86%) achieved uncorrected acuities of 20/40 or better, while only 2 of the 11 (18%) eyes with greater than −5 D of myopia obtained this level of improvement. Four of the 7 eyes (57%) with attempted corrections of −5 D or less were corrected to within 1 D of emmetropia, but only 2 of 11 eyes (18%) with attempted corrections greater than −5 D achieved this degree of accuracy.

Seiler and Wollensak published 1-year results on 26 sighted eyes that underwent PRK with the Summit system. Twenty-four (92%) were corrected to within 1 D of their intended correction, and (96%) attained an uncorrected visual acuity of 20/40 or better. This series is especially impressive because it included attempted corrections of up to 7.25 D. Of the 11 eyes with attempted corrections of −5 to −7.25 D, 9 (82%) were within 1 D of the target.

Sher and coworkers reported 6-month results from a multicenter trial of PRK with the Taunton excimer laser on 31 eyes with preoperative myopia between −4 and −12 D (spherical equivalent). Fifty-five percent were corrected to within 1 D of attempted correction, and 45% had an uncorrected visual acuity of 20/40 or better. The poorer results in this study are attributable to the larger corrections attempted by these investigators.

In the largest series to date, Gartry and coworkers reported the results of PRK with the Summit system on 120 sighted eyes divided equally into six treatment groups from −2 to −7 D in whole-diopter steps. Thus 20 patients had attempted corrections of 2 D, 20 others 3 D, 20 others 4 D, and so on through 7 D. The mean preoperative myopia for each of the treatment groups was as follows: 2.10 D for the 2 D group; 3.86 D for the 3 D group; 4.00 D for the 4 D group; 7.10 D for the 5 D group; 7.00 D for the 6 D group; and 10.26 D for the 7 D group. A complete correction was obviously not attempted in many of the eyes in the higher-treatment groups. All patients had a 4.0-mm-diameter treatment zone.

The accuracy of the target ablations within ± 1 D for each of the six groups was as follows: −2 D = 90%; −3 D = 75%; −4 D = 50%; −5 D = 45%; −6 D = 40%; −7 D = 20%. This study beautifully emphasizes the decreasing accuracy of PRK as larger corrections are attempted.

Since all the patients in this unique study were not targeted for full corrections, the uncorrected visual acuities are reported only for those eyes in which a full correction of the myopia was attempted. The percentage of eyes that achieved an uncorrected visual acuity of 20/40 or better for each treatment group was as follows (number of eyes targeted for full correction in parentheses): −2 D = 90% (20 eyes); −3 D = 78% (9 eyes); −4 D = 59% (17 eyes); −5 D = 50% (8 eyes); −6 D = 63% (8 eyes); −7 D = 25% (4 eyes).

Our own experience with the VISX at Cedars Sinai is limited. We have a 1-year follow-up on 12 eyes with preoperative myopia of −1.75 to −5.12 D. Eleven of the 12 eyes (92%) have an uncorrected visual acuity of 20/30 or better and are corrected to within 1 D of emmetropia. We have 6-month results on another 50 eyes with up to 6 D of myopia; these results show that approximately 80% are corrected to within 1 D of emmetropia and have uncorrected visual acuities of 20/40 or better.

Although there is not enough long-term data on any PRK series to draw any conclusions about stability, because the procedure does not produce a structural weakening of the cornea, a late refractive shift, especially in the direction of hyperopia, seems unlikely.

SAFETY AND SIDE EFFECTS

RADIAL KERATOTOMY

Although serious complications, such as endophthalmitis, have been reported following RK, fortunately they are rare. None of the three series discussed earlier reported any vision-threatening complications, and loss of more than one line of best-corrected visual acuity is uncommon in any of the published reports. Because RK does cause a structural weakening of the cornea, there have been several cases of late rupture of the cornea secondary to blunt trauma. The lack of complete wound healing in RK is also responsible for fluctuations in visual acuity throughout the day described by many patients and for the progressive hyperopic shift described earlier in the results section.

Although many RK patients are aware of the star bursting around lights, most of them do not find this troublesome enough to limit their night driving, and I do not consider this nighttime glare to be a major problem in RK unless the surgeon utilizes an excessive number of incisions or an optical zone smaller than 3.0 mm.

PHOTOREFRACTIVE KERATECTOMY

There were no serious vision-threatening complications reported in the four PRK series discussed earlier. Loss of more than one line of best-corrected visual acuity was reported in two eyes by McDonald et al., three eyes by Gartry et al., and no eyes by Sher et al. and Seiler and Wollensak. However the Seiler series included 225 eyes with less than 1-year follow-up, and 8 of these (2.8%) developed excessive corneal haze and a decrease in best-corrected vision of more than one line. Four of these eyes have had a second ablation with initially satisfying results.

In our own series at Cedars Sinai, we have one eye that has experienced a significant loss of best-corrected visual acuity at 6 months from 20/30 to 20/60 and 20/200 under glare testing secondary to excessive corneal haze (Figs. 5.5 and 5.6). This eye is also markedly undercorrected with a preoperative refraction of −5.5 D and a postoperative refraction of −3.75 D at one year. This eye underwent repeat PRK and at 1 month uncorrected visual acuity is 20/50 and corrected visual acuity is 20/40 with +1.00–2.25 × 180°. Figure 5.7 is a slit lamp photograph of this eye at one month demonstrating considerable clearing of the corneal haze.

RK PLUS PRK

The results of RK and the preliminary results of PRK show that both procedures seem to be most effective for patients with less than 6 D of myopia. Since an 8-incision RK can usually correct 4 to 8 D of myopia depending on patient age, the possibility of combining both procedures to extend the range of myopic corrections is an intriguing one.

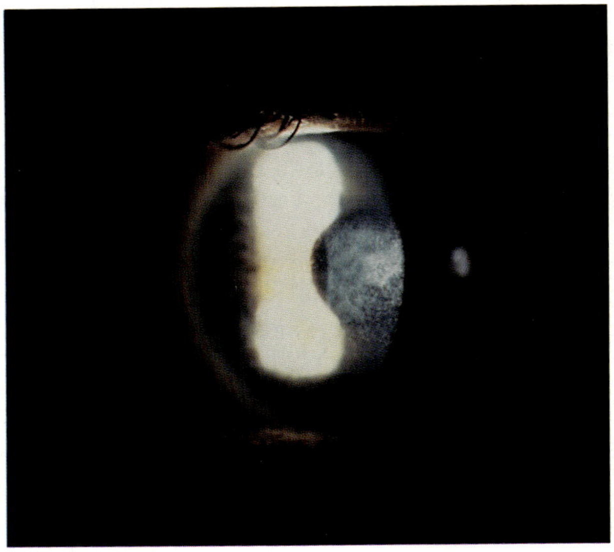

FIGURE 5.5. Slit lamp photograph of patient with excessive corneal haze post PRK.

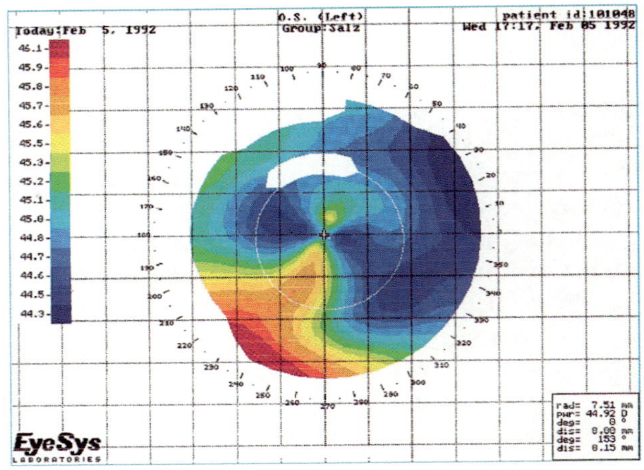

FIGURE 5.6. Computerized corneal map of patient with excessive corneal haze at 8 months postoperative. The white circle represents the pupil. The superior white patch represents an area that could not be interpreted. The blue ablated zone centrally along the 106° meridian is interrupted by a steeper astigmatic band, green and yellow along the 70° meridian.

For example, a −10 D myopic patient could have an 8-incision RK as an initial procedure. After stabilization, residual myopia of anywhere between 3 and 6 D could be corrected with a PRK.

We have treated three post-RK patients with residual myopia of 1.75 to 3.25 D with a PRK. All three patients had an 8-incision RK as an initial procedure. The results on these three patients are summarized in Table 5.2.

Figure 5.8 shows a clinical photograph taken at 1 month and Figure 5.9 shows the computerized corneal map at 6 months of patient J. V. S. The other two patients both experienced a late increase in corneal haze and loss of effect at 6 and 12 months that improved after another course of topical hydrocortisone drops. Figure 5.10 shows patient J. N. P. with the increased corneal haze causing a decrease in best-corrected vision to 20/50 at 1 year and Figure 5.11 shows his computerized corneal map 1 year post PRK. Only when other investigators report their results of PRK following RK will we be able to properly evaluate the success of these combined procedures.

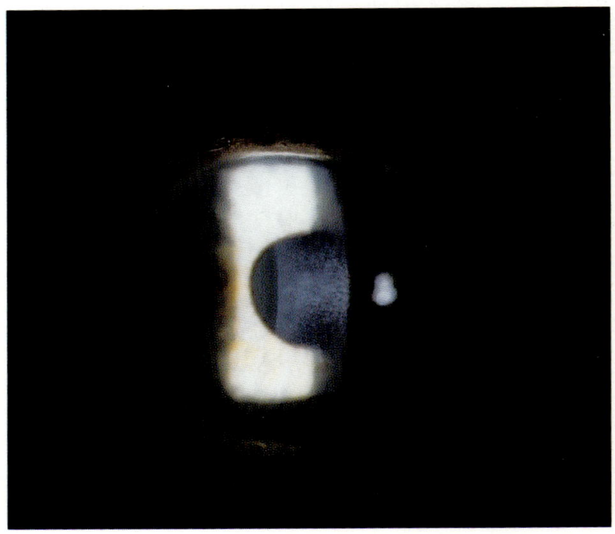

FIGURE 5.7. Slit lamp photograph of patient with excessive haze 1 month after repeat PRK demonstrating reduction in corneal haze.

TABLE 5.2. Results of PRK following RK*

Patient	*Pre-RK SE*	*Post-RK SE*	*Post-PRK SE*	*VA sc*	*Follow-up (months)*
J. V. S.	−3.75	−1.75	Plano	20/15	8
J. N. P.	−5.50	−3.25	−0.25	20/20	16
J. L. S.	−8.37	−3.25	Plano	20/50	13

*SE = spherical equivalent; sc = without correction; VA = visual acuity.

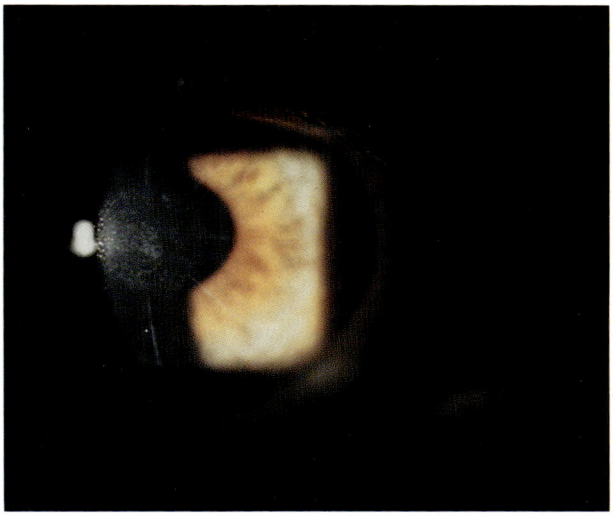

FIGURE 5.8. Slit lamp photograph of patient J. V. S. post-PRK following RK at 1 month postoperative.

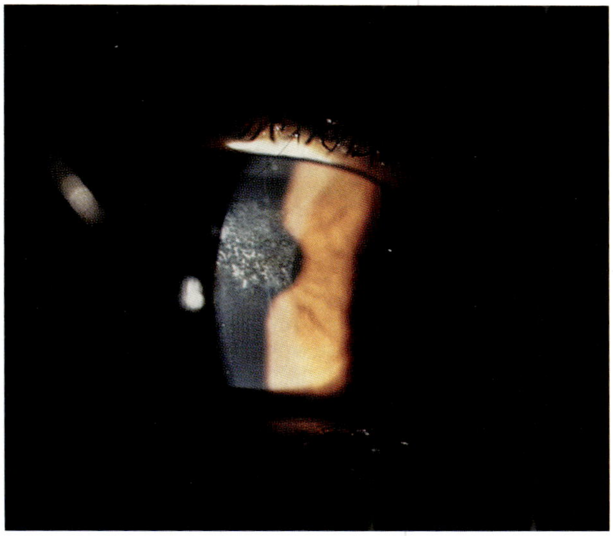

FIGURE 5.10. Slit lamp photograph of patient J. N. P. post-PRK following RK with excessive corneal haze at 1 year.

FINANCIAL CONSIDERATIONS

PATIENT

At Cedars Sinai Medical Center we have tried to keep the costs to the patient the same for PRK as they have been for RK. The usual charge for RK in our area including use of the operating room and follow-up surgery if necessary is $1500.

The fee for PRK is also $1500, with $750 to the surgeon and $750 to the hospital for use of the laser. Should a secondary treatment be necessary, the patient would still be required to pay the hospital fee. Fees for PRK at some of the other centers are between $2000 and $2500.

SURGEON

There is obviously an enormous difference in the financial obligations facing ophthalmic surgeons contemplating adding either RK or PRK to their practice. Assuming the surgeon has an operating microscope in the office, the major purchases necessary to begin performing RK are for an ultrasonic pachymeter ($4000), a micrometer diamond knife ($2000), and a set of optical zone markers ($1000). For less than $10,000 a surgeon can buy the equipment necessary to begin performing RK.

Contrast this to the investment necessary to be-

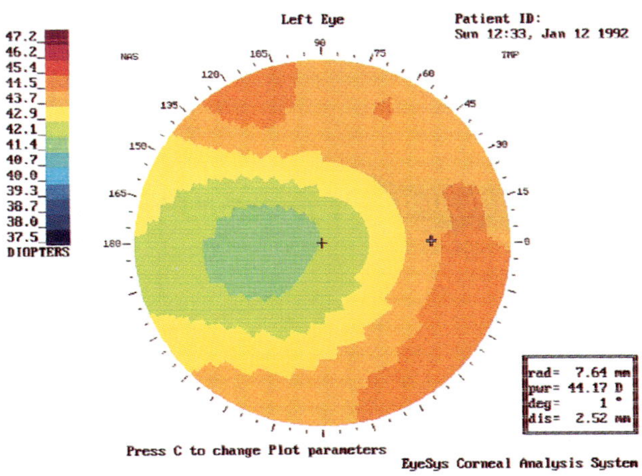

FIGURE 5.9. Computerized corneal map of patient J. V. S. post-PRK following RK at 6 months postoperative.

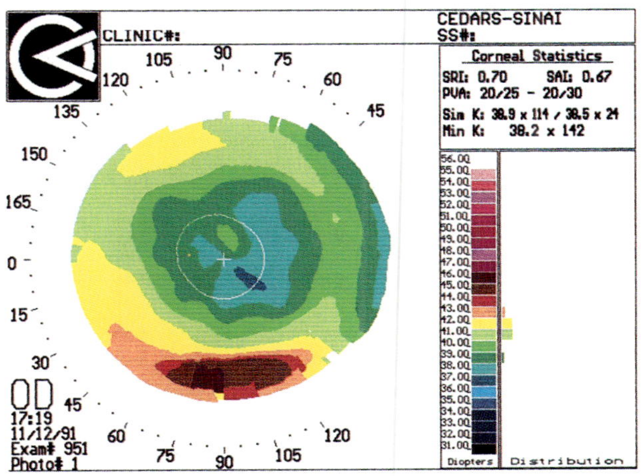

FIGURE 5.11. Computerized corneal map of patient J. N. P. post-PRK following RK at 1 year.

gin performing PRK. The current price quoted to me in June 1992 for excimer laser systems for correcting myopia, myopic astigmatism, and therapeutic applications were $475,000 for VISX and $401,000 for summit. With the summit system, there will be an additional charge for the ablatable mask required for astigmatic ablations. This includes a 1-year service warranty. After 1 year, a service contract must be purchased; typically this costs 10% of the purchase price of the laser. In addition, there is the cost of the various gases necessary to operate the laser. For the VISX system, this has been estimated to be approximately $50 per case if at least 10 patients per week have the procedure during a 1- or 2-day period. It is apparently very inefficient to turn on the laser for only one or two cases, and if this is done the gas costs will be even greater. It is also desirable to hire at least a part-time technician to assist with minor maintenance, start-up operations, gas fills of the excimer tube, gas tank exchanges, and plastic calibration procedures.

It is apparent that the substantial financial commitment required to purchase and maintain an excimer laser system virtually eliminates participation by most individual ophthalmologists. These expensive complicated laser systems will either have to be purchased by hospitals who can then make them available to all ophthalmologists on their staff or they will have to be purchased or leased by groups of ophthalmologists who will treat patients in a central location. Another alternative being publicized is purchase by commercial laser companies, who will place the lasers in laser centers and recoup their investment through patient charges. I have also seen advertisements promoting the idea of mobile excimer lasers that will be brought to the ophthalmologist's office. Unless there are significant improvements in the design of the delivery systems, I doubt that the accurate and delicate alignment of laser tube, mirrors, lenses, and iris diaphragm required for proper operation of the laser would stand up well to the bumps and turns of street travel.

CONCLUSIONS

As I discuss RK and PRK with prospective patients, I am constantly asked which is better. The honest answer at this stage of our knowledge is that I don't know. Both procedures seem to be very safe with a low incidence of vision-threatening complications, and both procedures seem to be most effective when the preoperative myopia is less than −6 D.

RK is attractive because of the simplicity of the equipment, sparing of the visual axis, and the rapid recovery of high-quality vision with minimal patient discomfort. The principal disadvantage of RK is the structural weakening of the cornea, which can result in progressive hyperopia in a significant percentage of patients, and rarely ruptured corneas in the event of significant blunt trauma. The presence of permanent corneal scars that can cause troublesome glare in some patients is also aesthetically unpleasing.

PRK is appealing because of the precision of the excimer laser and the mechanism of action, which removes less than 10% of the corneal surface, leaving a structurally sound eye that should maintain a stable result. The appearance of a perfectly clear cornea in many cases or one with only minimal corneal haze is aesthetically very appealing.

The most intimidating aspect of PRK is the fact that the laser works on the central cornea and involves removal of Bowman's membrane, causing a large central abrasion that produces considerable patient discomfort. PRK has already led to significant decreases in best-corrected visual acuity in a small number of patients due to excessive corneal scarring. If retreatment of these eyes can correct this complication, then working on the visual axis may turn out to be only a minor disadvantage. Probably the major disadvantage of PRK is the initial cost and ongoing expense required to purchase and maintain a high-tech, complicated, bulky piece of equipment.

Which technique is better? Time will tell, but as of now I think it will be PRK.

REFERENCES

1. Tenner A, Neyhann T, Schroder E, Salz JJ, Maguen, E: Excimer laser radial keratotomy in the living human eye: A preliminary report. *J Refract Surg* 4:5–8, 1988.
2. Waring GO: *Refractive Keratotomy for Myopia and Astigmatism*. St. Louis, Mosby-Year Book, 1992.
3. Seiler T, Wollensak J: Myopic photorefractive keratectomy with the excimer laser. *Ophthalmology* 98: 1156–1163, 1991.
4. McDonald MB, Liu JC, Byrd TJ, et al: Central photorefractive keratectomy for myopia. *Ophthalmology* 98:1327–1357, 1991.
5. Waring GO, Lynn MJ, Gelender H, et al: Results of the prospective evaluation of radial keratotomy (PERK) study one year after surgery. *Ophthalmology* 92:177–199, 1985.
6. Deitz MR, Sanders DR, Raanan MG: A consecutive series (1982–1985) of radial keratotomies performed

with the diamond blade. *Am J Ophthalmol* 103:417–422, 1987.

7. Salz JJ, Salz JM, Salz M, Jones DJ: Ten years experience with a conservative approach to radial keratotomy. *Refract Corneal Surg* 7:12–22, 1991.
8. Waring GO, Lynn MJ, Nizam A, et al: Results of the prospective evaluation of radial keratotomy five years after surgery. *Ophthalmology* 98:1164–1176, 1991.
9. Deitz MR, Sanders DR, Raanan MG: Progressive hyperopia in radial keratotomy. *Ophthalmology* 93: 1284–1288, 1986.
10. Damiano RE, Forstot SL: Extreme corneal flattening after radial keratotomy. *Am J Ophthalmol* (letter to the editor). 112:738, 1991.
11. Sher NA, Chen V, Bowers RA, et al: The use of the 193-nm excimer laser for myopic photorefractive keratectomy in sighted eyes. *Arch Ophthalmol* 109: 1525–1530, 1991.
12. Gartry DS, Muir MG, Marshall J: Photorefractive keratectomy with an argon fluoride excimer laser: A clinical study. *Refract Corneal Surg* 7:420–435, 1991.

CHAPTER 6

Photorefractive Keratectomy: High Myopia

FRANK B. THOMPSON
MAURO CAMPOS
PETER J. MCDONNELL

Myopia can be defined as the state of refraction in which parallel rays of light entering the eye are brought to a focus at a point in front of the retina. Consequent to this anterior focusing distance, vision is impaired.

The refraction of the eye is determined by four factors:

1. Corneal power
2. Anterior chamber depth
3. Lens power
4. Axial length of the eye

Refractive myopia, a condition in which the corneal curvature or human lens power is responsible for the degree of refractive error, is frequently associated with lower levels of myopia. A larger percentage of highly myopic individuals have axial myopia, a condition whereby the refractive error is associated with an increase in axial length.

Roughly 25% of people in the United States between the ages of 12 and 60 are myopic. This figure holds true for most European nations as well. There may be a higher incidence of myopia in Asia, particularly in Japan and China, where the prevalence of myopia has been estimated to be over 50%.[1] As the percentage of myopic individuals in a particular grouping increases, the incidence of high myopia increases as well. It has been estimated that perhaps 3 to 5% of the population fall within the highly myopic range.[2]

Highly myopic individuals whose visual acuity is correctable with glasses or contact lenses frequently suffer from significant aberrations and distortions of their perceptual space.

In addition, some cases of high myopia can lead to uncorrectable visual acuity and consequent blindness, for which only a few treatment modalities, such as scleral reinforcement, are available.

HIGH MYOPIA

HIGH MYOPIA VERSUS PATHOLOGIC MYOPIA

Myopia has been divided into low, moderate, and high degrees. The low and moderate ranges include those patients with a refractive error of under

Supported by a grant from the Autry Foundation, Los Angeles, CA.

TABLE 6.1. Thompson grading system for staphylomas

Type I—Inferior temporal staphylomas	
Grade I	Minimal inferior staphyloma with thinning of RPE, not involving macula; inferior to arcades
Grade II	More defined staphyloma with increased thinning of RPE, encroaching inside arcades, but not yet involving macula
Grade III	Definite staphyloma with thin RPE involving macula
Grade IV	Definite staphyloma involving macula with breaks in RPE and or possible "lacquer cracks"
Grade V	Definite staphyloma involving macula with small atrophic areas in RPE and choroid
Grade VI	Definite staphyloma involving macula with breaks in RPE, neovascular membrane, or Fuchs' spot
Grade VII	Sharply defined staphyloma with large atrophic areas in RPE, choroid, and retina ("whiteout") with sharply sloping staphyloma
Grade VIII	Complete loss of RPE, choroid, and retinal atrophy over posterior pole
Type II—Macular staphylomas	
Grade I	Macular staphyloma with thinning of RPE, contained within arcades and with possible breaks in RPE
Grade II	Macular staphyloma contained within arcades with atrophy of RPE and choroid; CAT scan and B scan reveal "nipple effect"

RPE = Retinal pigment epithelium.

−6.00 D or an axial length of under 26 mm. Those patients with myopia greater than −6.00 D or more than 26 mm in axial length fall into the high-myopia category.

High myopia may range from −6.00 D to greater than −40.00 D and from 26 mm to axial length measurements greater than 34 mm. High myopia may occur in patients in any age group, including infancy. In those patients whose refractive error or axial length reaches at least −8.00 D or greater than 27.00 mm, the myopia may continue to increase progressively throughout the patient's lifetime unless the increase in axial length is arrested.

The distinction between high myopia and pathologic myopia is somewhat ill defined. Pathologic myopia (malignant myopia, degenerative myopia, or progressive myopia) usually implies either a continued progressive increase in the measurement of myopia and axial length of the eye and/or pathologic changes that have occurred in the eye subsequent to these changes. The pathologic changes may include posterior and anterior staphylomata due to weakening of the thinned sclera with consequent deterioration of the choroid and retinal pigment epithelium, and thinning of the retina itself. This deterioration may result in blindness. Pathologic myopia may also be defined as myopia that occurs in one eye leading to uncorrectable anisometropia or myopia produced by injury or surgical intervention, such as encircling silicone bands for treatment of retinal detachment. Pathologic or high myopia constitutes the seventh leading cause of blindness in the United States and is the third or fourth leading cause of blindness in other countries around the world, particularly in Asia.[3]

The deterioration of the visual elements of the eye has been delineated in a number of grading systems including Curtin's and Thompson's.[4,5] These systems attempt to quantify the pathologic changes that occur in high degrees of myopia (see Table 6.1 and Figs. 6.1–6.4). In addition, we are now seeing pathologic changes occurring in eyes at lower levels of high myopia because of the continued aging of our population and the later development of staphylomas and deteriorative effects.

High myopia usually stabilizes during a patient's second or third decade. Progressive myopia patients may require surgical intervention with techniques such as scleral reinforcement or posterior scleral support surgery. Even if these patients are stabilized, their high degree of correction leads to numerous undesirable optical and sociological ef-

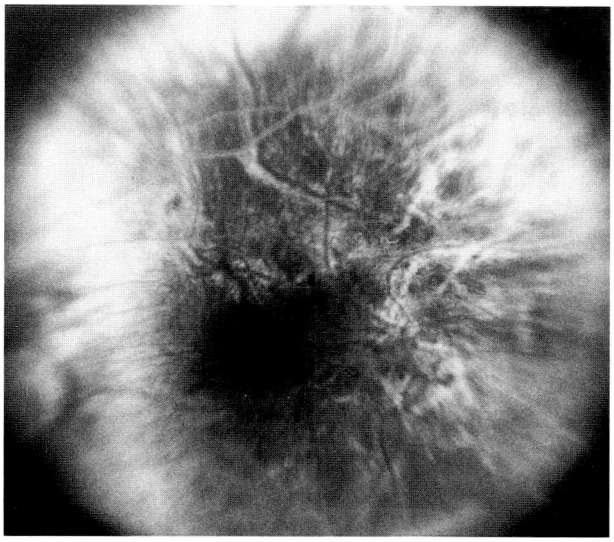

FIGURE 6.1. Fluorescein angiography of Figure 6.4 outlining lacquer cracks.

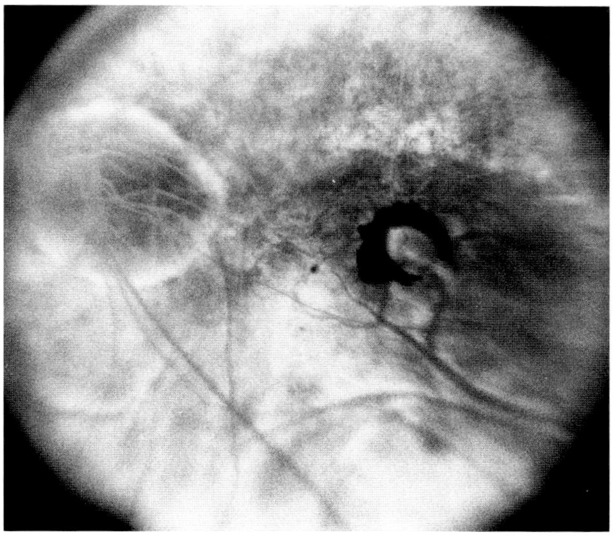

FIGURE 6.2. Fluorescein angiography of Figure 6.6 with neovascular membrane leading to macular hemorrhage.

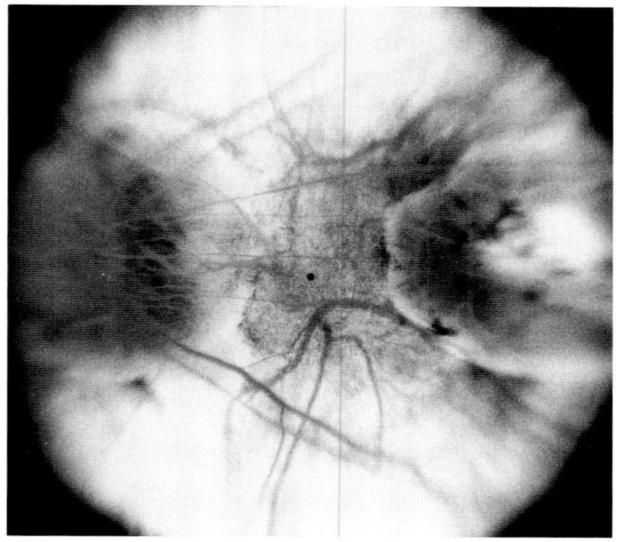

FIGURE 6.3. Fluorescein angiography of Figure 6.7 with central "white out."

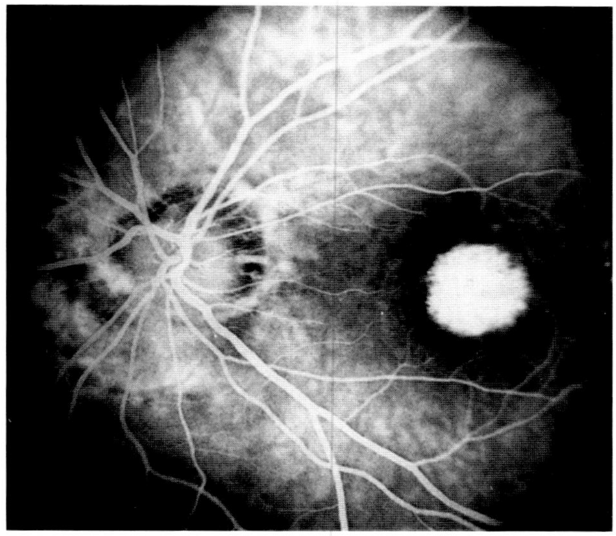

FIGURE 6.4. Fluorescein angiography of Figure 6.10 with central staphyloma with nipple.

fects. These negative aspects are discussed in a later section.

THE CLINICAL FEATURES OF THE HIGHLY MYOPIC EYE

The clinical features of the highly myopic eye are to a large extent genetically transmitted by either recessive, dominant, or X-linked means.

The anterior segments of the highly myopic eye are, in general, relatively normal, although there may be some increase in the corneal diameter but no concomitant decrease in corneal thickness. The anterior chamber may also demonstrate an increase in depth. In addition, atrophy of the anterior sclera allows the deeper uveal pigments to show through, causing the anterior sclera in certain cases to have a blue appearance. In some areas the sclera is very thin and the collagen fiber bundles, which make up the basic skeletal structure of this tissue, are also thinned and atrophic with individual fibers narrowed and widely separated.

There are frequently local areas of severe scleral abnormality leading to staphylomata in both the anterior equatorial regions and posterior segments of the globe.

There may be a reduction in the elastic fiber content and the number of melanocytes in highly myopic eyes. This is consistent with a disorganized tissue structure that can be complicated later by mechanical stretching forces.

Progressive myopia can lead to thinning and degenerative changes in the choroid, which can result in a marked loss of the choriocapillaris and the retinal pigment epithelium. This may appear as lacquer cracks and allow subretinal vessels to grow through as ingrowths, leading to hemorrhages and ultimately Fuchs' spots. The areas of choroidal tissue that seem to be most affected in high myopia are those within and adjacent to areas of posterior staphylomata.

The loss of the subretinal nutritive elements from the thinned choroid can lead to variable thinning in areas of the retina with changes usually found in the outer receptor segments. The inner neurosensory layers of the retina usually retain a fairly normal cellular structure.

VISUAL, PHYSIOLOGIC, AND SOCIOLOGICAL ASPECTS OF HIGH MYOPIA

Highly myopic patients who wear spectacles are faced with a large number of optical problems. Vision is reduced from distortions such as minification, peripheral aberrations, curvature of field, and coma, an aberration in which off-axis images appear comet-shaped. Additionally, spherical aberrations; "pincushion" effects; myopic rings and other associated reflections; and decreased contrast sensitivity disrupt vision. The instability of the vertex distance of a high-myopia patient's spectacles resulting from increased lens weight leads to visual fluctuations.

High myopia patients frequently have poor stereopsis secondary to a loss of binocular vision. Verzella has reported that in 237 of his patients with myopia greater than 15 D, 22% had no binocular vision. Another series of 348 patients showed that 21% were monocular.[6]

The visual field in these patients is frequently restricted from retinal deterioration in combination with smaller spectacle frame sizes. The retinal changes can also result in nyctalopia, poor color vision, and accommodation problems. If the retinal problems are macular or perimacular, image distortion or metamorphopsia results.

Bifocals are frequently unavailable in higher minus lenses. The increased weight of glasses also leads to nasal compression and adjustment problems.

Highly myopic patients have decreased mobility without correction, and, coupled with the esthetics of "Coke bottle" glasses, these two factors can be devastating to both their self-image and an outside observer's impression. The appearance of minification of ocular structure can lead to an improper evaluation of intelligence. These people are showing decreased levels of performance in their educational and vocational training as a result of their own self-image and society's expectations. A study in the *International Contact Lens Clinic,* May–June 1982, indicated that a majority of high-myopia patients studied held jobs in the unskilled labor category.[7]

Those patients who are fortunate to escape spectacles through contact lens wear face their own set of problems. These will be discussed in the next section.

NONSURGICAL TREATMENT MODALITIES

SPECTACLES

Until the mid-20th century, the only available treatment for myopic patients was corrective spectacles.

The refractive error in high myopia can be corrected in most instances with glasses. As the strength of the correction increases, however, the patient's vision is hampered by a series of optical aberrations as noted above. The thickness of the edge of the spectacles gives rise to loss of peripheral vision, occasional prismatic effects, and other visual abnormalities. Uncorrected visual acuity in patients with higher degrees of myopia is extremely poor and requires an almost complete dependence on the availability of spectacles for mobility. Fully corrected myopic patients frequently have abnormal perceptions of spatial relationships.

CONTACT LENSES

Contact lenses were originally developed earlier in this century but only became a practical reality after World War II. They do provide the more highly myopic patient with fewer visual aberrations but present special problems of their own.

Generally, high myopia patients exhibit larger eyes with an increased axial length, resulting in a decreased space between the superior bulbar conjunctiva and the palpebral conjunctiva.[8] High minus lenses have increased edge thickness and a decreased center thickness. These facts combine to adversely affect the lid–lens interaction. This results in poor lens centration, lens flexure, and an interruption of the normal tear pump mechanism. Because of these factors, hard contact lenses are frequently the lens of choice in high-myopia patients. These thicker lenses resist flexure, reducing induced astigmatic errors. On the other hand, these lenses are heavier, have thicker edges, and have smaller optic zones. They are consequently harder to keep centered due to lid–lens edge interaction and can be less comfortable than thinner lenses.

If centration, comfort, or corneal oxygen levels are inadequate, the practitioner can resort to either gas-permeable hard contact lenses or soft contacts. These lenses are thinner, have larger optic zones, are generally lighter, and transmit higher levels of oxygen to the cornea. The practitioner using either of these larger-diameter lens types faces an increased lid–lens interaction with the attendant problems mentioned above, an increase in flexure resulting in unstable acuity, and the added problem of potential GPC from deposits on these lenses. Compliance has been a perennial problem in contact lens care, and the anatomic factors noted above heighten the foreign body effect on the inner surface of the upper lid, leading to a greater incidence of GPC in high-myopia patients. The increased lid–lens edge interaction also reduces the rotational stability in fitting toric soft lenses.

Tear production frequently diminishes with age, and consequently lubrication becomes a significant problem. In many cases even the use of ocular lubrication becomes insufficient, and these patients may experience a decrease in wearing time.

In summary, contact lenses provide a more natural and true picture of the world while offering correction with reduced visual abnormalities in the high-myopia patient, considerable problems remain in fitting many of these patients comfortably and successfully.

SURGICAL MODALITIES FOR TREATMENT OF HIGH MYOPIA

RADIAL KERATOTOMY

Radial keratotomy (RK) is a surgical procedure consisting of radial incisions made in the cornea to cause central corneal flattening.

The history of RK goes back to Lans, who in 1897 first described the basic principles. Sato[9] in Japan reported in 1953 on radial corneal incisions in over 100 patients. These cases involved posterior incisions through the endothelium, and while they did reduce myopia, they eventually led to corneal decompensation and bullous keratopathy in many of the patients.

The first practical method of RK was described by Svyatoslav N. Fyodorov[10] in Russia in the early 1970s and since has become an extremely popular and a generally successful method for correcting lower degrees of myopia, that is, less than −8.00 D.

Radial keratotomy has been reported successful in cases of up to −12.00 D of myopia. Radial keratotomy in higher degrees of myopia necessitates deeper and more extensive incisions, which may lead to unpredictable results and an increase in complications from microperforations with possible corneal decompensation. Therefore, this refractive surgical technique is usually restricted to those myopic patients with refraction under −6.00 or −8.00 D and thus under 27 mm in axial length.

EPIKERATOPHAKIA

In 1979 Herbert Kaufman[11] first introduced epikeratophakia for the treatment of aphakia. In 1982 Werblin and Klyce[12] first described the design of a tissue lens to be used for myopia. The use of epikeratophakia for correction of myopia was pioneered by Kaufman and Marguerite McDonald at the LSU Eye Center.[13]

Epikeratophakia initially involved the freezing and lathing of donor corneal tissue to a precalculated dioptric power, followed by freeze-drying and storage under vacuum. Other methods for storing the tissue (i.e., in moist containers) have been developed, eliminating the need for lyophilization of the tissue. The use of fresh corneal tissue has also been investigated.

Epikeratophakia remains a method for the treatment of levels of myopia up to −40.00 D. However, epikeratophakia unfortunately has not proved as successful for the correction of highly-myopic patients as was initially hoped. The procedure still remains under careful investigation by McDonald, Kaufman, and others. Some of the same problems that produce the difficulties with contact lenses in highly myopic patients also seem to mitigate against the high success rate with epikeratophakia achieved in aphakia, keratoconus, or lower degrees of myopia. The necessity for increased thickness of the edge and the thinness of the center of the lathed tissue can reduce sutured tissue lens stability. Epikeratophakia, in contrast to radial keratotomy, remains a technique that may be useful for higher levels of myopia.

McDonald and others have recently experimented with lenticules of silicone and other artificial materials. These lenticules are larger than the tissue graphs and are tucked into a dissected peripheral lamellar corneal bed, thus requiring no sutures.

The lack of sutures causes less postoperative astigmatism, and, of course, no removal is required. The principal problem at this stage is the delay in reepithelialization of the artificial graft, but a suitable material may be found. When used with epithelial growth factor and fibronectin, these lenticules should offer a more stable graft, especially in highly myopic patients.

KERATOMILEUSIS

Keratomileusis was first described by Barraquer in 1964[14] and introduced to the United States by Troutman and Swinger in 1978.[15] Keratomileusis involves the removal of a piece of corneal tissue from the patient's own cornea with a microkeratome. This use of the patient's own tissue avoids the immune rejection response. The corneal tissue is then reshaped with a cryolathe and resutured to the cornea. The refractive correction for the removed corneal disc can be determined precisely with computer techniques.

Myopic keratomileusis can be used to correct myopia between −6.00 and −15.00 D, and in some cases it can actually be used to correct higher refractive errors. However, keratomileusis, despite its 25- to 30-year history and its general success rate, has never become as popular as some of the other refractive surgical techniques because of the expensive equipment required, the very precise computerization of corneal lathing techniques, and the extreme skill required of the surgeon. At the present time only a relatively few surgeons in the United States are performing myopic keratomileusis because of the above problems. Simpler and more predictable techniques have been developed in recent years, yet this surgery still remains relatively uncommon.

CLEAR LENS EXTRACTION

Clear lens extraction has been recommended by Verzella[16] and a number of other ophthalmologists around the world for the correction of high myopia.

Many highly myopic patients develop cataracts over a period of time and thus require lens extraction. However, the safety factor of the clear lens extraction must be greater than that for cataracts since one is theoretically removing a lens from a normal eye. In Dr. Verzella's patients, most of the relatively few complications have been retinal in nature.

Patient satisfaction has been excellent in highly myopic clear lens extractions, and the refractive error that can be corrected ranges up to −19.0 D. Still, as with cataract extraction, the retinal complications must be considered, and, since it is an invasive procedure, the possibility of infection or hemorrhage remains.

Clear lens extraction is increasing in popularity, yet it is still performed by relatively few surgeons in the United States.

The technique for clear lens extraction is essentially that of phacoemulsification or extracapsular cataract extraction. The patients are examined prior to surgery for peripheral retinal degeneration, and these areas are treated with either cryosurgery or laser to minimize the possibility of subsequent retinal detachments or tears. The pre- and postoperative management is basically the same. A low-power implant, usually of polymethyl methacrylate (PMMA), is utilized to correct the myopia to the degree the surgeon desires. It is important to note that the calculation of the implant strength becomes increasingly difficult toward the highly myopic end of the refractive spectrum. The final refraction may not always correspond to the expected results predicted by normal intraocular lens calculation techniques.

Finally, the lens of the myopic patient may have more fragile zonules, and the capsular tissue may be thinner, creating difficulties with lens extraction.

PHAKIC INTRAOCULAR LENS IMPLANTATION

A number of physicians, including Choyce[17] in England, Fyodorov[18] in Russia, and Kaufman[19] in the United States, have recommended the implantation of intraocular lenses in highly myopic phakic patients.

The initial results with phakic anterior chamber lens implantation were good with corrections to desired levels and a significant reduction in visual aberrations. However, recent reports have indicated a gradual increase in postoperative endothelial cell loss. Several ophthalmologists have recommended a lens design change with less vaulting of the implant, keeping the surface of the intraocular lens further away from the endothelial surface, thereby offering increased protection. The long-term efficacy of phakic intraocular lenses in myopia remains unclear.

Fyodorov recently has suggested the implantation of very thin posterior chamber intraocular lens in phakic patients (S. N. Fyodorov, personal communication). This lens design does not remain in contact with either the anterior lens surface or the iris. He states that there is a potential or theoretical space filled with aqueous material between the natural crystalline lens and the iris, particularly in highly myopic patients who have an increase in anterior chamber depth.

At the present time the question of phakic intraocular lenses for highly myopic patients remains controversial. An increasing number of physicians advocate them as the best long-term option, and certainly significant levels of correction of myopia can be obtained.

STUDY DESIGN FOR EXCIMER LASER THERAPY FOR HIGH MYOPIA

The problems associated with high myopia, even in those patients whose vision is correctable with spectacles or contact lenses, have been delineated above. Correcting or decreasing the refractive error in these patients should diminish visual abnormalities. In some cases this may enable a previously poor contact lens candidate to comfortably wear contact lenses, thus securing the benefits other lens wearers share.

Currently there is no satisfactory surgical procedure for correction of high myopia (Table 6.2). As discussed above, the upper limit of correction capable with RK is about −8.00 D. Myopic epikeratophakia has proved to be of limited accuracy, and irregular astigmatism is a major limiting factor with

TABLE 6.2. Comparison of surgical and nonsurgical treatment of high myopia

Treatment	*History*	*Correctable Levels*	*Complications*
Spectacles	Until mid-20th century the only available treatment.	All levels	As minus correction increases, increasing edge thickness leads to loss of peripheral vision, occasional prismatic effects, and abnormal perceptions of spatial relationships.
Contact lenses	Developed early 20th century, but only practical after WWII.	All levels	Poor lid–lens interaction resulting in poor lens centration, lens flexure, and decreased effectiveness of tear pump mechanism, leading to oxygen deficiency and corneal edema. GPC. Dry eye syndrome.
Radial keratotomy	Lans described basic principles in 1897. Sato in Japan 1953. Fyodorov early 1970s.	Up to −8.00 D	Microperforations with deeper cuts needed for higher levels of minus correction. Flare and glare.
Epikeratophakia	Herbert Kaufman 1979 as treatment for aphakia. Werblin and Klyce described design of tissue lens for myopia in 1982. Kaufman and McDonald pioneered procedure for myopia at LSU.	Up to −40.00 D	The grafts' thick periphery and thin center lead to poor graft stability.
Keratomileusis	Barraquer in 1964. Introduced in US by Troutman and Swinger in 1978.	Up to −15.00 D	Expensive equipment. High level of surgeon skill. Precise computerization of corneal lathing techniques.
Clear lens extraction	Versella	Up to −19.00 D	Possible retinal complications, infection, and hemorrhage. Fragile zonules and thinner capsular tissue makes lens extraction difficult.
Phakic IOL implantation	Choyce, Fyodorov, and Kaufman.	All levels	Unknown long-term results. Endothelial cell loss.

this procedure. Myopic lenticules are no longer available in this country.

The potential role of excimer laser photorefractive keratectomy (PRK), in which superficial layers of the cornea are removed so as to alter the curvature, remain unclear for high myopia. Initial trials in humans have demonstrated that the effects of the procedure are more predictable for individuals with 5.00 D or less of myopia; above −5.0 D, there appears to be a greater chance for regression and greater variability of final outcome. It is our assertion that some patients with pathologic myopia are so disabled by their very high refractive errors that even a partial correction would produce an appreciable improvement in visual function.

In addition, PRK in combination with a weakening procedure such as RK may lead to a more complete reduction in refractive error. In consideration of the numerous disadvantages faced by high-myopia patients, the authors have studied a group of these patients in order to examine the ability of PRK to reduce myopia and improve the patients' visual function as measured by both objective and subjective criteria.

The basic design of this PRK study for high myopia resembles the federally funded study designed to evaluate the safety and efficacy of radial keratotomy known as PERK (perspective evaluation of radial keratotomy). The study uses the VISX laser, and only one eye per patient is treated. If any occasion arises in which treatment of the second eye is recommended by the investigator, that particular case will require special FDA approval. The number of patients treated must be limited to no more than 25 at no more than five clinical sites. The study is nonrandomized, and therefore a formal control group has not been established. The study will be continued for a duration of 2 years or until the centers reach a total of 25 patients. At that point an assessment of the outcome and comparison to other alternative treatments will be made, and, if favorable, a request will be made to the FDA to proceed to the next phase, in which an additional 75 patients will be treated.

The trial hopes to address the following questions:

1. What is the upper limit of myopia that can be successfully treated with excimer laser and PRK?
2. What are the risks associated with PRK in high-myopia patients?
3. What are the effects of PRK on visual functioning as measured by both objective and subjective criteria?

Further studies need to address the following questions:

4. Will RK and PRK in combination safely reduce high myopia more effectively than PRK alone?
5. What are the risks associated with PRK alone and PRK in combination with RK in high-myopia patients?

PRETREATMENT EXAMINATION

Preoperative evaluation of the patient includes:

1. Uncorrected visual acuity examination
2. Manifest refraction examination
3. Cycloplegic refraction examination
4. Intraocular pressure examination
5. Biomicroscopic examination, including a corneal clarity evaluation
6. Complete ophthalmic dilated examination
7. Pachymetry of the central cornea
8. Keratometry
9. Contrast sensitivity examination
10. Corneal topographic evaluation

ELIGIBILITY CRITERIA

To be eligible for the study the candidates can be male or female of any race and at least 21 years of age. The patient must be intolerant to spectacles, medically unsuited to use contact lenses, and have rejected other refractive surgical procedures after an informed view of the surgical alternatives. In addition, the candidates must present with bilateral physiologic myopia without ophthalmoscopic signs of progressive pathologic myopia. Only patients between −10.0 and −20.0 D with 1.50 D or less of refractive astigmatism may be considered. Visual acuity must be correctable to better than 20/400 in the operative eye and better than 20/100 in the fellow eye.

The patient must have shown a change in the spherical portion of the refraction in each eye of no greater than 0.50 D during the year preceding the baseline examination and no more than 1.0 D during the preceding 3 years.

Before a candidate can be treated, he or she must have discontinued use of hard contact lenses for at least 3 weeks or soft or gas-permeable lenses for at least 2 weeks. If hard contact lenses have been used, there must be three central keratometry readings and manifest refractions taken at 1-week intervals following lens deprivation. The last two readings must not differ more than 0.50 D, and the last two manifest refractions taken at these times must also be within 0.50 D in both the spherical and cylindrical components of the refraction.

The patient must not have any active or residual ophthalmic disease or any systemic disease likely to affect wound-healing capability. A signed informed-consent document and agreement to be available for follow-up examination for the duration of the study must be obtained.

EXCLUSION CRITERIA

Those patients will be excluded from the study who show an inability to meet all the above listed eligibility criteria or have an inability to cooperate due to physical limitations or other predisposing factors including their overall physical and mental health.

Ocular changes that would eliminate patients from the study include poor visual acuity due to corneal pathologic lesions, uncontrolled uveitis, and rapidly progressing diabetic retinopathy. In addition, blepharitis, dry eye syndrome, and lagophthalmos would lead to exclusion if the patient is unwilling or unable to comply with medical therapy preoperatively.

Any history of previous corneal surgery or trauma would also exclude the patient from this study.

PROCEDURE AND SURGICAL TECHNIQUE

A 193 nm argon fluoride excimer laser (20/20 excimer laser, VISX, Sunnyvale, Cal.) is used for the treatment in all cases.

The patient is placed under the excimer laser, and topical proparacaine hydrochloride drops are instilled into the eye to be treated. A wire lid speculum is inserted, and the epithelium is removed with a blunt spatula. If the epithelium is difficult to remove, a sharp instrument may be utilized.

The remainder of the laser treatment is completed in a standard manner with a suction-held fixation ring applied to the globe to keep it centered after the patient has fixated on a flashing centration light. The fixation ring may be unnecessary with cooperative patients.

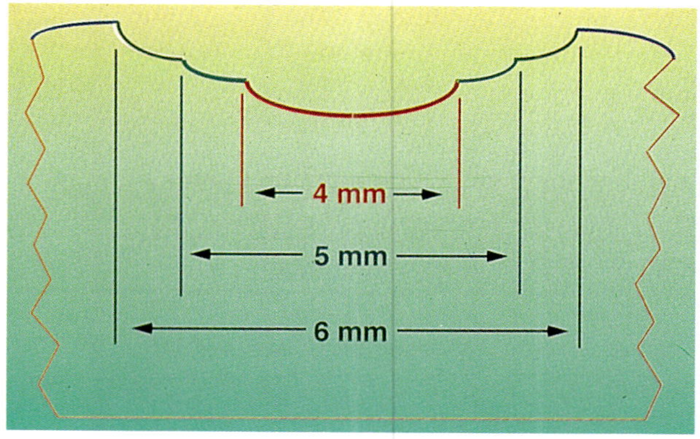

FIGURE 6.5. Drawing of multistep variable-diameter excimer laser spherical corneal ablation.

Some differences between the standard excimer treatment (PRK) for lower degrees of myopia do exist. The computer must be programmed for three different ablation zones and depths (Fig. 6.5). After each ablation zone is completed, the computer must be reset.

Since the treatment time is prolonged because of computer resetting, the patient must be reassured between each ablation zone treatment in order to avoid any movement of the patient's body or eye.

In addition, for the surgeon the extended treatment time means the eye will have to be held steady for a longer period of time with the fixation ring handle. Following each ablation zone treatment, the cornea becomes progressively hazier. Centration for successive treatments becomes more difficult as the patient has more difficulty visualizing the fixation light. The surgeon must maintain centration with the fixation ring, if the ring is used.

POSTTREATMENT MANAGEMENT

The patient is treated after surgery with tobramycin–dexamethasone sodium phosphate ointment and a pressure patch. Since there is considerable pain during the first 24 to 48 hours (much greater than with an RK), the patient should be warned, and systemic pain medication may be necessary.

Following the surgery the patients are treated exclusively with topical 0.1% fluoromethalone (FML®) drops four times a day for 3 weeks, two times daily for 3 weeks, and once per day for 4 weeks or longer if epithelial haze occurs.

The patient has a postoperative examination at 24 hours, 1 week, 1 month, 2 months, 3 months, 6 months, and 1 year. The postoperative clinical assessment evaluates both inflammation and healing response at each visit. The examinations at the 1- and 3-month visits include the preoperative test battery.

MULTISTEP VARIABLE-DIAMETER EXCIMER LASER SPHERICAL CORNEAL ABLATION

The technique for treatment of the highly myopic eyes in our study has been based on suggestions from Theo Seiler in Berlin.

A single-zone ablation may be suboptimal in highly myopic patients since the depth of the ablation would have to be excessive to produce the desired affect. Young myopic patients typically have relatively large diameter pupils; small-diameter ablations therefore result in postoperative halos. Large-diameter treatments, however, may require very deep ablations, as central depth is proportional to the square of the ablation zone diameter. The increased depth of a single large-diameter ablative treatment might increase damage to the underlying stroma and in turn cause increased fibrosis and subepithelial haze in the posttreatment healing process.

Because of the consistent undercorrection of myopia observed with PRK in initial studies and the tendency observed with phototherapeutic keratectomy (PTK) for reduction of corneal curvature with straight-down ablations not intended to alter refractive error, we have modified the PRK technique in this proposed study (Figs. 6.6 and 6.7). Three zones of 6.0, 5.0, and 4.0 mm are utilized. To determine the amount of ablation performed for each zone, the total target correction is divided among the three

Single Zone Ablation Technique		Multiple Zone Ablation Technique			

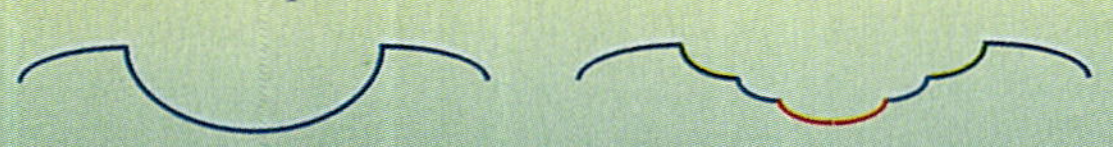

Correction (Diopters)	Central Depth (Microns)	6 mm Zone	5 mm Zone	4 mm Zone	Total
Minus 10	132	28	27	27	82
Minus 15	196	42	40	40	122
Minus 20	259	56	54	54	164

FIGURE 6.6. Comparison of overall ablation depth in single-step excimer laser spherical corneal ablation versus multistep variable-diameter excimer laser spherical corneal ablation.

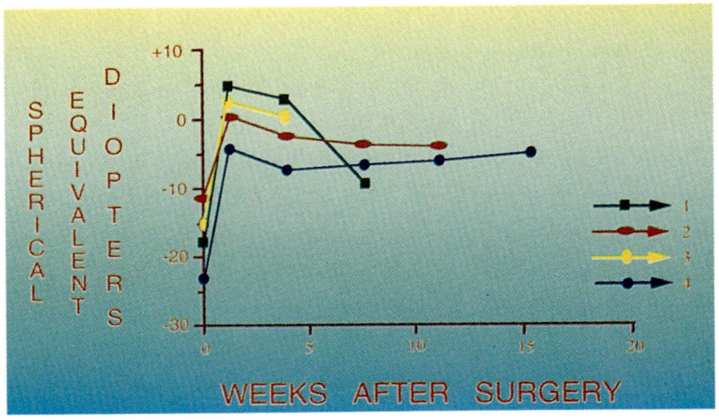

FIGURE 6.7. PRK refraction results. McDonnell-Thompson study involving multistep variable-diameter excimer laser spherical corneal ablation.

ablation diameters as follows: 6.0 mm = 20%; 5.0 mm = 30%; 4.0 mm = 50%.

Example 1:

Target correction of 10 D (after correcting for vertex distance). For the 6.0 mm zone do a 2.0 D ablation (28 μm); for the 5.0 mm zone do a 3.0 D ablation (27 μm); for the final 4.0 mm zone do a 5.0 D ablation (27 μm). The maximal (central) ablation depth is 82 μm, compared with 132 μm for a single 6.0 mm diameter ablation and 89 μm for a single 5.0 mm diameter ablation.

Example 2:

Target correction is 15.0 D (after correcting for vertex distance). For the 6.0 mm zone do a 3.0 D ablation (42 μm); for the 5.0 mm zone do a 4.5 D ablation (40 μm); for the final 4.0 mm zone do a 7.5 D ablation (40 μm). The maximal (central) ablation depth is 122 μm, compared with 196 μm for a single 6.0 mm diameter ablation and 132 μm for a single 5.0 mm diameter ablation.

Example 3:

Target correction is 20.0 D (after correcting for vertex distance). For the 6.0 mm zone do a 4.0 D ablation (56 μm); for the 5.0 mm zone do a 6.0 D ablation (54 μm); for the final 4.0 mm zone do a 10.0 D ablation (54 μm). The maximal (central) ablation depth is 164 μm, compared with 259 μm for a single 6.0 mm diameter ablation and 177 μm for a single 5.0 mm diameter ablation.

The purpose of this multilevel ablational pattern is to achieve the desired correction while avoiding excessive depth of ablation centrally.

TABLE 6.3. Comparison of four highly myopic eyes treated with the excimer laser

Date	*Days PO*	*Sph Eq*	*Spec Va*	*Haze*	*Pachymetry (mm)*	*Actual K*	*Refraction (sph/cyl)*
Case 1							
12/2/91	0	−17.75	0.5		0.54	42.50/44.62	−19.25/+1.75
12/9/91	7	+4.00	0.6	1.5			+4.00
12/27/91	25	+2.50	0.5	1.5			+1.00/+2.00
2/5/92	60	−10.50	0.3	2	0.5	41.50/43.50	−11.25/+1.25
Case 2							
10/21/91	0	−11.60	1.333		0.578	43.50/45.00	−12.50/+1.75
10/22/91	1	+2.00	0.333				
10/23/91	2	+2.00	0.4			33.00/35.00	
10/25/91	4	+2.00	0.666		0.456	35.00/36.00	
11/1/91	11	+0.50	1	0.5		36.25/38.50	−0.25/+1.50
11/22/91	30	−2.50	1.33	0.5	0.468	37.00/40.00	−4.25/+3.25
12/13/91	50	−5.13	1	0.5		38.37/40.37	−7.00/+3.75
1/17/92	85	−6.00	0.8	0.5	0.47	39.62/41.37	−7.75/+2.75
Case 3							
11/4/91	0	−15.50	0.25		0.0461	43.75/43.25	−15.25/+1.25
11/22/91	15	+2.35	1		0.389	39.62/40.75	+1.50/+1.75
12/4/91	30	+1.35	1	0.5	0.39	34.00/36.25	+0.50/+1.75
Case 4							
8/27/91	0	−23.25	0.4		0.544	45.12/47.00	−24.00/+1.50
8/28/91	1						
8/30/91	3						
9/4/91	8	−3.75	0.33	0.5		38.62/41.00	
9/25/91	29	−8.25	0.33		0.46	39.25/40.75	
11/27/91	90	−8.35	1	0.5	0.473	39.75/41.50	−9.00/+0.75
12/11/91	105	−7.13	0.66	0.5			−9.00/+1.75

DISCUSSION OF RESULTS

Our results with patients treated using the multilevel ablation technique at the Doheny Eye Institute are still in the preliminary stage and will need considerably longer follow-up (Table 6.3 and Figs. 6.8–6.12).

The findings on these few patients indicate an initial marked drop in myopia, which appears to persist for approximately 1 month. During the 2- to 3-month period, these patients begin to show a significant regression of the initial refractive correction, dropping to a level 60 to 70% of the original value. This level of correction is encouraging, as it would enable many patients to successfully wear contact lenses or spectacles with much less degradation of the visual image and fewer visual symptoms than experienced prior to correction.

It remains to be seen whether the current level of correction will persist in the months to come. If

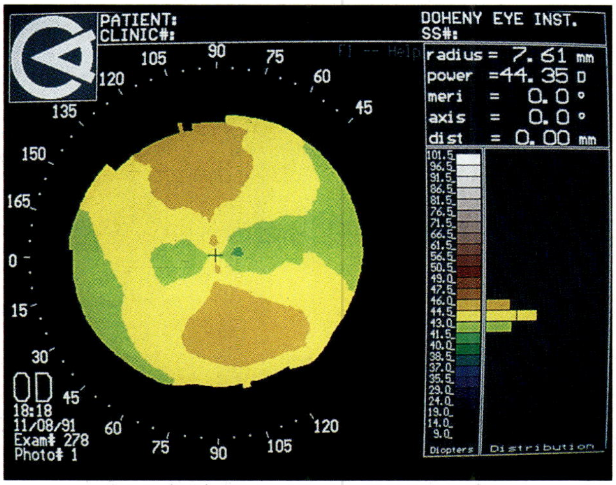

FIGURE 6.8. Color-coded keratograph of patient 1 before multistep spherical ablation of −14.50 D.

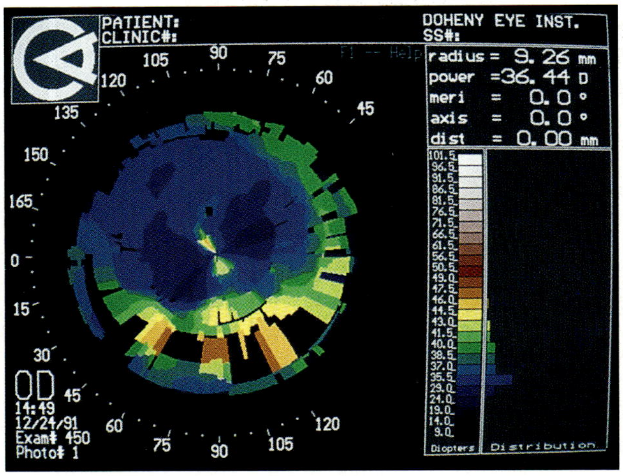

FIGURE 6.9. Color-coded keratograph of patient 1 2 months after multistep spherical ablation. A significant overall flattening of the cornea was achieved.

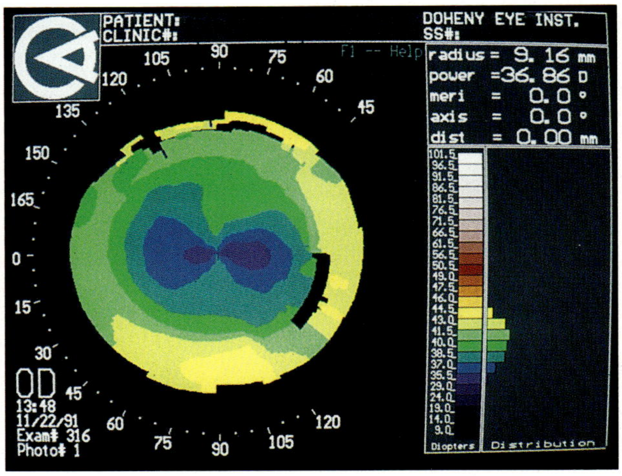

FIGURE 6.11. Color-coded keratograph of patient 2 1 month after multistep spherical ablation. A well-centered ablation is noted here.

the regression of the refractive error continues, then the results would be quite discouraging in the absence of further refractive surgery such as RK.

One of the patients developed a considerable corneal opacification within a week after treatment, and it has persisted through the 3-month postoperative period (Figs. 6.13 and 6.14). The opacification has not cleared, and it is possible that further treatment with the excimer laser may be necessary to both reduce the amount of myopia and further ablate the corneal opacification that has developed. This patient also developed an unrelated retinal hemorrhage 2 months following ablation (Fig. 6.15). She has had a history of hemorrhagic episodes during pregnancy and trauma, in addition to two spontaneous hemorrhages over an 18-year period. A fifth patient who had laser ablation performed shortly before publication had his myopia decreased from −24.00 D to −8.00 D at one month following treatment. The cornea was clear from one week after surgery.

Other studies involving excimer laser treatment for the correction of high myopia include those of M. Piovella from Monza, Italy. Piovella used both a single optical zone of 6.0 mm with a 180 μm depth ablation and a PTK involving multiple optical zones

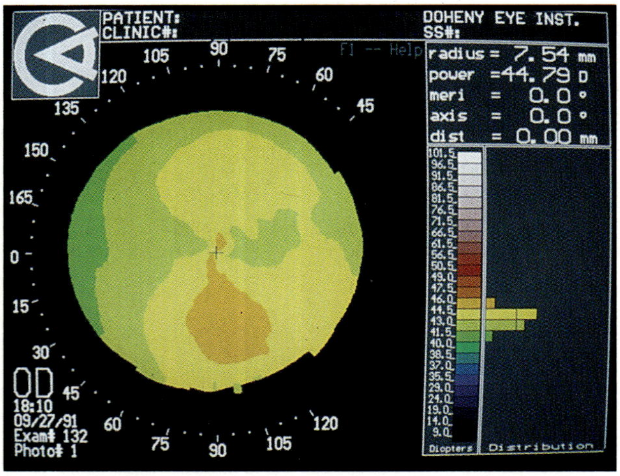

FIGURE 6.10. Color-coded keratograph of patient 2 before multistep spherical ablation of −10.75 D.

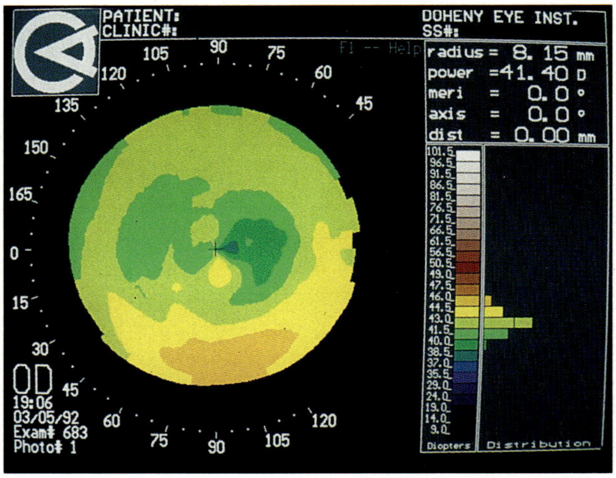

FIGURE 6.12. Color-coded keratograph of patient 2 5 months after multistep spherical ablation. A slight regression of the achieved flattening of the cornea is apparent at this point.

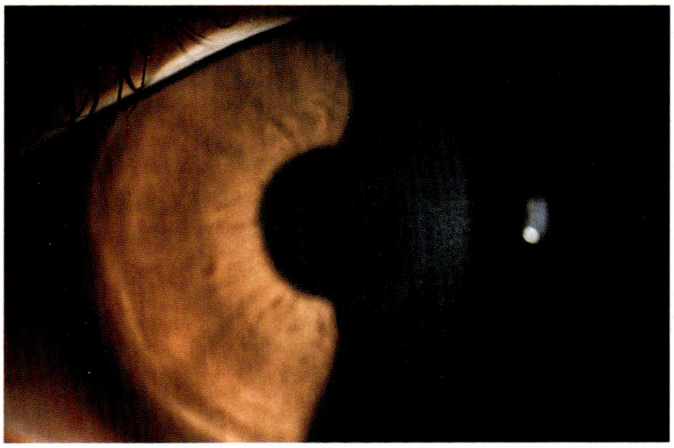

FIGURE 6.13. Slit-lamp optic section of patient 4 3 months post-PRK. Minimal corneal haze.

of 6.0, 5.0, and 4.0 mm generating a total ablation of 128 μm.

Using both the single-zone and the multiple-zone techniques, Piovella achieved the desired refractive correction of 15.0 D with a slightly greater stabilization of correction in the multiple-zone modality. His report is based on an average follow-up of 8.3 months with a range of 6 to 13 months.

David Leach and Marguerite McDonald at Louisiana State University (LSU) have done a study of multizone excimer laser ablation for high myopia in African green monkeys using the VISX excimer laser. Multizone ablations consisted of three concentric zones with diameters of 4.0, 5.0 or 5.5, and 6.0 mm. Six of the monkey corneas received 8.0 D, five received 12.0 D, and three received 16.0 D of attempted correction. The treatment depths were 95, 115, and 135 μm, respectively. The postoperative corneal thickness measurements agreed with the prescribed treatment depths, the posttreatment examinations being performed at 1, 2, 3, 5, 8, and 13 weeks.

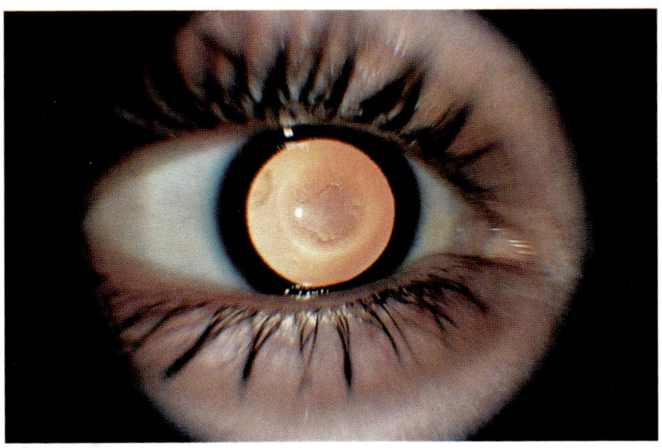

FIGURE 6.14. Dilated picture of corneal opacification in patient 1 at 3 months.

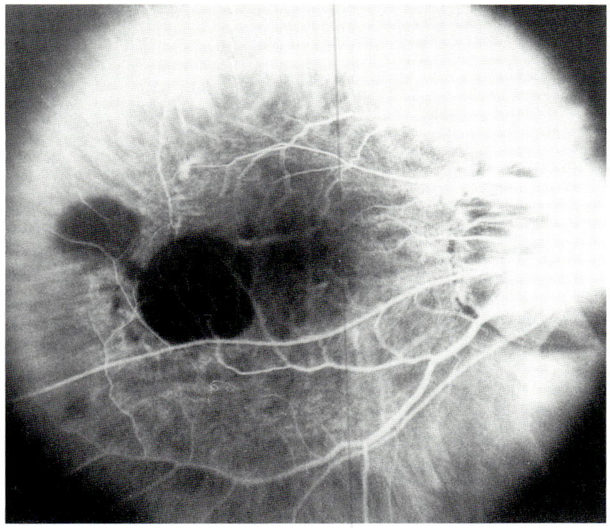

FIGURE 6.15. Fluorescein angiography of unrelated spontaneous retinal hemorrhage in patient 1.

The multizone ablations used in the LSU study resulted in undercorrections that remained stable throughout the 13-week period. Retinoscopy showed a spherical equivalent correction of 66.6% in the 8.0 D range, 50% in the 12.0 D range, and only 46.4% in the 16.0 D range at 3 weeks.

Corneal topography revealed central corneal flattening with marked surface irregularities at 1, 2, 3, and 5 weeks. The keratometry and pachymetry measurements showed an initial flattening and thinning of the cornea with no significant regression during the first 13 weeks following treatment. Corneal clarity averaged from trace haze to a one-plus haze.

Frank L. Lavery from Dublin, Ireland,[20] has treated a number of highly myopic patients with the double-ablation technique pioneered in Germany and Italy. In the first step, Lavery applied the laser to an optical zone of between 4.0 and 4.3 mm in an attempt to obtain the desired level of refractive correction. After achieving a stable refractive end point, a subsequent 5.0 mm zone ablation was performed to correct the residual error. Dr. Lavery stated that he had treated nine patients with refractive errors ranging from −6.5 to −9.5 D using the two-step technique. At least two patients have been followed for 3 months post-PRK and had visual acuities of 20/20 and 20/10 with only traces of subepithelial reticular haze. As Lavery pointed out,

"When looking at the results, one should remember that we were not always aiming for zero in these patients. If we had been our results would have been even better." He also noted that age and sex appeared to have some influence over the patient's outcome.

Lavery recommends a substantial topical steroid dosage to the patients, particularly those who develop a "second wave" subepithelial reticular haze, which occasionally spontaneously occurred some months after the laser treatment.

In a multicenter study, Neal Sher at the Phillips Eye Institute in Minneapolis and others have treated 11 eyes ranging from −8.17 to −14.50 D of myopia with a mean of −11.23 D.[21] Their mean postoperative refraction was −0.06 D. All these patients have been followed for 6 months, all the patients have at least 20/40 uncorrected vision, and all are within 2.0 D of the attempted correction. Only one patient had two lines of decreased vision. None of the patients have shown a significant amount of regression during the follow-up period. These patients were treated with a single-level ablation modality. Dr. Sher feels that the previous failures in treating high myopia were due to an insufficient aperture size. He suggests at least a 6.0 mm diameter aperture and ablation depth of up to 200 μm. He is currently using a 6.5–6.9 mm aperture on lower myopes. He also notes that the high myope takes much longer to both regain their best corrected vision and for complete epithelial re-structuring.

Sher and others in the multicenter group have published a study on excimer laser treatment in moderate myopia ranging from −4.00 to −12.00 D (mean −6.49 D).[22]

At 6 months the average residual refractive error was −1.85 D. There was only minimal corneal haze, which was not visually significant in any patient, and 68% of these eyes were corrected to within 2.0 D while 55% were corrected to within 1.0 D of attempted correction. The Taunton Technology LV2000 laser was used in all the moderate-myopia cases.

FURTHER SURGICAL CONSIDERATIONS OF HIGH MYOPIA

PRK may or may not prove effective in the treatment of high myopia. The long-term evaluation still needs to be made. The multilevel ablation technique offers a means of minimizing the total depth of ablation.

The two principal undecided factors at this point appear to be whether even multilevel ablation can achieve the desired correction of high myopia and whether the deeper levels of ablation will produce more corneal scarring and corneal opacification, leading to a diminution of best-corrected visual acuity.

If increased corneal scarring, opacification, or haze occurs, then further excimer laser treatment may be efficacious in removing the opacified tissue, as Theo Seiler in Berlin suggests. This may produce a further decrease in the eventual myopic correction.

The combination of excimer laser photocoagulation (PRK) and RK, as suggested by James Salz, may offer an additional reduction in the long-term myopic correction.

If the excimer laser alone or in combination with RK does not achieve long-term effective results with high myopia, then other treatment modalities may need to be considered. Intrastromal wide-area treatments with the double yttrium-aluminum-garnet (yag) laser with its longer wavelength may enable the ophthalmologist to ablate the corneal stroma without damage to the epithelium or Bowman's membrane. The consequent collapse of the cavities created by the ablative treatment could have a larger effect in highly myopic patients. A number of these machines have been described and developed over the past several years, but currently there appears to be very little hard data from either animal or human studies.

The proponents of the double yag laser expect minimal thermal effects from this technique, allowing treatment of the corneal stroma. The initial problem with the double yag involves the precise delivery of the laser energy to the designated areas in the corneal tissue without precipitating thermal damage. The technology is currently in its developmental stage, and practical usage may be 5 to 10 years away.

Another possible use for the excimer laser in high myopia is a technique for myopic keratomileusis with the excimer laser as reported at the American Society of Cataract and Refractive Surgery in San Diego in 1992 by L. Buratto from Italy. Several doctors, in a multicenter study led by Steven F. Brint from New Orleans, treated 10 patients utilizing the UV 200 LA excimer laser to carve the disc for myopic keratomileusis and reported that the results on all 10 patients had compared favorably to those of traditional cryolathe keratomileusis. This new technique may offer a resurgence of interest in keratomileusis since it should be more predictable and less complicated than the use of the cryolathe.

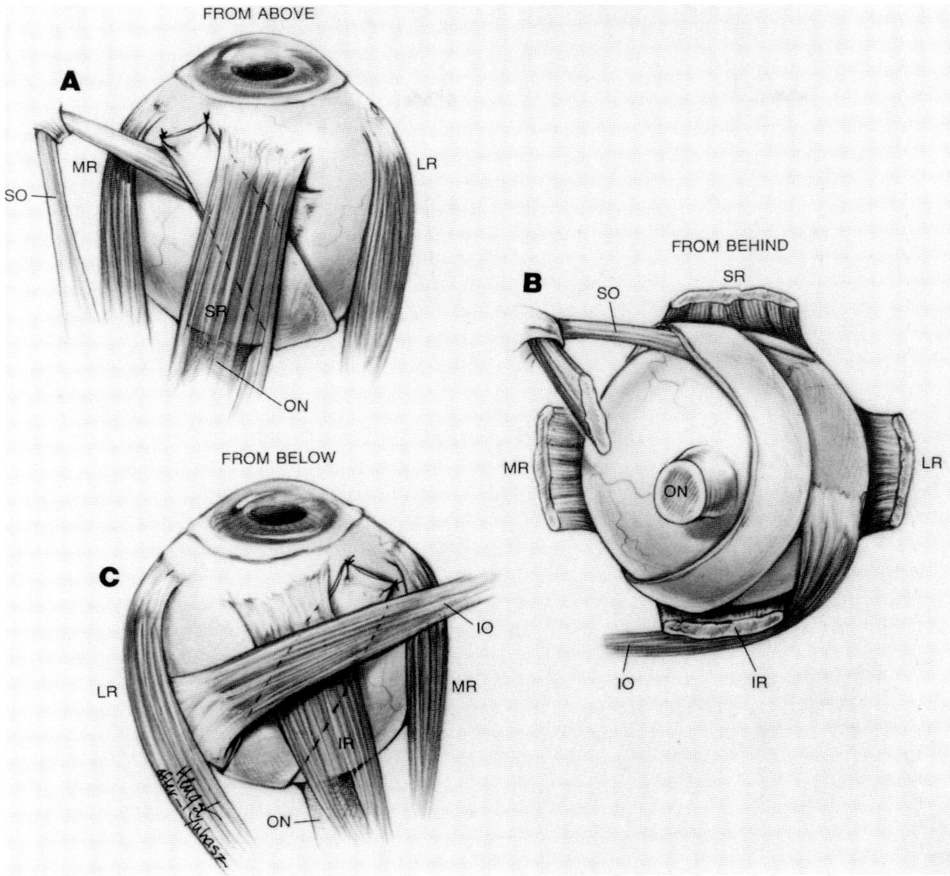

FIGURE 6.16. Diagram of scleral reinforcement technique.

The refractive correction of high myopia in any form, whether with current techniques such as radial keratotomy or the excimer laser, or with future techniques such as the double yag laser, only reduce the degree of refractive error. These techniques do not address the high-myopia patient's increased axial length and frequent development of posterior staphylomas. These physiologic changes lead to deterioration of the retinal pigment epithelium, choroid, and retinal elements.

Scleral reinforcement, a procedure to reinforce the posterior staphylomatous pole of the highly myopic eye with either human sclera or artificial materials, has been available for a number of years and, in conjunction with the correction of the highly myopic refractive error, may not only enable the patient to use a weaker refractive correction but may also protect the visual elements in the posterior pole of the eye and thus preserve long-term visual acuity (Fig. 6.16).

Scleral reinforcement has a track record of over 20 years. Most of the published studies indicate that the efficacy of scleral reinforcement in the prevention of axial elongation and posterior staphylomatous development in adult eyes is in the 85 to 87% range.

The future for the highly myopic patient may entail correction of the refractive error with one of the treatment modalities discussed above and the protection of the posterior pole of the eye with scleral reinforcement or other procedures both to improve current visual acuity and to protect long-term vision.

REFERENCES

1. Thompson FB: *Myopia Surgery*. New York, MacMillan, 1989, p 8.
2. Thompson FB: *Myopia Surgery*. New York, MacMillan, 1989, p. 8.
3. Curtin BJ: *The Myopias*. Philadelphia, Harper & Row, 1985, p 7.
4. Curtin BJ: *The Myopias*. Philadelphia, Harper & Row, 1985, p 303.
5. Thompson FB: *Myopia Surgery*. New York, MacMillan, 1989, p 271.

6. Verzella F: P.E. and transparent lenses. In Verzella F (ed): *Atlas of Extracapsular Technique, Phacoemulsification and Intraocular Lenses*. Bologna, Italy, Lens Editions, 1981, pp 98–108.
7. Friedman DM, Ciuffreda, KJ: Changes in the spatial horopter of myopes with contact lenses and spectacles. *Int Contact Lens Clin* 9 (May/June):174–183, 1982.
8. Waring GO: The Lans distinguished refractive surgery lecture (editorial). *J Refractive Surg* 3:115–116, 1987.
9. Sato, T: Posterior incision of cornea. Surgical treatment for conical cornea and astigmatism. *Am J Ophthalmol* 33:943–948, 1950.
10. Fyodorov SN, Durnev VV: Operation of dossaged dissection of corneal circular ligament in cases of myopia of mild degree. *Ann Ophthalmol* 11:1885–1890, 1979.
11. Kaufman HE: The correction of aphakia. *Am J Ophthalmol* 89:1–10, 1980.
12. Werblin TP, Klyce SD: Epikeratophakia: The surgical correction of myopia: I. Lathing of corneal tissue. *Cher Eye Res* 1:591–597, 1981/1982.
13. McDonald MB, Klyce SD, Kaufman HE: Epikeratophakia for myopia correction: *Ophthalmology* 92: 1417–1422, 1985.
14. Barraquer JI: Keratomileusis. Para la correction de la myopia. *Arch Soc Am Oftalmol Optomol:* 27, 1964.
15. Troutman RC, Swinger CA: Refractive keratoplasty: Keratophakia and keratomileusis. *Trans Am Ophthalmol Soc* 76:329, 1978.
16. Verzella F: P.E. and transparent lenses. In Verzella F (ed): *Atlas of Extracapsular Technique,* Phacoemulsification and intraocular lenses. Bologna, Italy, Lens Editions, 1981, pp 98–108.
17. Choyce DP: Recollections of the early days of intraocular lens implantation. *J Cataract Refract Surg* 16: 505–508, 1990.
18. Fyodorov SN: Personal communication, 1990.
19. Kaufman HE. Study on anterior chamber lenses for myopia. *Ocular Surg News* 9:23, 1991.
20. Lavery F: Irish center reports single and double PRK treatment results. *Ocular Surg News* 10:46, 1991.
21. Sher NA: Personal communication, 1991.
22. Sher NA, Chen V, Bowers RA, et al: The use of the 193 nm excimer laser for myopic photorefractive keratectomy in sighted eyes: A multicenter study. *Arch Ophthalmol* 109:1525–1530, 1991.

CHAPTER 7

Photorefractive Keratectomy: Astigmatism

MAURO CAMPOS

PETER J. McDONNELL

Astigmatism, naturally occurring or postoperative, has challenged ophthalmic surgeons for decades. Recent advances in cataract surgical techniques, including the use of intraocular lenses and multifocal intraocular lenses, has stimulated interest in minimizing the period required for recovery of excellent postoperative vision, minimizing postoperative astigmatism, and maximizing postoperative unaided acuity. Similarly, there is great emphasis on identifying those surgical variables (e.g., trephination technique, suture placement) that contribute to postkeratoplasty astigmatism, so that such astigmatism, a major limitation of keratoplasty surgery, can be minimized.

The pathogenesis of congenital astigmatism remains unclear, while postoperative astigmatism is the consequence of asymmetric corneal deformation by the surgery. The spherical cornea has radially symmetric topography with a single keratometric end point in all meridians, circular photokeratoscope images, and excellent acuity when corrected with spherical lenses. With computer-assisted topographic analysis (Fig. 7.1), one can see that the central cornea is steepest, with concentric rings of color illustrating gradual flattening toward the periphery. With the astigmatic cornea, the refractive power of the eye varies with the orientation of incident light rays. Astigmatism is said to be regular when two principal or major meridians are identifiable by refraction and keratometry, the meridians are 90° apart, the end point of keratometry is distinct, the photokeratoscope mires are regular circles or ovals, and excellent acuity is obtained with spectacle correction. With computer-assisted topographic analysis, regular astigmatism typically has a figure-of-eight pattern that is symmetric about the two principal meridians, which are oriented 90° apart (Fig. 7.2). Astigmatism is irregular if the principal meridians are separated by an angle other than 90°, the end point of keratometry is indistinct, the circular mires of the photokeratoscope are distorted (Fig. 7.3), excellent acuity is not obtained with spectacle correction, and refraction over a hard or gas-permeable contact lens does result in excellent acuity. With computer-assisted topographic analysis, the topography is seen to be asymmetrically distributed about the corneal apex. The two steep hemimeridians, which should be oriented 180° apart, may be separated by 170°, 160°, or less. Also, the amount of steepening in the two hemimeridians may not be symmetric about the center of the cor-

Supported by a grant from the Autry Foundation, Los Angeles, CA.

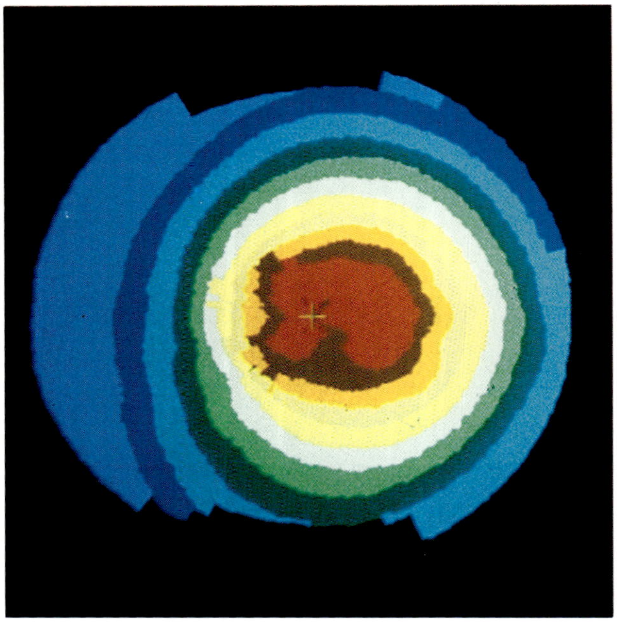

FIGURE 7.1. Computer-assisted topographic map of normal spherical human cornea. The central cornea is steepest, with gradual flattening toward the limbus, reflecting the asphericity of the cornea.

neal apex, with one steep hemimeridian being substantially steeper than the opposite steep hemimeridian. Similarly, the flat hemimeridians may be separated by an angle other than 180° and exhibit asymmetry about the corneal apex. Occasionally seen in unoperated astigmatic corneas (Fig. 7.4), this topography is typical after trauma or surgery (Fig. 7.5). Appreciation of the sometimes complex topography of astigmatic corneas has been long in coming; of all the papers that describe surgery for astigmatism, only one or two have taken the preoperative topography into account when planning the placement of incisions or sutures.

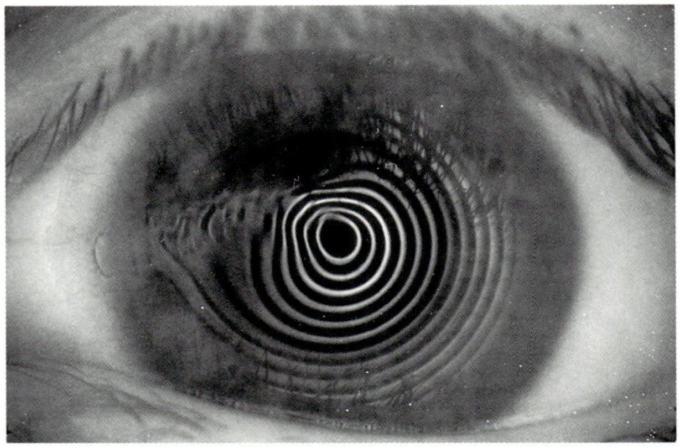

FIGURE 7.3. Photokeratoscope mires are distorted in a patient with irregular corneal astigmatism resulting from corneal laceration.

A BRIEF HISTORY OF SURGICAL CORRECTION OF ASTIGMATISM

The search for a surgical technique to correct astigmatism began almost a century ago with Bates,[1] and currently available techniques are still unsatisfactory because of relative unpredictability and operative and postoperative complications. Many surgical procedures, including relaxing incisions (radial,

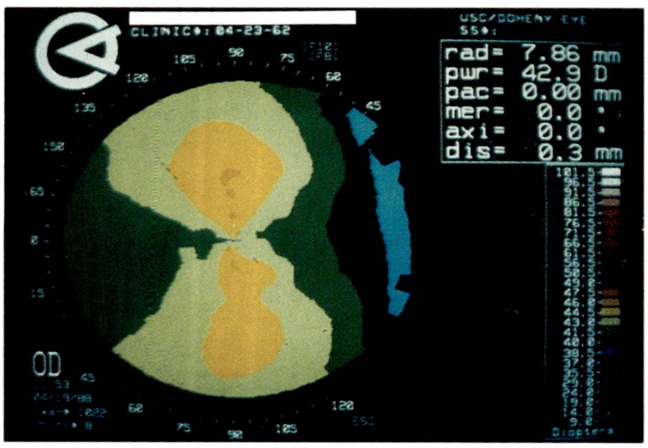

FIGURE 7.2. Computer-assisted topographic map of unoperated human cornea with naturally occurring regular astigmatism. A figure-of-eight pattern is symmetric about the two principal meridians, which are oriented 90° apart.

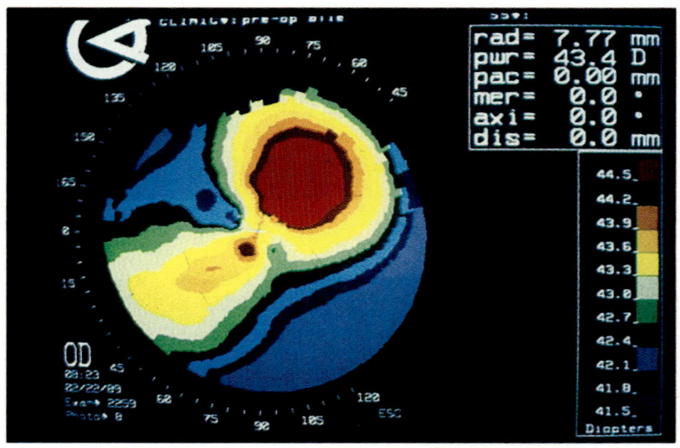

FIGURE 7.4. Computer-assisted topographic map of unoperated human cornea with naturally occurring oblique astigmatism. The figure-of-eight pattern is asymmetrically distributed about the corneal apex and the two principal meridians are not oriented 90° apart.

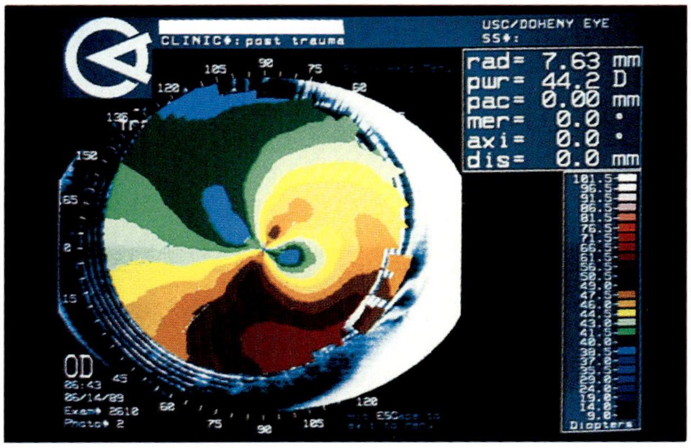

FIGURE 7.5. Computer-assisted topographic map of human cornea with irregular astigmatism following inferior corneal laceration. A figure-of-eight pattern is not recognizable, but rather a steep inferonasal quadrant is located about 180° away from a flat superotemporal quadrant.

transverse, and arcuate), trapezoidal astigmatic keratotomy (Ruiz procedure), and wedge resection, have been described for the correction of naturally occurring and postoperative astigmatism.[2-14] The number and variety of techniques reflect the inability of any particular approach to predictably eliminate astigmatism in all patients, and great variability in outcome is reported in most series.[2-6] All reported techniques are based on the possibility of inducing changes in the corneal curvature by incising the paracentral and peripheral cornea. Presumably, inter-individual variability in corneal wound healing and an unpredictable corneal response to the mechanical stresses induced by the surgery might play a role in the variability of the final results. In the case of intersecting corneal incisions, touted at one time for the correction of astigmatism, poor healing, epithelial ingrowth into the stroma at the site of intersection, and excessive corneal scarring almost invariably result in irregular astigmatism with loss of best-corrected spectacle acuity. Incisional procedures will continue to have limited predictability until we discover a method for preoperative in vivo measurement of the biomechanical properties of the corneal tissue layers and the distribution of stress and stress-induced strain within the individual human cornea.

Initially, the excimer laser was used in an attempt to correct corneal astigmatism by creating straight or arcuate linear excisions into the corneal stroma. This technique involved the use of a mask placed over the cornea, into which had been cut the appropriate opening so that the desired excision was created. Despite initial enthusiasm for this procedure, experience determined that it did not, in most hands, represent a substantial improvement over the diamond knife in terms of accuracy or wound healing, and this approach has been abandoned.

In early 1990, we initiated studies at the Doheny Eye Institute, University of Southern California, using the excimer laser to perform superficial toric ablations of the cornea. Just as myopic photorefractive keratectomy (PRK) differs from radial keratotomy in that the former procedure does not involve creation of deep stromal incisions, our approach to astigmatism using the excimer laser has been to correct the refractive error by performing a superficial ablation of tissue in the shape of a cylindrical lens, rather than creating deep incisions (or excisions) into the stroma. Based on the ability of the laser to induce flattening of the central cornea to eliminate myopic refractive errors,[15] we developed a nonradially symmetric approach to tissue ablation, with selective flattening of the steep meridian.[16] An expanding slit was created, with no refractive change intended parallel to the slit opening, and central flattening was induced in the meridian in which the slit was expanded. We first tested the newly developed computer-controlled iris diaphragm in polymethyl methacrylate (PMMA) blocks, plastic corneas, and rabbit corneas.[16] The induced change in cylinder agreed closely with the desired change, and the induction of cylinder was demonstrated by computer-assisted topographic analysis (Figs. 7.6 and 7.7). These encouraging experimental results stimulated us to clinically investigate the technique

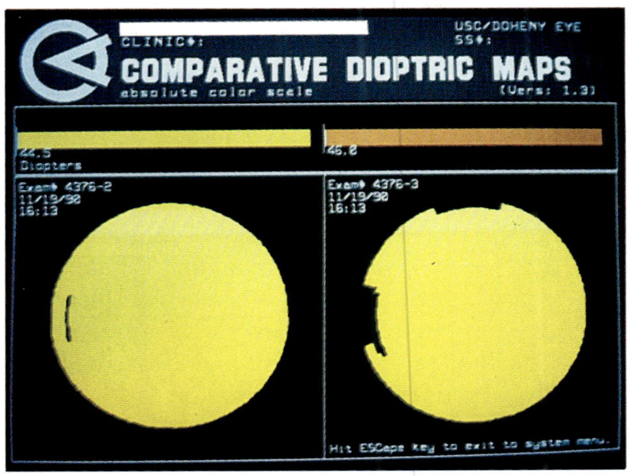

FIGURE 7.6. Pair of computer-assisted topographic maps of PMMA simulated spherical cornea before ablation with the excimer laser. The maps demonstrate good reproducibility and lack of toricity.

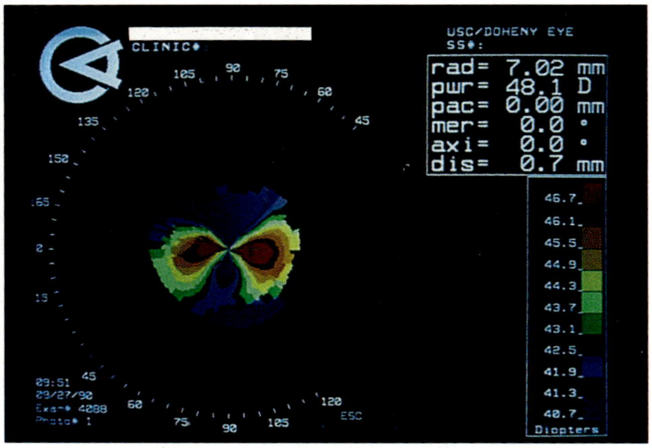

FIGURE 7.7. PMMA simulated cornea shown in Fig. 7.6 after toric excimer laser ablation, with resulting induction of cylinder in the horizontal meridian.

in humans.[17] Like superficial ablation for myopia, this represents a new approach to the surgical correction of astigmatism, one that does not rely on creation of deep corneal incisions, excisions, or compression sutures.

PREOPERATIVE PREPARATION

SELECTION OF PATIENTS

Candidates for PRK for astigmatism should have healthy corneas and stable refractive errors. We have operated on patients who have had naturally occurring astigmatism and those who have postoperative (after keratoplasty and cataract extraction) astigmatism. Patients with postsurgical astigmatism should have had all sutures removed, with stable topography and refraction documented by repeat examinations performed at least 1 month apart. Our patients are primarily young adults who lead active lives, but no restrictions have been placed on their activities or participation in sports following surgery. Just as with surgery for myopia, underlying eye diseases, such as dry eye or chronic blepharitis, represent contraindications to the surgery and should be looked for carefully and treated preoperatively. Preoperative examination consists of measurement of visual acuity with and without correction, refraction, keratometry, biomicroscopic evaluation, pachometry, funduscopy, tonometry, measurement of pupil diameter, and computer-assisted corneal topographic analysis. Patients with mild keratoconus appreciated only by topographic examination are excluded from the surgery.[18,19]

INFORMED CONSENT

All the patients are informed fully about the investigational nature of excimer laser surgery of the eye, and of the risks and alternatives to this procedure. Patients are also informed that their surgery is being carried out under an investigational protocol approved by the federal Food and Drug Administration and the Institutional Review Board of the University of Southern California. We carefully differentiate this procedure from radial keratotomy and review the potential implications of superficial ablations versus deep incisions.[20]

PLANNING THE SURGERY

The amount of correction desired is based on the patient's preoperative refraction. The computer is programmed to perform cylindrical ablations equal to the patient's cylindrical error, and the desired refractive change is programmed into the computer in minus cylinder form. If the patient has compound myopic astigmatism, we will typically correct that at the same time as the astigmatism by performing a myopic ablation. In general, we "err" on the side of undercorrecting any coexisting myopia, with the understanding that residual myopia can be addressed, if necessary, with a subsequent spherical ablation.

DESCRIPTION OF THE PROCEDURE AND SURGICAL TECHNIQUE

LASER OPERATION

We use a 193 nm argon fluoride excimer laser (20/20 excimer laser, VISX, Sunnyvale, Calif.). To correct myopia, this laser uses a computer-controlled iris diaphragm to vary the diameter of the ablation beam so as to ablate more tissue centrally than peripherally, thereby flattening the cornea. To correct astigmatism, the same large-diameter excimer beam is passed through a set of parallel blades. The separation of the blades is under computer control, and the resultant variable slit is used to control the laser delivery much as the iris diaphragm used for myopia ablations.[21] In the case of the slit, however, the cornea should be flattened only in the meridian perpendicular to the long axis of the slit (termed the mechanical axis); no refractive change is intended along the mechanical axis (long axis of the slit). Thus, if the mechanical axis is oriented horizontally (in the 180° meridian), a flattening of the cornea will

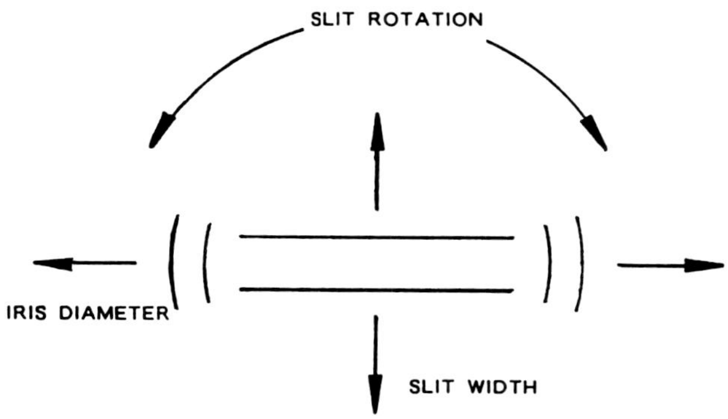

FIGURE 7.8. Schematic illustration of the method of creating toric ablations by progressively widening the separation between blades during the ablation. Variables that can be controlled include depth of ablation, width of ablation zone, and orientation of the slit.

occur in the vertical (90°) meridian. Primarily, this technique is designed to eliminate myopic astigmatism. The slit mechanism can be rotated, also under computer control, such that the mechanical axis can be aligned with the astigmatic axis of the patient (Fig. 7.8). The blades are oriented by the computer to be parallel to the axis of refractive cylinder expressed in minus cylinder form, thereby flattening the cornea in the appropriate (steep) meridian. With this approach, a vertical "wall" equal to the astigmatic ablation depth would appear at the two ends of the resultant rectangular ablation, along the mechanical axis. For this reason, a "transition zone" of 0.3 mm is generated at the ends of the slit to form a sigmoidal transition between unoperated and ablated cornea (Fig.7.9).

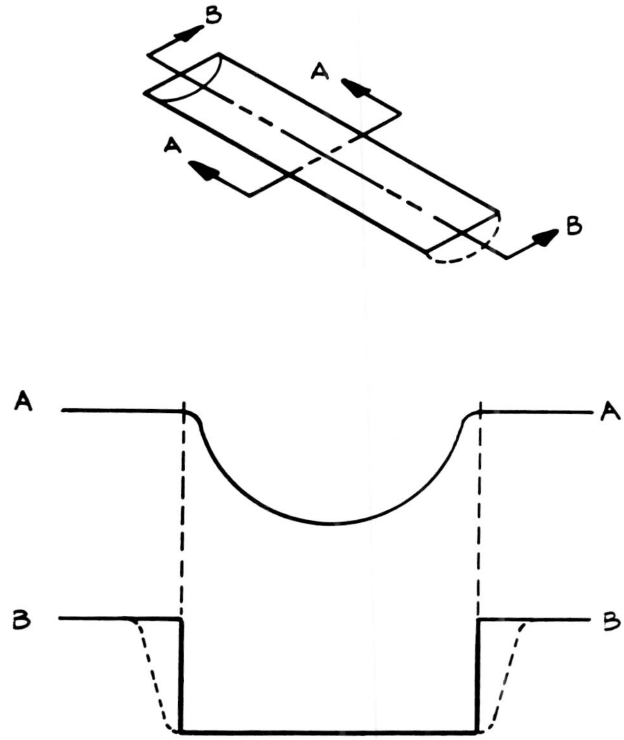

FIGURE 7.9. Schematic illustration of toric superficial ablation using a beam that begins as a narrow slit (mechanical axis perpendicular to the corneal meridian to be flattened) and widens gradually to the ablation zone of 4.5 mm in diameter. (A) A cross section of the ablation zone perpendicular to the mechanical axis shows a curved ablation profile with greater tissue ablation centrally than peripherally, flattening the cornea in this meridian. (B) A cross section of the ablation zone parallel to the mechanical axis of the slit shows straight-edged ablation with 0.3 mm transition at the ends, with no intended refractive change in this meridian.

PREPARATION OF THE PATIENT

The patient is placed under the excimer laser, topical proparacaine hydrochloride is instilled into the eye, and a circular protractor is placed on the globe at the limbus and oriented using a limbal landmark observed at the slit lamp before surgery. A few pulses of laser are then applied with the slit maximally narrowed in order to confirm proper orientation of the slit relative to the corneal cylinder and to acquaint the patient with sensations associated with the laser ablation. The patient's preoperative topographic corneal map is positioned so that the surgeon can readily double-check that the laser slit is properly oriented. The corneal epithelium is then removed with a blunt spatula. The eye is fixated with a vacuum fixation ring, and the area for laser treatment is centered over the entrance pupil while the patient fixates on a flashing centration light.[22] We do not mark the center of the entrance pupil with any instrument. We attempt to minimize corneal dehydration during the treatment,[23] as our studies in vitro and in living animal eyes suggest that maintaining corneal hydration during the procedure may lead to faster postoperative reepithelialization and perhaps to a smaller amount of postoperative superficial corneal haze. Because we use no pharmacologic sedation as part of our surgical routine, we attempt to put the patient at ease before and during the procedure by maintaining surgeon–patient physical contact, explaining the steps of the procedure and constantly reassuring the patient as these steps are performed, and desensitizing the patient to the noises and other sensations associated with the laser treatment. Failure to adequately calm the patient and acquaint him or her with the procedure will invariably result in sudden movement in response to the first few laser pulses. When the patient is adequately prepared, the laser treatment is begun. Should the patient make any movements during the procedure that result in loss of proper centration, the procedure is immediately interrupted, the centration is reestablished, the patient is reassured, and the procedure is completed.

INTRAOPERATIVE CONSIDERATIONS

The patient fixates on the fixation light during the entire procedure. The surgical assistant reports the number of pulses remaining to be delivered. The surgery can be stopped by the surgeon, if necessary, at any time during the procedure. We have had no intraoperative complications to date.

POSTOPERATIVE CONSIDERATIONS

POSTOPERATIVE CARE AND FOLLOW-UP

Patients are treated after surgery with a combination tobramycin sulfate–dexamethasone sodium phosphate ointment and semipressure patching and are examined daily or every other day until reepithelialization is complete. The patient is then treated with topical 1% prednisolone acetate (patients with postkeratoplasty astigmatism) or 0.1% fluorometholone (patients with naturally occurring astigmatism) four times daily for 2 weeks, three times daily for 4 weeks, and twice daily for the following 4 weeks. Prednisolone acetate is used in the postkeratoplasty patients because of our perceived need to use a penetrating corticosteroid to minimize the risk of allograft reaction. We perform refraction, keratometry, and computer-assisted corneal topographic analysis as early as 2 weeks after the procedure. Patients are seen 1, 3, 4, 6, and 12 months after surgery and thereafter on yearly basis.

WOUND HEALING AND COMPLICATIONS

Corneal reepithelialization is usually complete within 3 days. We did have one patient operated on for correction of postkeratoplasty astigmatism who had delayed reepithelialization, but in this case the keratoplasty had been done following an alkali burn. In general, patients who undergo surgery for postkeratoplasty astigmatism experience less discomfort and pain than do the patients operated on for correction of naturally occurring astigmatism. Oral narcotic analgesic therapy is given to all patients immediately after surgery, and many patients experience fairly severe pain for the first 24 hours. Herpes simplex keratitis can be reactivated by ultraviolet light,[24] and we had one patient who developed a recurrent herpetic dendrite 4 weeks after the laser surgery; this process cleared rapidly after topical trifluoridine therapy was started.[17] A mild corneal haze develops at about 1 month after surgery, but this usually decreases markedly within 6 months postoperatively. The intensity of the corneal haze after PRK for compound myopic astigmatism does not appear to differ from that observed after PRK for postoperative astigmatism. None of our patients have experienced disturbances in visual acuity that we could attribute to the corneal haze. We have not observed other wound-healing complications, recurrent epithelial erosions, or episodes of corneal graft rejection. We have specifically warned all patients with postkeratoplasty ametropias of the risk of allograft reactions but have seen no such events, perhaps related to the use of a relatively intensive course of topical prednisolone acetate once the graft has reepithelialized after the procedure. Furthermore, we have observed that corneal sensitivity after the excimer laser corneal surgery for astigmatism is mildly compromised for a short period of time and returns to normal levels within the first 3 months after surgery (Fig. 7.10).[25]

Computer-assisted corneal topographic analysis has demonstrated that an unintended variable flattening of the flattest meridian may occur concomitantly with the flattening of the steepest meridian. We do not consider this to be an adverse effect in patients who have compound myopic astigmatism,

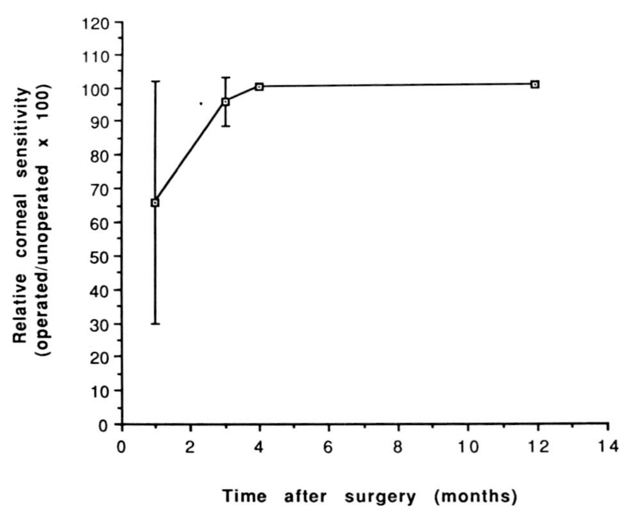

FIGURE 7.10. Recovery of central corneal sensitivity in patients following PRK.

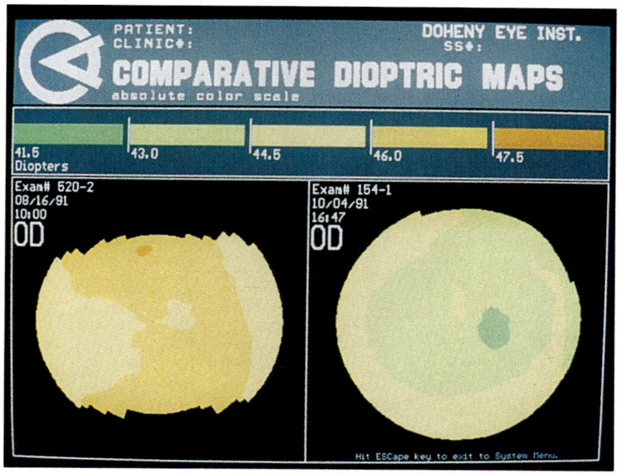

FIGURE 7.11. Color-coded keratograph of patient 1 before (left) and 2 months after (right) toric ablation to correct a refractive error of −5.00 −1.00 × 41°. Postoperative keratograph shows an overall symmetric flattening of the cornea in both meridians.

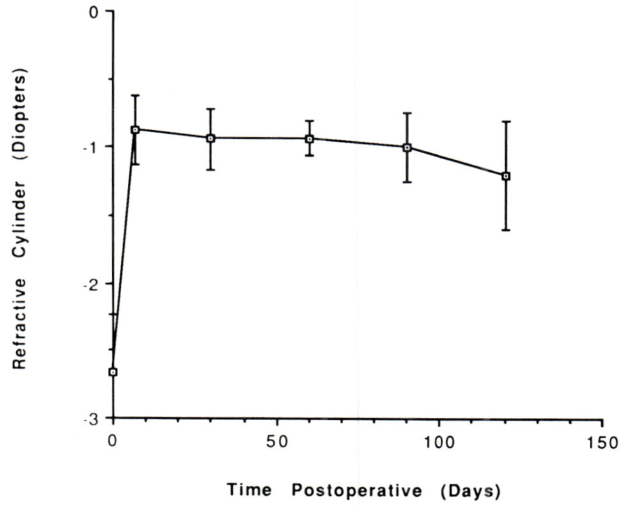

FIGURE 7.12. Graph of refractive cylinder (mean ± standard error) over time following superficial ablation for compound myopic astigmatism.

in which an associated treatment for the myopic component of the refractive error is desired.

RESULTS

NATURALLY OCCURRING ASTIGMATISM

Case illustration:

Patient 1, a 43 year-old woman with naturally occurring compound myopic astigmatism who was contact lens–intolerant. Her preoperative examination revealed a manifest refraction of −5.00 −1.00 × 41°, keratometric readings of 44.87/45.50 at 86°, uncorrected visual acuity of 20/200, and best-corrected visual acuity of 20/20. Preoperative corneal topography revealed an asymmetric steepening of the 106° meridian (Fig. 7.11, left). The excimer laser was programmed for a target correction of −4.50 −1.00 × 41°. Examination at 1 month postoperative revealed an uncorrected visual acuity of 20/50, manifest refraction of −0.50 −0.75 × 107° and keratometric readings of 41.75/42.25 at 58°. Four months after surgery, the uncorrected visual acuity was 20/80, manifest refraction was −2.00 −0.50 × 14°. Corneal topography revealed an overall symmetric flattening of the cornea (Fig. 7.11, right). A barely detectable stromal haze was observed by biomicroscopic examination.

The results of the first nine eyes on which we operated to correct compound myopic astigmatism with the excimer laser, shown as follows, represent a follow-up ranging from 4 to 11 months (mean, 5 months). Based on previous studies,[17] in which an overall flattening of the cornea was observed after astigmatic ablations alone, in all nine patients we attempted to correct the full cylindrical error, but to only partially correct the total spherical component of the refractive error. Figure 7.12 shows the mean reduction of the refractive cylinder. The correction of the cylindrical error ranged from 33 to 80%. One eye had a paradoxical increase of 50% of the preoperative cylindrical error. The spherical equivalent changed from a preoperative value (mean ± standard deviation) of −3.40 ± 1.6 D to −0.75 ± 1.4 D (Fig. 7.13). The uncorrected visual acuity improved in all patients from a mean of 20/300 to 20/40. Four months after surgery only two of the patients showed corneal haze that was barely detectable.

POSTKERATOPLASTY ASTIGMATISM

Case illustration:

Patient 2, a contact lens–intolerant 45 year-old man, had a corneal transplant performed in his left eye 2 years ago for removal of a corneal scar. This patient had a preoperative manifest refraction of −4.75 −5.25 × 65°, keratometric readings of 51.25 at 152°/46.62 at 62°, uncorrected visual acuity of 20/400, and best-corrected visual acuity of 20/20. Corneal topography revealed a regular oblique astigmatism present with the steeper portion in the 145° axis meridian and steepness also present in the inferior portion of the graft (Fig. 7.14, right). The contralateral eye examination was unremark-

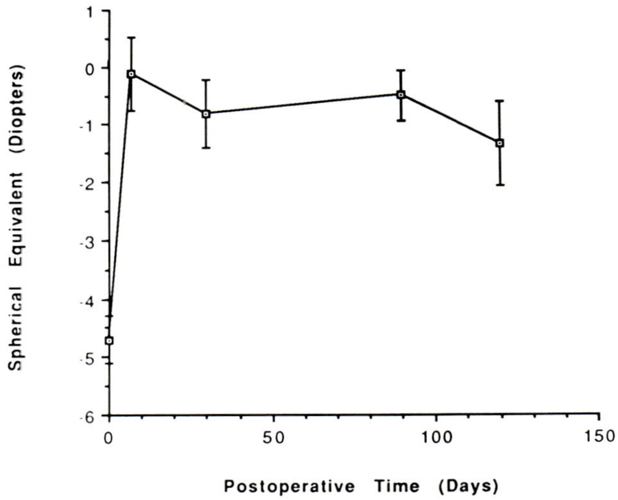

FIGURE 7.13. Graph of spherical equivalent (mean ± standard error) over time following superficial ablation for compound myopic astigmatism.

able. The excimer laser was programmed to perform a target correction of −1.00 −4.25 × 65°. One month postoperative, the manifest refraction was −0.25 −0.75 × 157°, and uncorrected visual acuity was 20/25. Corneal topography revealed an overall flattening of the cornea and a remaining irregular astigmatism (Fig. 7.14, left). Two months after surgery, the uncorrected visual acuity was 20/40, manifest refraction was +1.75 −3.00 × 173° and keratometric readings were 42.37/42.62 at 98°. Biomicroscopy revealed a barely detectable haze (Fig. 7.15).

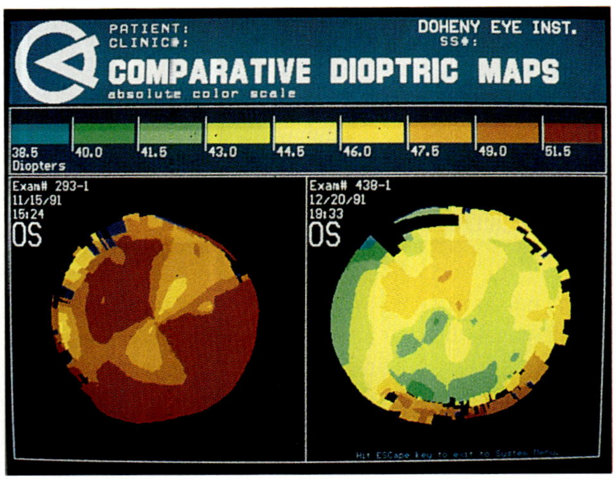

FIGURE 7.14. Color-coded keratograph of patient 2 before (left) and 1 month after (right) toric ablation to correct a refractive error of −1.0 −4.25 × 65°. A moderate residual irregular astigmatism is present after surgery (right).

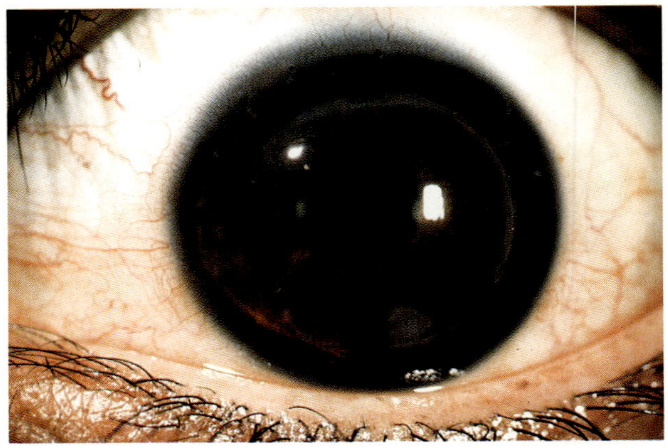

FIGURE 7.15. Biomicroscopic photograph showing different intensity stromal haze in two patients 2 months after PRK for correction of postkeratoplasty astigmatism.

We operated on 12 eyes of 12 patients with high disabling postkeratoplasty astigmatism. All patients were contact lens–intolerant and were unable to tolerate the high cylindrical prescription in their glasses. The results shown represent a minimum of 3 months after the surgery. Surgery was performed based on the refractive cylinder corrected to the corneal plane. Half the patients had programmed undercorrections as consistent with our conservative approach (see comments). An overall reduction of 53% was achieved on the preoperative cylindrical error, and the maximum effect was observed in the first 3 months after surgery (Fig. 7.16). The spherical equivalent revealed a hyperopic shift within the

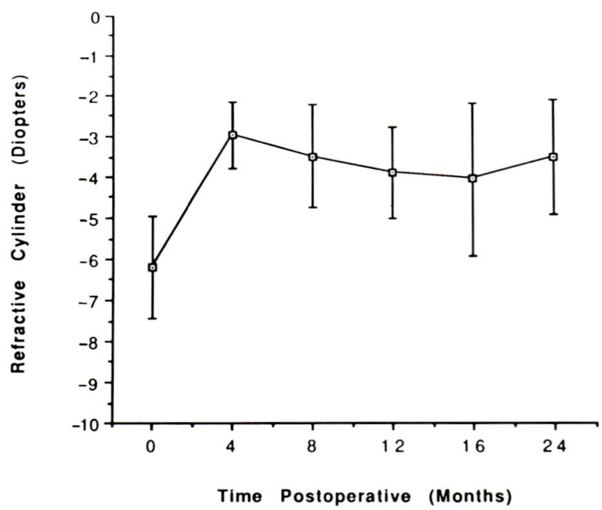

FIGURE 7.16. Graph of refractive cylinder (mean ± standard error) over time following toric ablation with the excimer laser for correction of postkeratoplasty astigmatism.

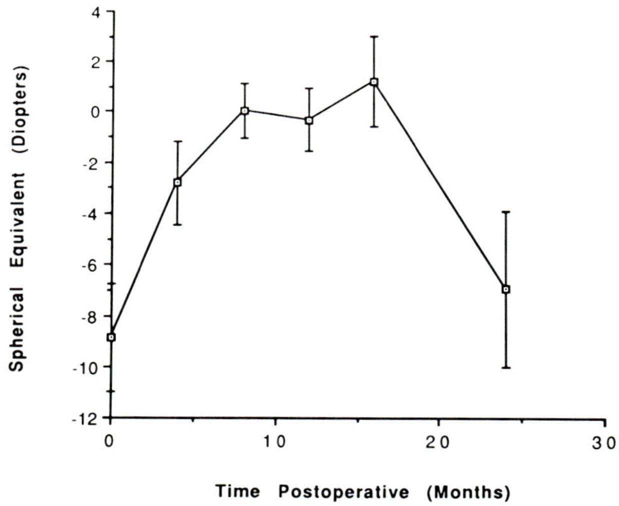

FIGURE 7.17. Graph of spherical equivalent (mean ± standard error) over time following toric ablation with the excimer laser for correction of postkeratoplasty astigmatism.

first 16 weeks after surgery, with a slight reduction of the effect thereafter (Fig. 7.17). Uncorrected visual acuity improved by at least one line in nine patients, did not change in one patient, and decreased one line in another patient. Five patients improved the best-corrected visual acuity by at least two lines. One patient had a delayed epithelial healing related with his underlying disease (chemical burn). The amount of haze detected in these patients was slightly more intense than in the other group of naturally occurring astigmatism patients but was barely detected in almost all the patients (Fig. 7.15). One patient had an easily detectable haze that did not interfere with retinoscopy or visual acuity. This group of patients had milder postoperative pain than the naturally occurring astigmatism patients, presumably due to incomplete reinnervation of the grafts.[26]

POSTULCER ASTIGMATISM

Case illustration:

Patient 3, a 43 year-old man with simple myopia for which he wore soft contact lenses on an extended-wear basis, developed a central corneal ulcer due to *Psuedomonas aeruginosa*. After prompt diagnosis and aggressive antibiotic therapy, the patient was left with a mild superficial stromal opacity about 5.0 mm in diameter and high compound myopic astigmatism with an irregular component (Fig. 7.18A). This patient had a preoperative manifest refraction of −2.25 −6.75 × 82°, keratometric readings of 43.62/47.62 at 78°, uncorrected visual acuity of 20/

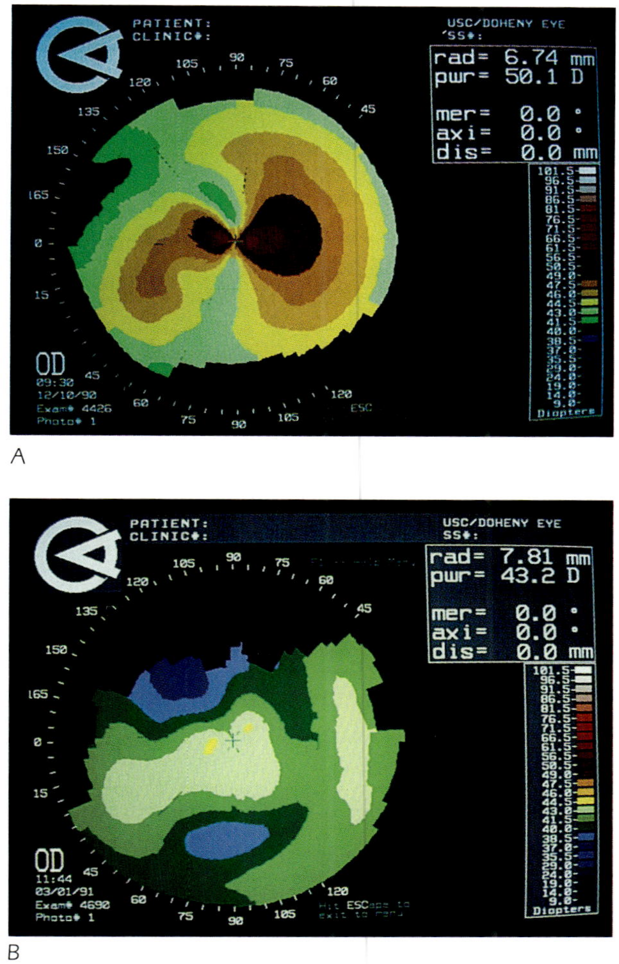

FIGURE 7.18. Color-coded keratograph of patient 3 (A) before and (B) after cylindrical ablation for astigmatism. Preoperative astigmatism resulted from *Pseudomonas* corneal ulcer and is moderately irregular. Surgery resulted in reduction of refractive astigmatism from 6.75 to 0.5 D.

200, and best-corrected visual acuity of 20/25. Corneal topography revealed an against-the-rule astigmatism that was moderately irregular. The contralateral eye examination was remarkable only for simple myopia. The patient's acuity improved to 20/25 with a gas-permeable contact lens, but he was unable to tolerate this due to discomfort, and he could not tolerate the high cylindrical correction in his spectacles. The excimer laser was programmed to perform a target correction of plano −6.75 × 82°. Four months postoperatively, the manifest refraction was plano −0.50 × 76° and uncorrected visual acuity was 20/30. Corneal topography revealed an overall flattening of the cornea and a remaining irregular astigmatism (Fig. 7.18B). Keratometric readings were 40.62/41.87 at 74°. Biomicroscopy revealed a barely detectable haze.

COMMENTS

Naturally occurring astigmatism and postoperative astigmatism are common problems in general ophthalmic practice. The extensive list of different approaches published in the literature indicates that the optimal means for surgical correction of astigmatism remains to be determined. Incisional procedures have limited precision but are technically simple, and the instrumentation is relatively inexpensive. Excimer laser surgery of the cornea, by contrast, is an expensive and technology-intensive instrument with unknown long-term complications.

The technique described here was designed for regular astigmatism, with symmetric steepening in the two steep hemimeridians. We know, however, that not all astigmatism is regular. Irregular astigmatism is frequently encountered after penetrating keratoplasty,[27] after refractive surgical procedures such as epikeratophakia,[28] with intersecting corneal incisions,[29] or even in unoperated corneas.[30] Thus, patients with substantial irregular astigmatism will have limitation of uncorrected or spectacle-corrected acuity after reduction of the regular astigmatism with the technique described here. At this time, therefore, the most appropriate candidate for cylindrical ablation with the excimer laser has primarily regular astigmatism, with reasonable improvement in visual acuity with spectacle correction. Additional work will be required before we can confidently deal with the irregular component of the astigmatism using this approach.

The ideal patient for this technique also has a myopic spherical refractive error in addition to the myopic astigmatism. In our studies to date we have utilized a conservative approach when programming the amount of desired correction in almost all the patients so as to avoid rendering patients hyperopic. We did, in fact, leave most of our patients substantially undercorrected (i.e., with residual myopia). Using this conservative approach, we did not observe a progressive effect of the surgery in flattening the cornea even on the greater corrections performed on postkeratoplasty patients. Thus, we avoided a hyperopic shift in these operated patients. Currently, an overly flattened cornea resulting in hyperopia cannot be subsequently resteepened with the laser. With the excimer laser, a subsequent myopic photorefractive keratectomy can be performed to treat residual myopic refractive errors.

Although we substantially undercorrected the astigmatism in many of our early patients using a conservative approach, we have been impressed by patient satisfaction and good improvement in unaided visual acuity. It would appear that the requirement for correction of nearly all refractive error, typical with surgery for myopia, may not apply as much in surgery to correct myopic astigmatism. For example a patient with 3 D of myopia would likely be disappointed with a 50% correction, while we have many patients who are delighted with the 50% reduction of this amount of astigmatism. In fact, Sawusch and Guyton have demonstrated that some degree of postcataract extraction astigmatism may actually be preferred by patients, affording them a greater level of visual acuity over a range of defocus, thereby allowing some patients to avoid the need for correction at both distance and near.[31] It may be that elimination of all corneal cylinder will not ultimately prove to be the ideal end point of this surgery; preservation of some predetermined amount of astigmatism may increase patient satisfaction by minimizing symptoms of presbyopia.

Another approach to the correction of astigmatism with the excimer laser is the use of a premanufactured "ablatable mask" having a toric geometry. The laser is used to ablate through the mask, with the underlying cornea subsequently being ablated when the laser breaks entirely through the mask. In this fashion, the underlying cornea is differentially ablated according to the thickness of the mask material overlying each portion of the cornea. The use of this approach is described in greater detail in chapter 4.

We have recently begun a series of patients in whom we are performing elliptical ablations to correct compound myopic astigmatism. This technique involves a single ablation having an elliptical shape, instead of performing two ablations (one cylindrical ablation for astigmatism and a second ablation for the spherical myopia). While the initial results using this elliptical ablation technique look encouraging, the numbers allowed under FDA guidelines have been relatively small and the follow-up is short, so we cannot yet determine whether this new approach constitutes a substantial improvement over the technique described in this chapter.

It is clear at this point that the excimer laser can successfully treat corneal astigmatism by ablating superficial stroma in the shape of a cylindrical lens. The problems of interindividual variability in wound healing and correction of irregular astigmatism remain. Elsewhere in this text we discuss research efforts currently underway or needed in these areas.

REFERENCES

1. Bates WH: A suggestion of an operation to correct astigmatism. *Arch Ophthalmol* 23:9–13, 1894.

2. Lavery GW, Lindstrom RL, Hofer LA, et al: The surgical management of corneal astigmatism after penetrating keratoplasty. *Ophthalmic Surg* 16:165–169, 1985.
3. Troutman RC, Swinger C: Relaxing incision for control of postoperative astigmatism following keratoplasty. *Ophthalmic Surg* 11:117–120, 1980.
4. Lindstrom RL, Lindquist TD: Surgical correction of postoperative astigmatism. *Cornea* 7:138–148, 1988.
5. Villaseñor RA, Stimac GR: Clinical results and complications of trapezoidal keratotomy. *J Refract Surg* 4:125–131, 1988.
6. Krachmer JH, Fenzl RE: Surgical correction of high postkeratoplasty astigmatism: Relaxing incisions vs wedge resection. *Arch Ophthalmol* 98:1400–1402, 1980.
7. Franks JB, Binder PS: Keratotomy procedures for the correction of astigmatism. *J Refract Surg* 1:11–17, 1985.
8. Sugar J, Kirk AK: Relaxing keratotomy for post keratoplasty high astigmatism. *Ophthalmic Surg* 14: 156–158, 1983.
9. Lavery GW, Lindstrom RL: Clinical results of trapezoidal astigmatic keratotomy. *J Refract Surg* 1:70–74, 1985.
10. Rowsey JJ: Review: Current concepts in astigmatic surgery. *J Refract Surg* 2:85–94, 1986.
11. Arciniegas A, Amaya LE: Corneal curvature modification by scleral surgery: Preliminary results. *Ann Ophthalmol* 17:221–226, 1985.
12. Troutman RC: Corneal wedge resections and relaxing incisions for postkeratoplasty astigmatism. *Int Ophthalmol Clin* 23(4):161–168, 1983.
13. Duffey RJ, Jain VN, Tchah H, et al: Paired arcuate keratotomy: A surgical approach to mixed and myopic astigmatism. *Arch Ophthalmol* 106:1130–1135, 1988.
14. McCluskey DJ, Villaseñor R, McDonnell PJ: Prospective topographic analysis in peripheral arcuate keratotomy for astigmatism. *Ophthalmic Surg* 21: 464–471, 1990.
15. McDonald MB, Frantz JM, Klyce SD, et al: Central photorefractive keratectomy for myopia: The blind eye study. *Arch Ophthalmol* 108:799–808, 1990.
16. McDonnell PJ, Moreira H, Garbus J, et al: Photorefractive keratectomy to create toric ablations for correction of astigmatism. *Arch Ophthalmol* 109:710–713, 1991.
17. McDonnell PJ, Moreira H, Clapham TN, et al: Photorefractive keratectomy for astigmatism: Initial clinical results. *Arch Ophthalmol* 109:1370–1373, 1991.
18. Maguire LJ, Bourne WM: Corneal topography of early keratoconus. *Am J Ophthalmol* 108:107–112, 1989.
19. Rabinowitz YS, Garbus J, McDonnell PJ: Computer-assisted corneal topography in family members of patients with keratoconus. *Arch Ophthalmol* 108:365–371, 1990.
20. Campos M, Cuevas K, Lee M, et al: Ocular integrity after photorefractive keratectomy and radial keratotomy. *Invest Ophthalmol Vis Sci* 33(suppl):999, 1992.
21. Marshall J, Trokel SL, Rothery S, et al: Photoablative reprofiling of the cornea using an excimer laser: Photorefractive keratectomy. *Lasers Ophthalmol* 1:21–48, 1986.
22. Uozato H, Guyton DL: Centering corneal surgical procedures. *Am J Ophthalmol* 103:264–275, 1987.
23. Campos M, Cuevas K, Lee M, et al: Photorefractive keratectomy for myopia: Effects of the nitrogen gas blower. *Ophthalmology,* in press.
24. Laycock KA, Lee SF, Brady RH, et al: Characterization of a murine model of recurrent herpes simplex viral keratitis induced by ultraviolet β radiation. *Invest Ophthalmol Vis Sci* 32:2741–2746, 1991.
25. Campos M, Garbus J, McDonnell PJ: Corneal sensitivity after photorefractive keratectomy. *Am J Ophthalmol,* 114:51–54, 1992.
26. Rao GN, John T, Ishida N, et al: Recovery of corneal sensitivity in grafts following penetrating keratoplasty. *Ophthalmology* 92:1408–1411, 1985.
27. Maguire LJ, Bourne WM: Corneal topography of transverse keratotomies for astigmatism after penetration keratoplasty. *Am J Ophthalmol* 107:323–330, 1989.
28. Reidy JJ, McDonald MB, Klyce SD: The corneal topography of epikeratophakia. *Refract Corneal Surg* 6:26–31, 1990.
29. McDonnell PJ, Caroline PJ, Salz J: Irregular astigmatism after radial and astigmatic keratotomy. *Am J Ophthalmol* 107:42–46, 1989.
30. Bogan SJ, Waring GO III, Ibraham O, et al: Classification of normal corneal topography based on computer-assisted videokeratography. *Arch Ophthalmol* 108:945–949, 1990.
31. Sawusch MR, Guyton DL: Optimal astigmatism to enhance depth of focus after cataract surgery. *Ophthalmology* 98:1025–1029, 1991.

CHAPTER 8

Therapeutic Keratectomy: Corneal Opacities

WALTER J. STARK
WALLACE CHAMON
DIMITRI T. AZAR
MARY T. KAMP
CHERYL L. ENGER

TREATMENT OF CORNEAL SCARS: A BRIEF HISTORY

The treatment of corneal scars began in the 18th century when St. Yves introduced superficial keratectomy, and Pellier de Quengsy the use of artificial implants.[1] Since that time surgeons have tried a variety of procedures, such as the creation of an artificial opening in the sclera and total or partial penetrating keratoplasty.[1-5] By the 1840s the interest in lamellar keratoplasty began to increase, because of the poor results obtained with other techniques.[2] It was not until 1906 that Edward Zirm reported the first successful penetrating keratoplasty in humans.[3] Further developments and improvements continued into the 1940s,[4] because of refinements in original instrumentation and sutures rather than changes in the original concepts.[1,2,4] Superficial keratectomy and penetrating or lamellar keratoplasty were the mainstays in the treatment of corneal opacities until the introduction of the excimer laser.

After the first report of corneal effects of the 193 nm argon fluoride excimer laser in 1981,[6] Trokel and colleagues demonstrated that precise corneal ablations could be achieved in bovine eyes using the same type of apparatus.[7] Further studies in animals[8-15] and in vitro[16-20] as well as clinical and histopathologic studies in humans[21-36] have now established the preciseness and safety of the argon fluoride excimer laser in performing ablations of the cornea with minimal damage to surrounding tissue.

In argon-fluoride excimer laser phototherapeutic keratectomy (PTK), laser energy is used to ablate corneal tissue for the purpose of removing opacities and/or smoothing irregular surfaces.[37]

Supported in part by grants from Margaret Mosher, Ralph O'Connor, and The George R. Brown Endowed Fund for Corneal Research.

PREOPERATIVE PREPARATION

PATIENT SELECTION

Patients with opacities in the anterior third of the cornea (approximately 160 μm in depth) or surface irregularity who do not have functional vision with spectacles or contact lenses should be evaluated for PTK. Current contraindications to treatment include blepharitis, dry eye, lagophthalmus, active inflammation of the eye, decreased corneal thickness, and systemic immunosuppression. Patients are excluded from treatment if the postoperative corneal thickness is predicted to be less than 250 μm. There are no age restrictions; however, younger patients

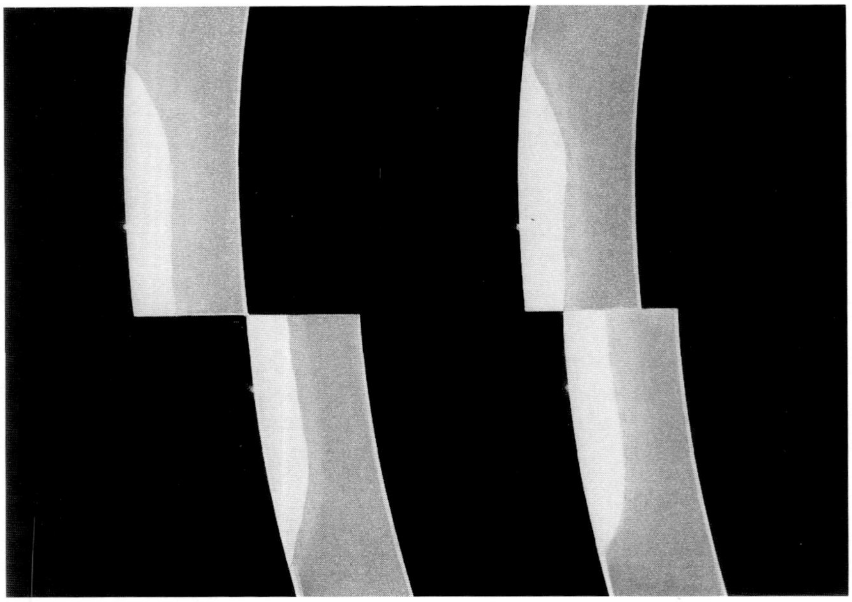

FIGURE 8.1. The use of an optical pachometer to determine the depth of a stromal scar. After aligning the posterior surface to the anterior surface (left), the thickness of the scar is measured by aligning the anterior corneal surface with the posterior limit of the scar (right). (From Stark et al: *Arch Ophthalmol* 108:12–13, 1990, with permission.)

are preferred because of their willingness to try a contact lens postoperatively if induced hyperopia occurs. Patients unwilling to consider contact lens correction for postoperative hyperopia should be discouraged from undergoing the laser ablation procedure.

Currently, all patients must meet the eligibility criteria approved by the U.S. Food and Drug Administration (FDA), must be informed of the investigational nature of the laser procedure, and must provide written informed consent prior to the surgery.

PREOPERATIVE EXAMINATION

Preoperative evaluations are performed on all patients and include external, slit lamp, and dilated fundus examinations. Visual acuity is evaluated without correction, with manifest refraction, with pinhole, and with a hard contact lens. Pneumotonometry, keratometry, ultrasonic pachymetry, and topographic analysis of the cornea are also attempted.

The thickness of the affected cornea is measured using a Haag-Streit optical pachometer (Bern, Switzerland), modified by S. Mishima.[38] The full thickness of the cornea is measured by aligning the posterior surface of the endothelium in the upper field with the anterior surface of the epithelium in the lower field. The anterior surface is then aligned with the posterior limit of an optically distinct corneal opacity to measure the thickness of the scar (Fig. 8.1).

PLANNING THE SURGERY

The depth of the treatment is determined by the thickness of the affected cornea. The diameter is determined by the size of the scar as it relates to the optical zone of the cornea.

SURGICAL TECHNIQUE

Oral analgesic and sedative are administered to the patient prior to surgery. Peribulbar and retrobulbar anesthesia have been replaced by topical anesthesia. The patient is positioned beneath the surgical microscope, the lids are prepared and draped, and the lid speculum is applied. The patient is asked to fixate on the blinking light of the microscope. Centration of the image of the pupil (entrance pupil)[39] within the ablating laser beam is facilitated by a reticule with concentric rings, placed in the right ocular of the surgeon's microscope.

The microscope is initially focused at the plane of the corneal surface using a magnification of 18X; however, the treatment is performed at a magnification of 12X to ensure exact correlation of the measurements on the surgeon's eyepiece with corneal dimensions. Initiation and termination of ablation are achieved using foot-pedal control.

The decision whether to ablate through the intact epithelium with the laser or to remove the epithelium mechanically is based on the smoothness of the epithelial surface. If the anterior surface of the cornea is smooth, the epithelium is ablated with the laser; if irregular, it is removed manually with a platinum spatula or Bard-Parker blade with minimal pressure on the cornea. The treatment surface is maintained meticulously clear of debris and cellular remnants to avoid irregularities. A combination of 1% methylcellulose and Tears Naturale II® (Alcon, Fort Worth, Texas) (1:2) is used to fill the base of microscopic roughness,[40] thus promoting a regular surface for treatment.

In the initial cases, a suction ring was used over the limbus to stabilize the eye during the laser exposure. More recently, whenever possible, we ask the patient to fixate on the blinking light located in the center of the microscope's objective lens. The initial technique utilized a nitrogen flow system set at 10 standard cubic feet per hour (SCfh) and an aspiration port to remove ablated fragments and any ozone formed during the laser procedure. We no longer use the nitrogen system, however, because of potential desiccation of the cornea. The pattern of ablation (diameter of the beam for each pulse) is determined by the computer software that controls an iris diaphragm capable of producing up to 300 steps with a resolution of 25 μm per step. Initially this pattern consisted of a treatment zone of up to 6.0 mm diameter and a 0.5 mm taper to the peripheral zone. This was associated with an induced hyperopia of 7.2 D at the 6-month follow-up.[36] More recently treated patients did not receive the standard 0.5 mm taper; instead we have used a modified taper with the intention of minimizing the hyperopic effect. The surgeon attempts to decrease the induced central corneal flattening by moving the eye under the laser in a circular fashion and treating the edge of the ablation zone with a 2.0 mm diameter beam.

Sub-Tenon's injections of an antibiotic and a steroid are given after the surgery, topical antibiotic and cycloplegic are applied, and the eye is pressure-patched. Analgesics are prescribed postoperatively as needed.

POSTOPERATIVE CARE AND COMPLICATIONS

Patients are observed at two day intervals during the immediate postoperative period until reepithelialization occurs, and all patients return at 1 and 3 months after treatment as required by the FDA protocol. Additional follow-up is requested of all patients at 6, 9, 12, 18, and 24 months; the compliance rate is high. The measurements taken at the preoperative evaluation are repeated at each visit from 1 month onward. The initial patients were treated with 1% prednisolone acetate drops four times daily for 1 week, tapered down to once daily by 1 month and continued for 6 months, unless steroid responsiveness was noted. More recently we have used 0.1% fluorometholone with a similar tapering manner. Five percent sodium chloride ointment is prescribed at bedtime as needed.

WOUND HEALING AND COMPLICATIONS

Potential postoperative complications include recurrent erosions, infectious corneal ulceration, and persistent epithelial defects.

Reepithelialization usually occurs within 1 week. Two of the 28 eyes in our series required bandage contact lenses to heal and reepithelialized completely in 3 and 4 weeks, respectively.[36] No subsequent infections, epithelial defects, or recurrent erosions were observed.

We monitor corneal haze during the slit lamp examination and grade it as follows: 0 = clear; 0.5 = barely detectable; 1.0 = mild, not affecting retinoscopy; 1.5 = mildly affecting retinoscopy; 2.0 = moderate, retinoscopy possible but difficult; 3.0 = opacity preventing retinoscopy, anterior chamber easily viewed; 4.0 = impaired view of anterior chamber; and 5.0 = inability to see the anterior chamber. The cornea is divided into five hypothetical layers (superficial and deep epithelium, and anterior and posterior stroma and endothelium); each layer is graded separately. In all our patients, postoperative corneal clarity scores were lower than preoperative scores.

HISTOPATHOLOGIC STUDIES

The ultimate success of excimer laser therapy depends on corneal healing, and variability in the rate of wound healing may determine the predictability of the final visual outcome. Because the ablation process depends on the breakdown of molecular bonds and on achieving an energy level greater than these bond energies, some tissue damage is inevitable. Histopathologic studies (Figs. 8.2–8.6) show, however, that the degree of damage is minimal, especially with the currently used wavelength of 193 nm and energy of 160 mJ/cm^2.[41] Heat transmission is minimal beyond a fraction of a micrometer from the treated zone with a repetition rate of 5 pulses per second.[41]

The variability in wound healing thus results from the postoperative events as evidenced histopathologically.

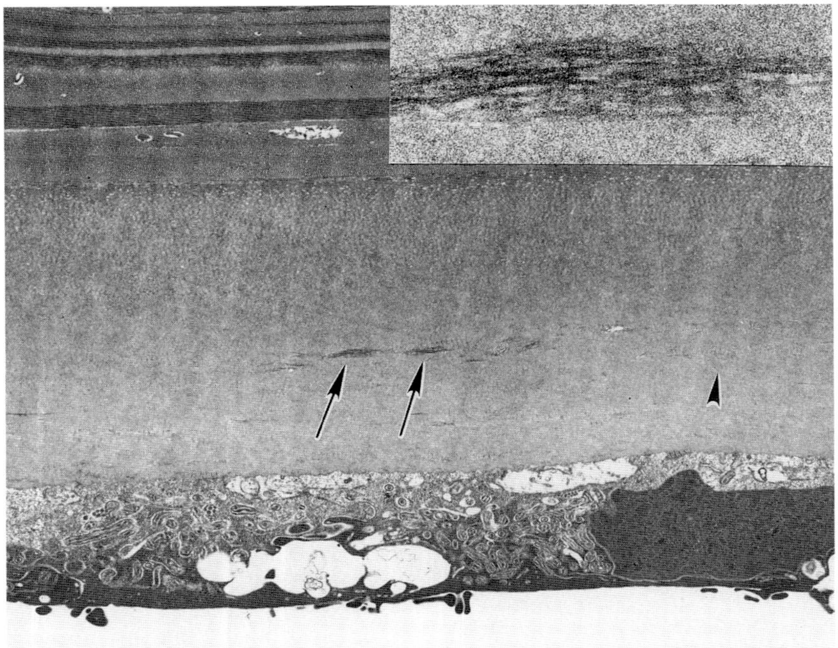

FIGURE 8.2. Electron-dense fibers in Descemet's membrane underlying ablated zone (arrows and inset) 11 months post-PTK (original magnification, 6000×; inset, 60,000×). (From Wu et al: *Arch Ophthalmol* 109:1426–1432, 1991, with permission.)

1. Epithelial hyperplasia may occur and is probably more pronounced in nontapered ablations.[24]
2. Reformation of the epithelial basement membrane adhesion structures may be delayed.[34] We have studied histopathologically three human corneas that required penetrating keratoplasties following PTK.[33,34] Reductions in the number of epithelial cells having normal adhesion complexes were noted as late as 6 and 11 months after PTK. These patients, however, did not have delayed wound closure, recurrent erosions, or persistent epithelial defects.
3. Stromal wound healing may be complicated initially by the absence of an epithelial barrier and later by the activation of keratocytes and possible deposition of abnormal type III collagen.[13] These factors may contribute to the subepithelial haze that is frequently seen clinically, and to the mild scarring observed beneath the ablated area in histopathologic examinations.[11,33]
4. Evidence of clinically significant endothelial damage is lacking despite the presence of ill-defined changes in Descemet's membrane in some monkey and human specimens.[12,33]

RESULTS

Since 1989, 30 eyes of 28 patients with diverse corneal pathologic conditions have undergone PTK performed by a single surgeon (W. J. S.) at The Wilmer Institute. Follow-up ranged from 3 to 30 months. Results are presented as mean plus or minus standard error.

The mean preoperative visual acuity (logarithmic) was 20/99 with manifest refraction. The mean postoperative visual acuity was 20/46 using manifest refraction in 25 eyes (83%) and contact lenses in 5 eyes (17%) (Fig. 8.7). One patient (3%) had lost two lines, and 20 patients (66%) had improved two lines or more of spectacle-corrected visual acuity at the most recent follow-up. All patients were contact lens–intolerant before the surgery, either from lack of visual improvement or discomfort. Five patients became contact lens–tolerant after PTK. Three eyes did not achieve significant visual improvement and subsequently underwent corneal transplantation at 6, 11, and 14 months post-PTK, respectively.

We could not obtain keratometric readings in seven eyes preoperatively and in an additional number at different postoperative visits. Those eyes for which readings were obtainable (Fig. 8.8) had an average keratometric reading before surgery of 45.1 ± 0.66 D. The keratometric reading decreased by 5.7 ± 0.93 D at 3 months ($p < .001$), and by 3.9 ± 1.30 D from baseline at 24 months ($p < .05$).

The change in spherical equivalent (Fig. 8.9) reflects the induced hyperopic shift caused by PTK. Those eyes treated with the standard 0.5-mm taper had an average of 5.5 ± 1.12 D of induced hyperopia at 3 months postoperatively ($p < .001$), 6.8 ± 1.17 D at 6 months ($p < .001$), and 5.0 ± 2.20 D at 24 months ($p < .05$). The seven eyes that were

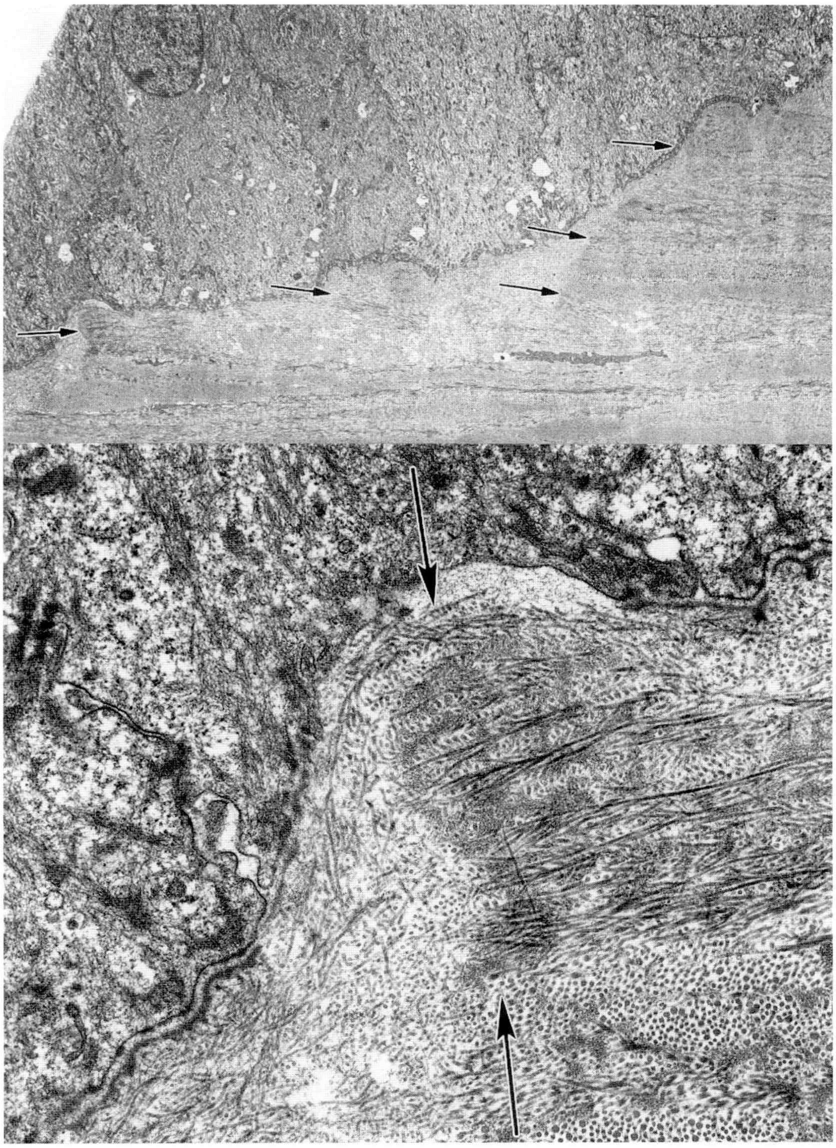

FIGURE 8.3. Eleven months following PTK, little reparation of the stroma occurs at the margin of laser ablation (top: original magnification, 2250×; bottom: original magnification, 22,000×). (From Wu et al: *Arch Ophthalmol* 109:1426–1432, 1991, with permission.)

more recently treated with the modified taper had an initial shift of induced hyperopia of 5.8 ± 2.28 D at 3 months postoperatively ($p < .05$), and 3.7 ± 2.15 D at 6 months ($p > .10$). Figure 8.9 suggests a possible trend in reducing the amount of induced hyperopia with the modified taper, but the numbers are too small and do not demonstrate a statistically significant difference between tapering procedures.

Correlation between depth of stromal ablation and amount of induced hyperopia was evaluated at 3 months postoperatively (Fig. 8.10). No eye treated with less than 95 μm had more than 10 D of induced hyperopia, whereas 50% of those treated with more than 95 μm had 10 D or more of induced hyperopia ($X^2 = 11.25$, $p < .001$).

Sher and colleagues[35] reported that 15% of their patients lost two lines or more of spectacle-corrected visual acuity following PTK. Their results may be due to different criteria for patient selection.

DISCUSSION

The success of PTK in treating patients with superficial corneal dystrophies or scars relates to the resulting postponement or prevention of keratoplasty. Corneal dystrophies are known to recur in the graft,[42-44] and four of the eyes in our series were treated for recurrent corneal dystrophy in the graft

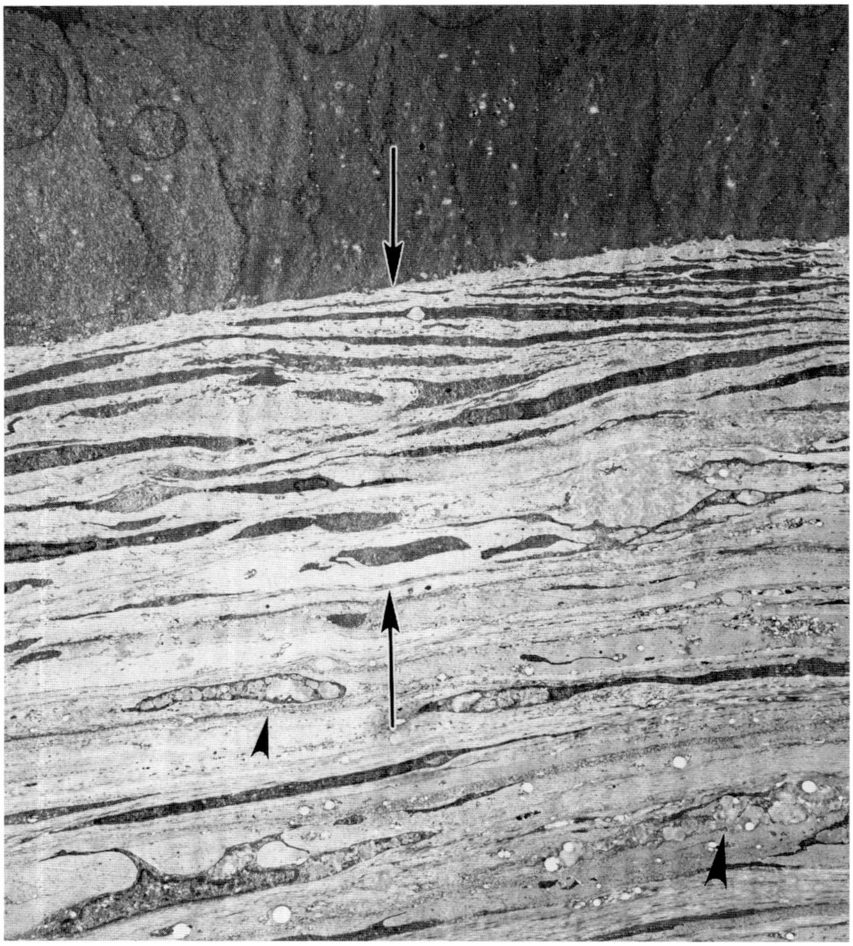

FIGURE 8.4. Elongated fibrocytes (arrowheads) and loss of lamellar structures (between arrows) are seen in the superficial stroma 6 months following PTK (original magnification, 2000×). (From Wu et al: *Arch Ophthalmol* 109:1426–1432, 1991, with permission.)

(lattice dystrophy in three; granular dystrophy in one).

Minimal complications were observed in our patients. One patient with Salzmann's nodular degeneration and one patient with a history of significant alcohol intake experienced delayed wound healing (3 and 4 weeks, respectively). In another review of PTK[35] 1 of 33 patients had delayed reepithelialization. Although rating the corneal clarity is a subjective evaluation, it does allow us to report that no significant additional scarring occurred postoperatively and that haze remained minimal compared with the preoperative level.

Central flattening of the cornea (hyperopic effect) appears to be the principal undesirable effect of PTK. This flattening can be caused by the change in the angle of incidence of the beam across the corneal surface, such that the beam is delivered at a 90° angle to the surface at the center of the treatment area and at less than a 90° angle at the periphery. The laser ablates the same amount of tissue per pulse when tested on a planar surface. At the corneal periphery, where the incidence angle is not perpendicular to the surface, the depth of ablation will be less than that in the center, creating a flatter surface of curvature. Epithelial hyperplasia and flattening of the tear meniscus at the periphery of the ablation area may also account for the induced flattening of the central cornea.

This flattening may be unacceptable to patients who are not myopic preoperatively. Because our patients were awaiting penetrating keratoplasty, they tolerated the induced hyperopia as an alternative to more invasive surgery. Attempts at rectifying this surgically induced hyperopia, such as the modified taper, warrant further investigation.

Of those patients with induced hyperopia and anisometropia after PTK, a contact lens has been fitted in five cases. Therefore, both the surgeon and the patient must consider the patient's potential for a significant hyperopic shift in refraction and the possibility of wearing a contact lens postopera-

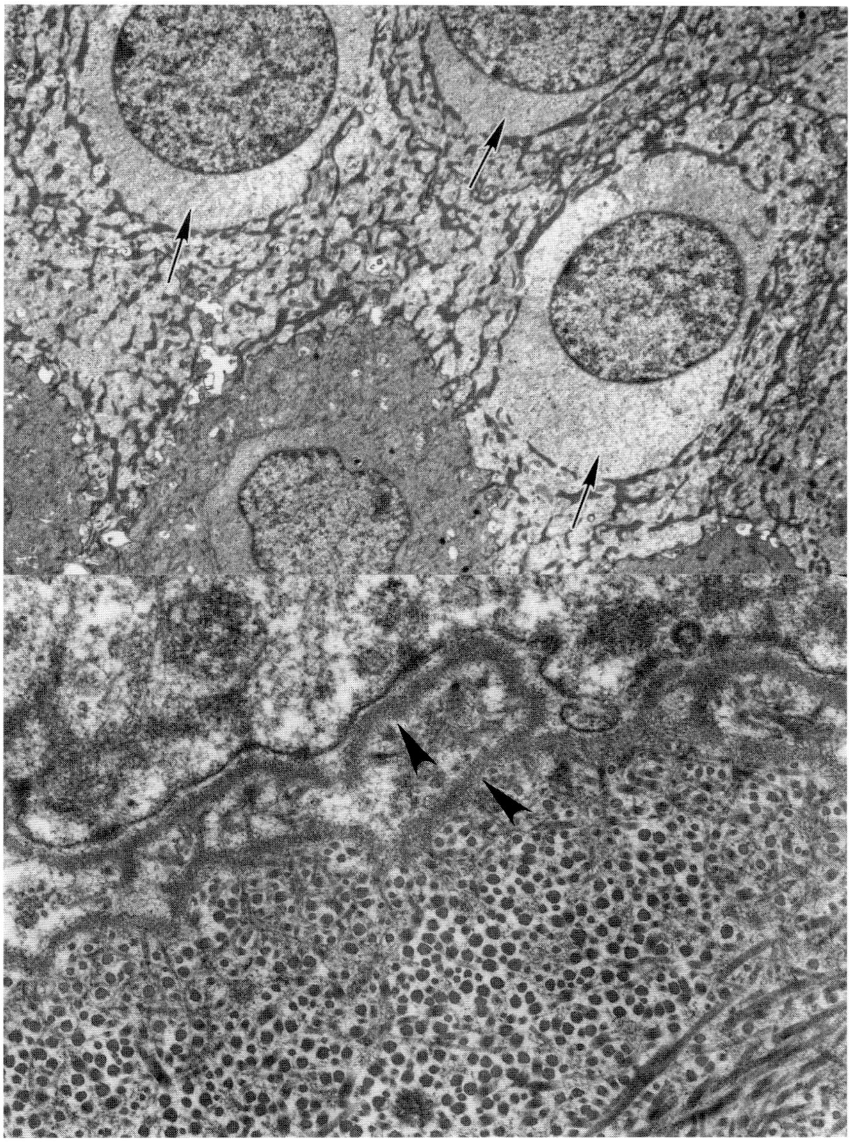

FIGURE 8.5. Top, epithelial cells (arrows) superficial to the basal cells contain granular material around the nucleus 11 months post-PTK. Bottom, epithelial basement membrane duplication (arrowheads) is also noted (original magnification, 44,000×). (From Wu et al: *Arch Ophthalmol* 109:1426–1432, 1991, with permission.)

tively. A patient unwilling to accept this situation should not be considered for the procedure.

A number of patients with recurrent corneal erosions or primary band keratopathy have been referred for PTK. Normally, we recommend alternative treatment in such cases. Patients with recurrent corneal erosion respond well to 5% sodium chloride ointment at night and as needed during the day. Primary band keratopathy should be removed from the cornea by debridement with ethylenediaminetetraacetic acid (EDTA).[45-47] As we gain additional experience with the excimer laser, it may be appropriate to treat specific eyes unresponsive to these more conservative therapies. However, neither of these alternative procedures is associated with corneal flattening or refractive shift, and they should be attempted before considering PTK.

CASE STUDIES

CASE 1. A 31 year-old man with a history of corneal lattice dystrophy in both eyes underwent treatment in the left eye (75 μm stromal depth after epithelial ablation). Reepithelialization occurred within 7 days. The patient's preoperative best-corrected visual acuity (20/200) improved to 20/25 at the 30-month follow-up. Significant hyperopic shift (+10.00 D of spherical equivalent induced hyperopia) was noted in the first 2

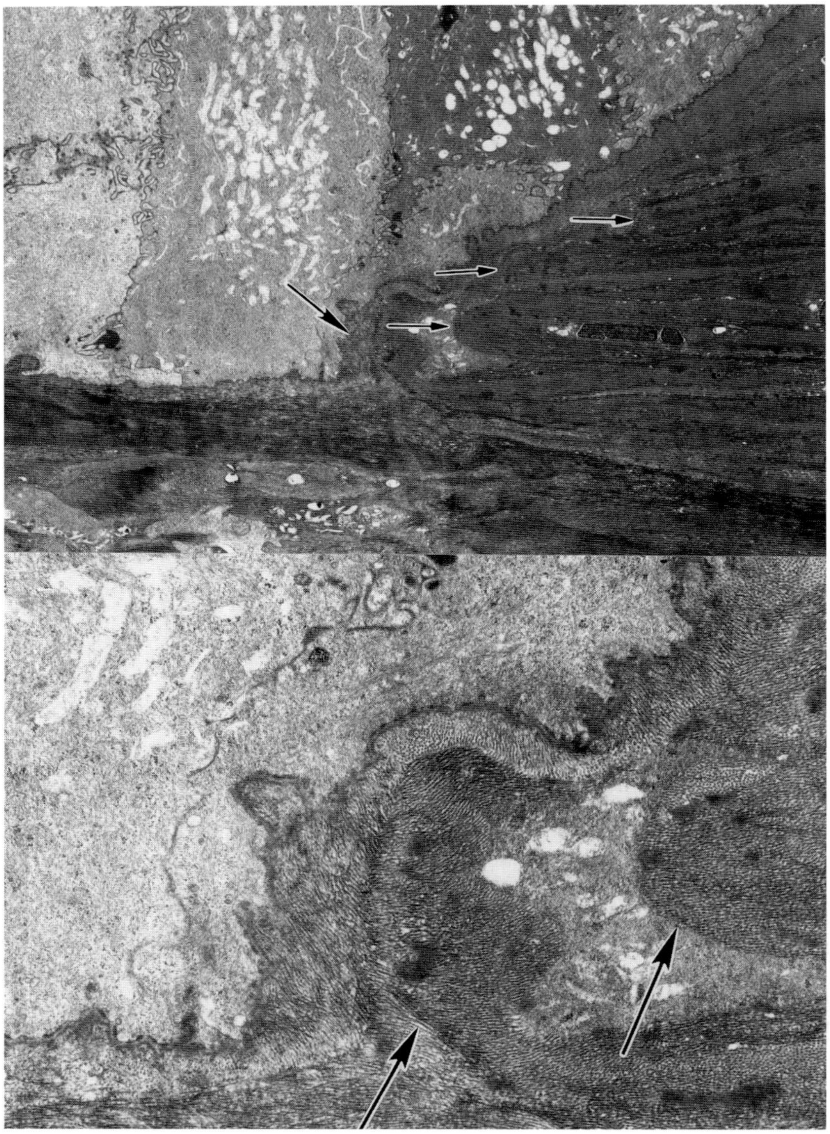

FIGURE 8.6. Fifteen months following PTK, collagen bundles are discontinuous near the margin of laser ablation (top: original magnification, 3100×; bottom: original magnification, 11,000×). (From Wu et al: *Arch Ophthalmol* 109:1426–1432, 1991, with permission.)

months; this decreased to a final net hyperopic effect of +3.00 D (Fig. 8.11).

CASE 2. A 47 year-old man, who had undergone penetrating keratoplasty in the right eye for corneal lattice dystrophy 8 years previously, presented with recurrent superficial dystrophy in the graft. He received a superficial PTK (7.29 μm stromal ablation after mechanical epithelial removal). Reepithelialization occurred in 5 days. The patient's best-corrected preoperative visual acuity (20/25) showed some improvement (20/20) by 1 month and stabilized thereafter. His refraction at the latest visit (12 months) was −1.50 spherical diopters (Fig. 8.12).

CASE 3. A 29 year-old man underwent PTK in the right eye (120 μm stromal ablation) for corneal lattice dystrophy. Reepithelialization occurred in 7 days. He developed a significant corneal haze at 3 months that gradually diminished. At this most recent visit (12-month follow-up) the patient's best-corrected visual acuity had improved from 20/200 to 20/30 with +3.50 D of spherical equivalent induced hyperopia (Fig. 8.13).

CASE 4. A 73 year-old woman with a history of granular dystrophy was treated in both eyes with a 9-month interval between the procedures. The right eye received 100 μm of central stromal ab-

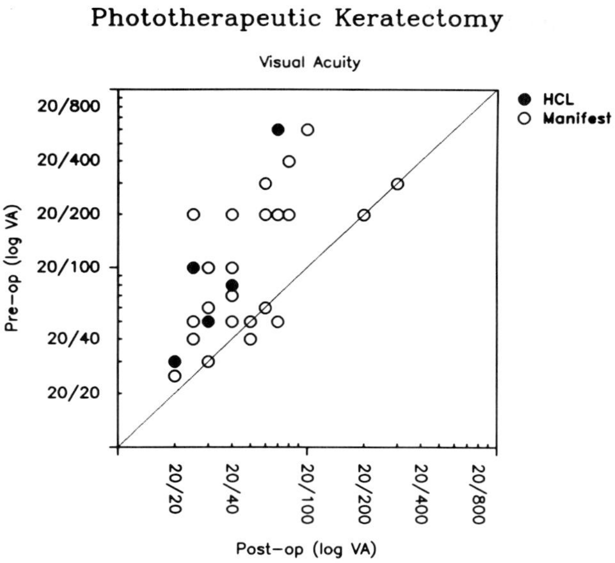

FIGURE 8.7. Comparison between the preoperative and postoperative visual acuity shows marked improvement in the vast majority of the patients. HCL: hard contact lens; log VA: logarithmic visual acuity.

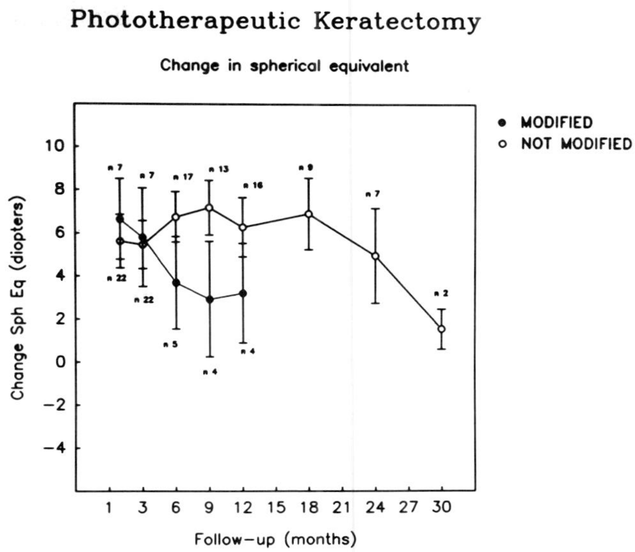

FIGURE 8.9. Relationship between the induced refractive change and time following PTK. In those patients with modified treatment, the refractive change stabilizes at a level of reduced hyperopia (full circles) when compared with the standard treatment (empty circles).

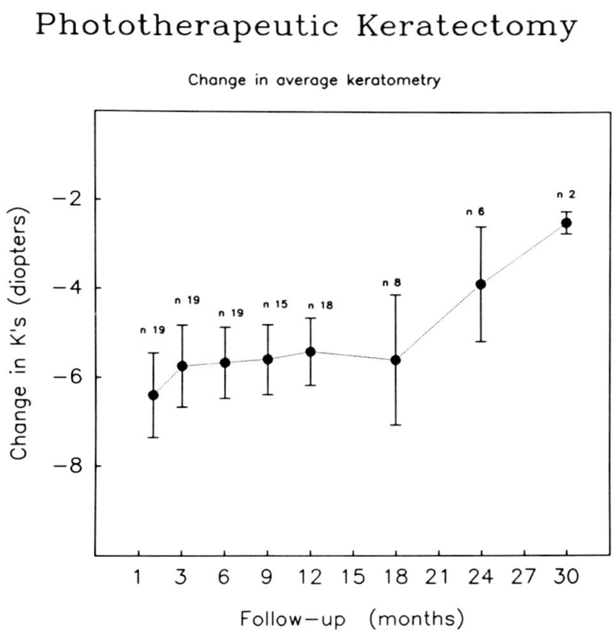

FIGURE 8.8. Temporal relationship of keratometric change following PTK. Note that the hyperopic shift (approximately 6 D) partially reverted after 18 months.

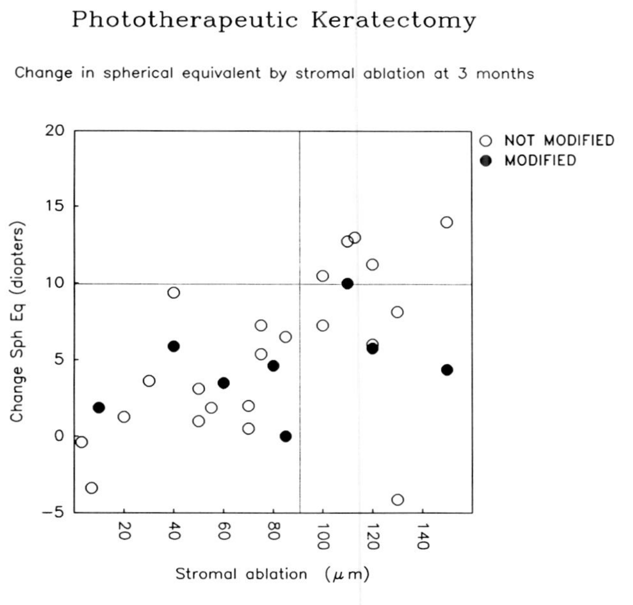

FIGURE 8.10. At 3 months post-PTK, a direct relationship between the induced hyperopia and the depth of ablation is suggested. This is more apparent with the standard (empty circles) compared with the modified (full circles) technique.

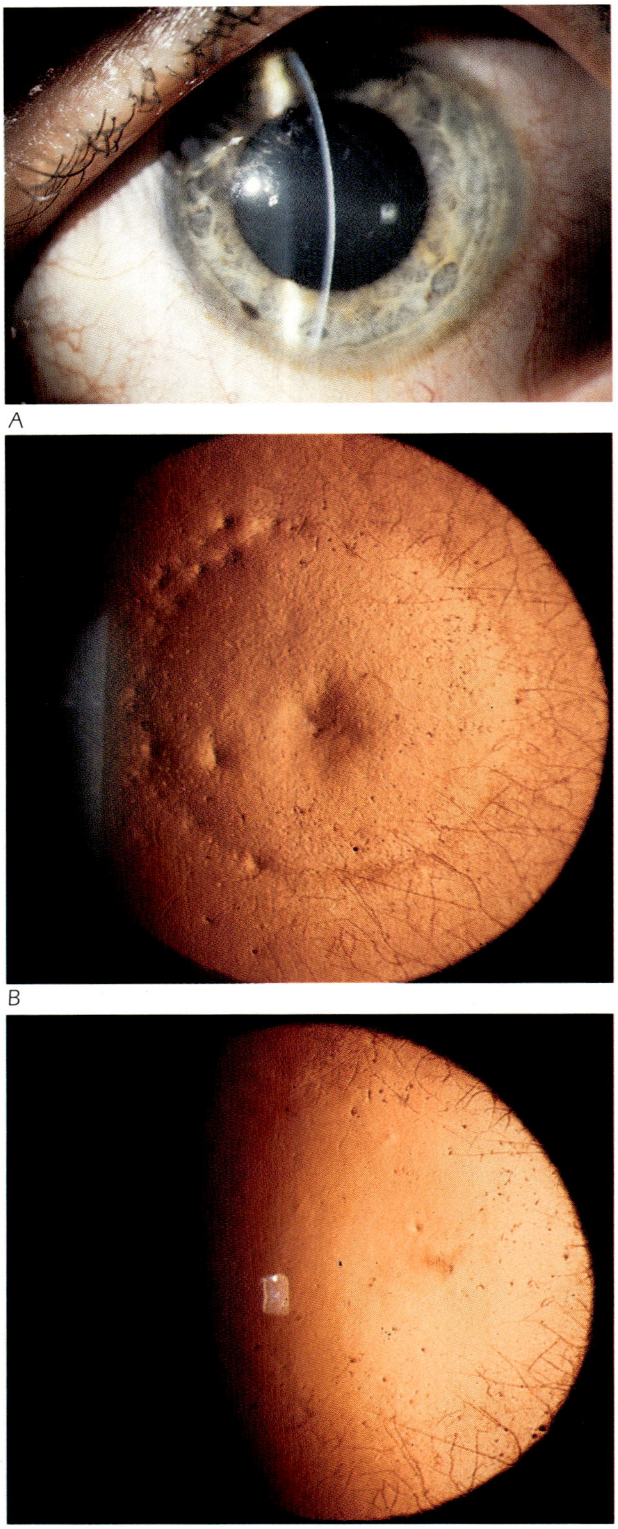

FIGURE 8.11. Case 1. (A) Lattice dystrophy preoperatively. (B) Appearance of cornea 3 months after PTK by retroillumination. (C) Marked improvement 24 months postoperatively.

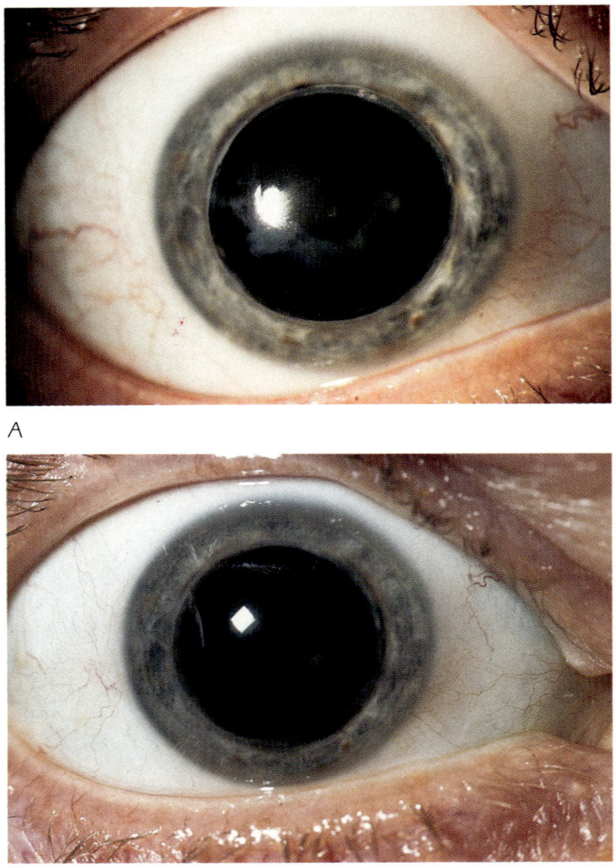

FIGURE 8.12. Case 2. Recurrent lattice dystrophy clinical appearance (A) prior to superficial laser ablation and (B) 3 months postoperatively.

lation and reepithelialized in 4 days (Fig. 8.14). The left eye was treated with 40 μm of stromal ablation combined with a modified tapering procedure, and reepithelialized within 13 days (Fig. 8.15). This patient also developed a hyperopic shift in the right eye (+8.50 D of spherical equivalent induced hyperopia) associated with an improvement in best-corrected spectacle visual acuity from 20/50 (preoperative) to 20/25 (18-month follow-up). The spherical equivalent induced hyperopia in the left eye was +5.00 D at the 9-month follow-up, with an improvement of best-corrected visual acuity from 20/50 to 20/30.

CASE 5. A 44 year-old man with a history of Reis-Buckler's dystrophy in both eyes received treatment in the right eye (85 μm central stromal ablation with modified tapering). Reepithelialization occurred in 3 days. The patient's preoperative best-corrected visual acuity (20/50) improved to 20/25 following PTK with +4.50 D of

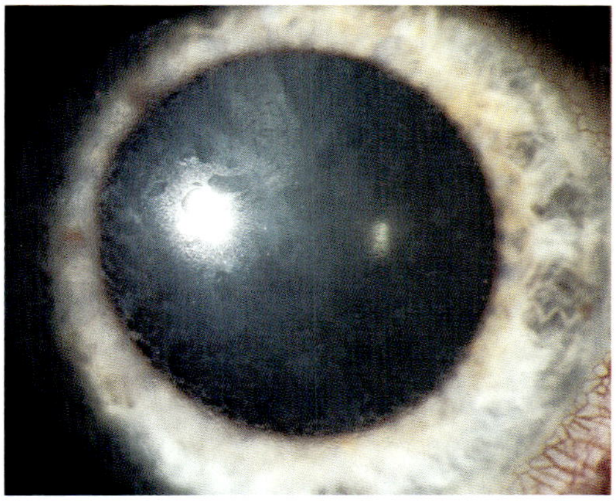

A

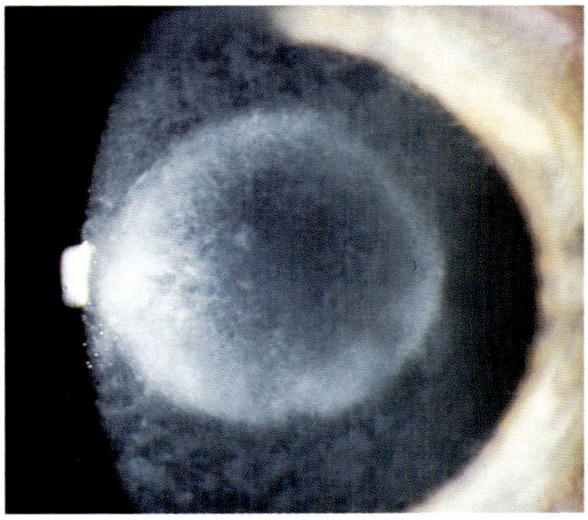

B

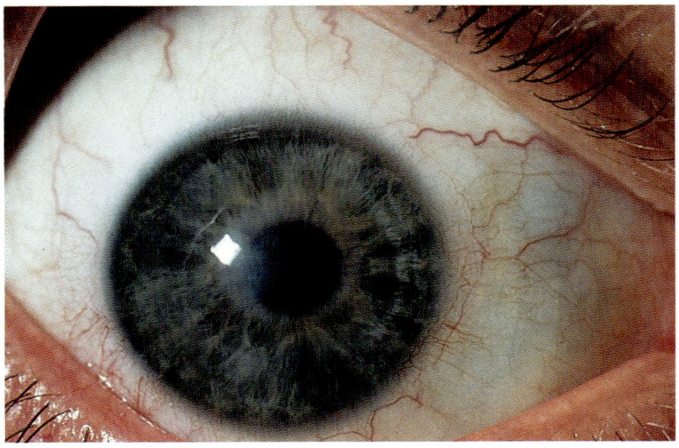

C

FIGURE 8.13. Case 3. Lattice dystrophy. Clinical appearance (A) prior to, (B) 3 months, and (C) 9 months following PTK. Note that the induced haze decreases at 9 months.

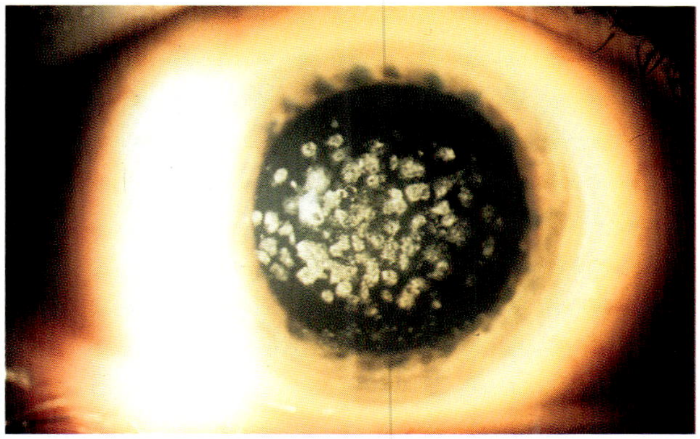

A

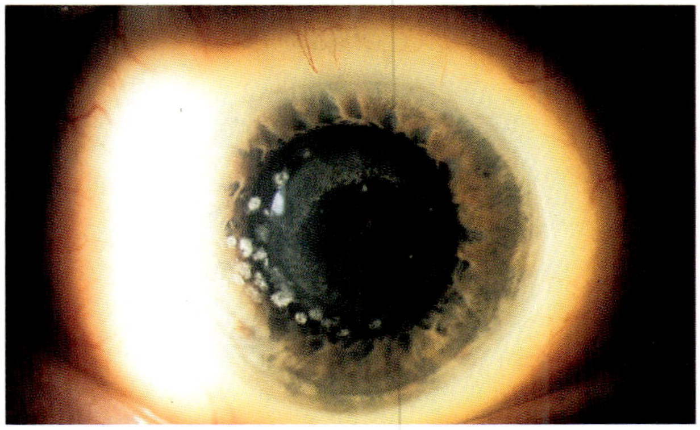

B

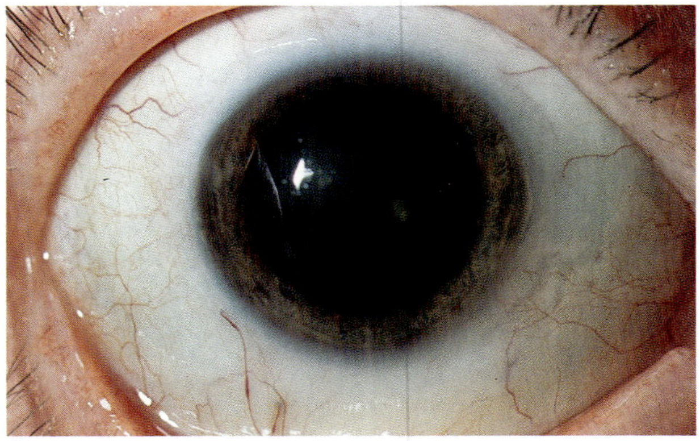

C

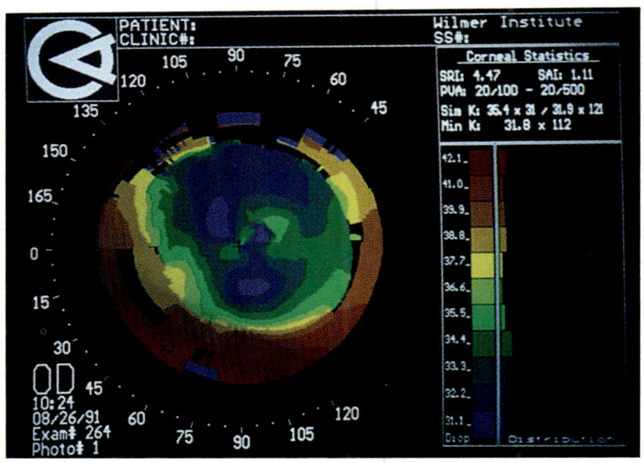

D

FIGURE 8.14. Case 4. Granular dystrophy in the right eye (A) preoperatively, (B) 3 months, and (C) 9 months following standard PTK. (D) The corneal topographic map illustrates the flattening of the central cornea.

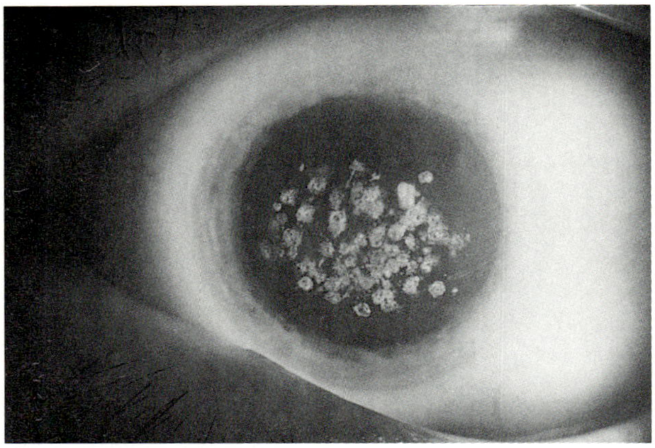

A

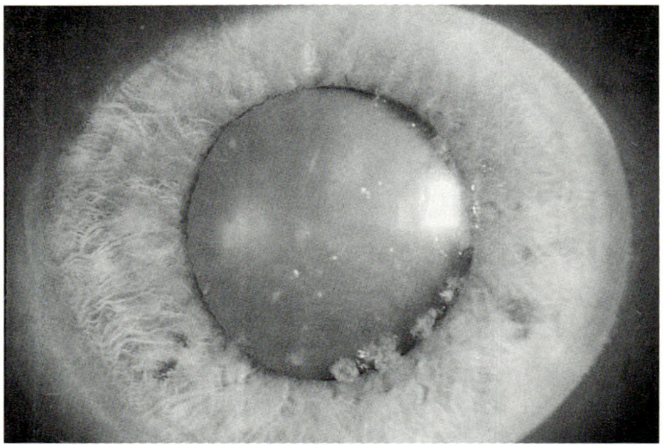

B

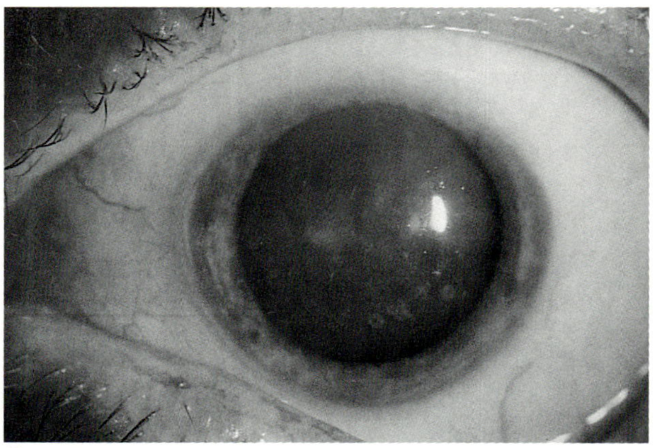

C

FIGURE 8.15. Case 4. Granular dystrophy left eye (A) preoperatively, (B) 6 months, and (C) 9 months follow modified PTK.

spherical equivalent induced hyperopia at the 6-month follow-up. His uncorrected visual acuity improved from 20/400 to 20/50 (Fig. 8.16).

CASE 6. A 61 year-old woman, who had undergone penetrating keratoplasty in the right eye for

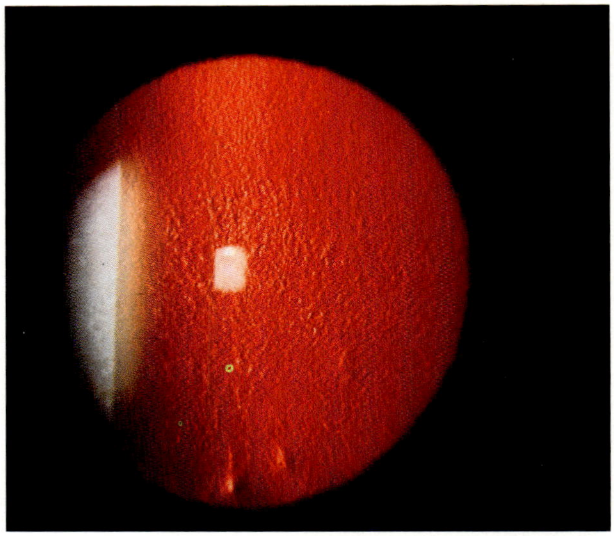

A

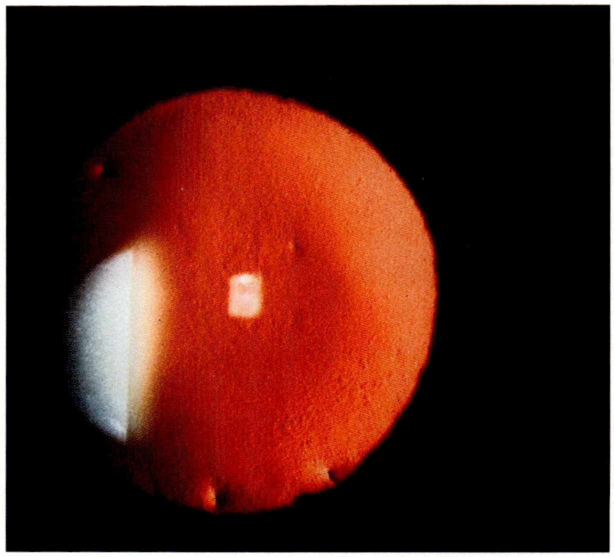

B

FIGURE 8.16. Case 5. Reis-Buckler's dystrophy (A) before and (B) 3 months following PTK. Retroillumination demonstrates a beneficial effect of the treatment.

lattice dystrophy 8 years previously, was treated with superficial PTK (10 μm of stromal ablation with modified taper). Reepithelialization occurred in 5 days. At the 6-month follow-up her best-corrected visual acuity had improved from 20/50 to 20/25, and her uncorrected visual acuity remained at 20/60 (Fig. 8.17).

CASE 7. A 47 year-old man with a history of granular dystrophy in both eyes was treated in the right eye (100 μm central stromal ablation). Reepithelialization occurred in 4 days. The pa-

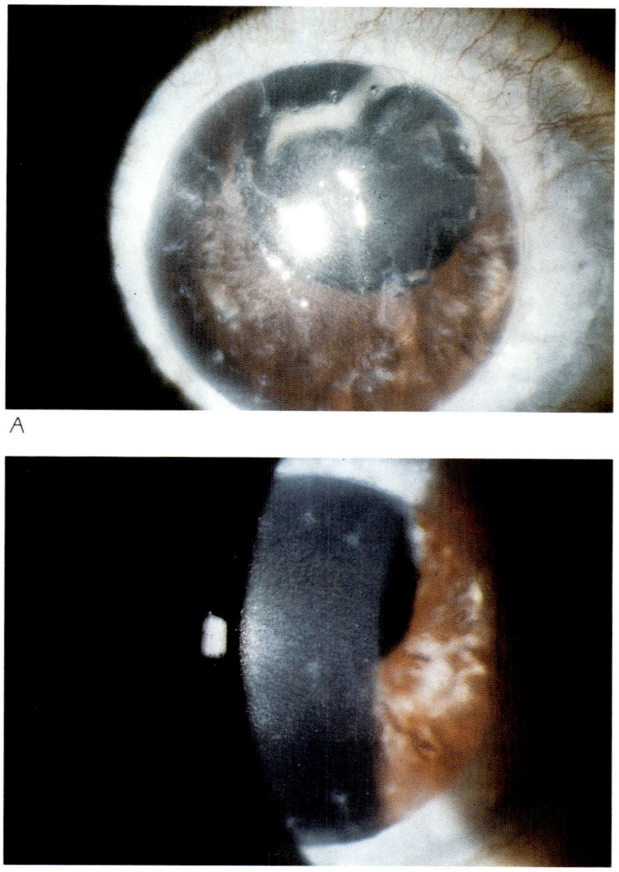

FIGURE 8.17. Case 6. (A) Recurrent lattice dystrophy in a graft prior to superficial excimer PTK (B) shows marked improvement 3 months postoperatively.

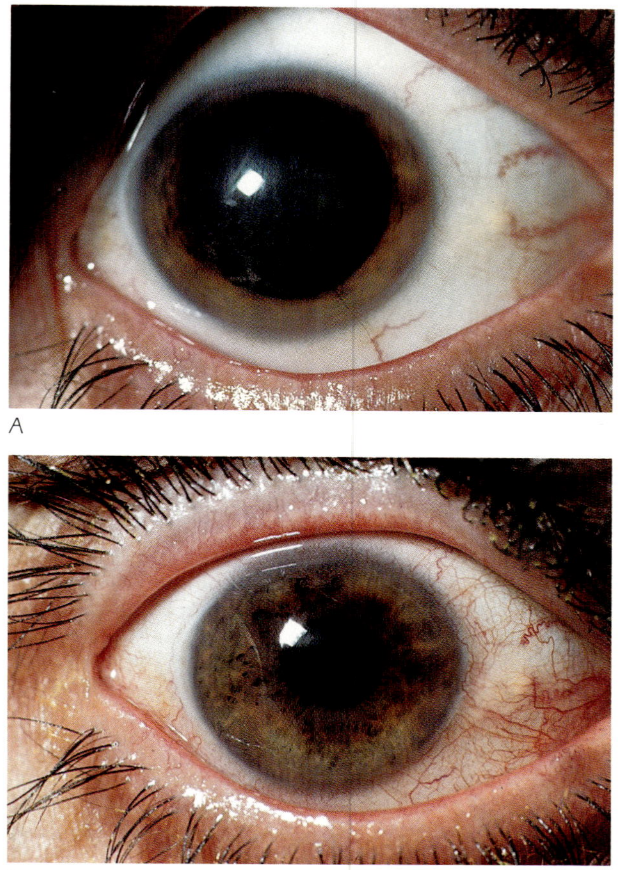

FIGURE 8.18. Case 7. Clinical appearance of granular dystrophy (A) before and (B) 4 months following 100 μm central PTK.

tient was wearing a hard contact lens at his most recent visit (18-month follow-up). Best-corrected visual acuity improved from 20/30 to 20/20 postoperatively, and he had a significant reduction in glare disability, permitting him to maintain his occupation as a driver. A net spherical equivalent hyperopic effect of +6.75 D was induced (Fig. 8.18).

ANTICIPATED CHANGES IN THE PROCEDURE

Centration is a problem with laser treatment. Because photoablation creates a new surface on the cornea, it is important that all light rays focusing at the retina pass through the treated corneal area. Two improvements are possible: enlarging the treatment zone and improving the alignment devices. Currently, the maximum treatment zone diameter with the VISX 20/20 excimer laser is 6.0 mm, which still imposes the need for care in centration procedures. The use of computerized corneal topographic analysis in the laser microscope, as well as a coaxial fixation light in the monocular eyepiece during the treatment, would also be helpful in achieving centration.

It is impossible to determine the amount of tissue ablated per pulse for each individual patient. We currently use a piece of flat polymethyl methacrylate as a standard to test the depth of ablation per pulse. Measurement of the refractive change is performed using a lensometer. This is an indirect measure of the thickness of ablation per pulse. Additionally, the use of a flat surface as a standard for refractive measurements is not the most appropriate model for the cornea.[48]

The 193 nm argon fluoride excimer laser ablates a constant amount of tissue per pulse when a fixed repetition rate and a fluence of 160 mJ/cm^2 are used. This stability depends on a surface that is free of debris and with constant water content. Better control of these parameters would further improve the reproducibility of the treatment results.

REFERENCES

1. Paton RT: *Keratoplasty*. New York, McGraw-Hill, 1955.
2. Castroviejo R: *Atlas of Keratectomy and Keratoplasty*. Philadelphia, WB Saunders, 1966.
3. Zirm E: Eine erfolgreiche totale Keraroplastik. *Graefes Arch Clin Exp Ophthalmol* 64:580–593, 1906.
4. Olson RJ. Corneal transplantation techniques. In Kaufman HE, McDonald MB, Barron BA, Waltman SR (eds): *The Cornea*. New York, Churchill Livingstone, 1988, pp 743–785.
5. Magitot A: Recherches expérimentales sur la survie possiblie de la cornée conservée en dehours de l'organisme et sur la kératoplastie différée. *Ann d'Ocul* 146:1–34, 1911.
6. Taboada J, Archibald CJ: An extreme sensitivity in the corneal epithelium to far UV ArF excimer laser pulses. In *Proceedings of the 52nd Annual Meeting of Aerospace Medical Association*. Washington DC, Aerospace Medical Association, 1981, pp 98–99.
7. Trokel SL, Srinivasan R, Braren B: Excimer laser surgery of the cornea. *Am J Ophthalmol* 96:710–715, 1983.
8. Munnerlyn CR, Koons SJ, Marshall J: Photorefractive keratectomy: A technique for laser refractive surgery. *J Cataract Refract Surg* 44:46–52, 1988.
9. McDonald MB, Beuerman R, Falzoni W, et al: Refractive surgery with the excimer laser (letter). *Am J Ophthalmol* 103:469–470, 1987.
10. Berns MW, Liaw L-H, Oliva A, et al: An acute light and electron microscopic study of ultraviolet 193 nm excimer laser corneal incisions. *Ophthalmology* 95:1422–1433, 1988.
11. Marshall J, Trokel SL, Rothery S, et al: Long term healing of the central cornea after photorefractive keratectomy using an excimer laser. *Ophthalmology* 95:1411–1421, 1988.
12. Fantes FE, Hanna KD, Warring Go III, et al: Wound healing after excimer laser keratomileusis (photorefractive keratectomy) in monkeys. *Arch Ophthalmol* 108:665–675, 1990.
13. Malley DS, Steinert RF, Puliafito CA, et al: Immunofluorescence study of cornea wound healing after excimer laser anterior keratectomy in the monkey eye. *Arch Ophthalmol* 108:1316–1322, 1990.
14. Hanna KD, Poulliquen YM, Savoldelli M, et al: Corneal wound healing in monkeys 18 months after excimer laser photorefractive keratectomy. *Refract Corneal Surg* 6:340–345, 1990.
15. Seiler T, Wollensak J: In vivo experiments with excimer laser: Technical parameters and healing processes. *Ophthalmologica* 192:65–70, 1986.
16. Thompson KP, Trentacoste J, Parrish RK, et al: Corneal photoablation by far ultraviolet lasers (letter). *Am J Ophthalmol* 105:312–313, 1987.
17. Hanna KD, Chastang JC, Pouliquen YM, et al: Excimer laser keratectomy for myopia with a rotating-slit delivery system. *Arch Ophthalmol* 106:245–250, 1988.
18. Seiler T, Bende T, Winckler K, et al: Side effects in excimer corneal surgery: DNA damage as a result of 193 nm excimer laser radiation. *Graefes Arch Clin Exp Ophthalmol* 226:273–276, 1988.
19. Bende T, Seiler T, Wollensak J: Side effects in excimer corneal surgery: Corneal thermal gradients. *Graefes Arch Clin Exp Ophthalmol* 226:277–280, 1988.
20. Gebhardt BM, Salmeron B, McDonald MB: Effect of excimer laser energy on the growth potential of corneal keratocytes. *Cornea* 9:205–210, 1990.
21. Aron-Rosa DS, Boerner CF, Bath P, et al: Corneal wound healing after excimer laser keratectomy in a human eye. *Am J Ophthalmol* 103:454–464, 1987.
22. L'Esperance FA, Taylor DM, Warner JW: Human excimer laser keratectomy: Short term histopathology. *J Refract Surg* 4:118–124, 1988.
23. Taylor DM, L'Esperance FA, Del-Pero RA, et al: Human excimer laser lamellar keratectomy: A clinical study. *Ophthalmology* 96:654–664, 1989.
24. Goodman GL, Trokel SL, Stark WJ, et al: Corneal healing following laser refractive keratectomy. *Arch Ophthalmol* 107:1799–1803, 1989.
25. Tuft SJ, Zabel RW, Marshall J: Corneal repair following keratectomy: A comparison between conventional surgery and laser photoablation. *Invest Ophthalmol Vis Sci* 30:1796–1777, 1989.
26. Seiler T, Kriegerowski M, Schnoy N, et al: Ablation rate of human corneal epithelium and Bowman's layer with the excimer laser (193 nm). *Refract Corneal Surg* 6:99–102, 1990.
27. L'Esperance FA, Warner JW, Telfair WB, et al: Excimer laser instrumentation and technique for human corneal surgery. *Arch Ophthalmol* 107:131–139, 1989.
28. McDonald MB, Frantz JM, Klyce SD, et al: Central photorefractive keratectomy for myopia: The blind eye study. *Arch Ophthalmol* 108:799–808, 1990.
29. Seiler T, Kahle G, Kriegorowski M: Excimer laser (193 nm) myopic keratomileusis in sighted and blind human eyes. *Refract Corneal Surg* 6:165–173, 1990.
30. Liu JC, McDonald MB, Varnell R, et al: Myopic excimer laser photorefractive keratectomy: An analysis of clinical correlations. *Refract Corneal Surg* 6:321–328, 1990.
31. Zabel RW, Sher NA, Ostrov CS, et al: Myopic excimer laser keratectomy: A preliminary report. *Refract Corneal Surg* 6:329–334, 1990.
32. Seiler T, Wollensak J: Myopic photorefractive keratectomy with the excimer laser: One year follow-up. *Ophthalmology* 98:1156–1163, 1991.
33. Wu WCS, Stark WJ, Green WR: Corneal wound healing after 193 nm excimer laser keratectomy. *Arch Ophthalmol* 109:1426–1432, 1991.
34. Fountain TR, Azar DT, de la Cruz J, Green WR, Stark WJ: Reassembly of corneal epithelial adhesion

structures following human excimer laser keratectomy. *Invest Ophthalmol Vis Sci,* 33:1106(suppl), 1992.

35. Sher NA, Bowers RA, Zabel RW, et al: Clinical use of the 193 nm excimer laser in the treatment of corneal scars. *Arch Ophthalmol* 109:491–498, 1991.
36. Stark WJ, Chamon W, Kamp MT, et al: Clinical follow-up of 193nm ArF excimer laser photokeratectomy. *Ophthalmology,* 99:805–812, 1992.
37. Warring GO III: Classification and terminology of laser corneal surgery: Making sense of keratospeak III. *Refract Corneal Surg* 6:318–320, 1990.
38. Stark WJ, Gilbert ML, Gottsch JD, et al: Optical pachometry in the measurement of anterior corneal disease: An evaluative tool for phototherapeutic keratectomy (letter). *Arch Ophthalmol* 108:12–13, 1990.
39. Uozato H, Guyton DL: Centering corneal surgical procedures. *Am J Ophthalmol* 103:264–275, 1987.
40. Kornmehl EW, Steinert RF, Puliafito CA: A comparative study of masking fluids for excimer laser phototherapeutic keratectomy. *Arch Ophthalmol* 109:860–863, 1991.
41. Steinert RF, Puliafito CA: Lasers in corneal surgery. *Ophthalmol Clin North Am* 2:611–623, 1989.
42. Herman SJ, Hughes WF: Recurrence of hereditary corneal dystrophy following keratoplasty. *Am J Ophthalmol* 75:689–694, 1973.
43. Meisler DM, Fine M: Recurrence of the clinical signs of lattice corneal dystrophy (type I) in corneal transplants. *Am J Ophthalmol* 97:210–214, 1984.
44. Klintworth GK, Ferry AP, Sugar A, et al: Recurrence of lattice dystrophy type 1 in the corneal grafts of two siblings. *Am J Ophthalmol* 94:540–546, 1982.
45. Breinin GM, DeVoe AG: Chelation of calcium with edathamil calcium-disodium in band keratopathy and corneal calcium affections. *Arch Ophthalmol* 52:846–851, 1954.
46. Wood TO, Walker GG: Treatment of band keratopathy. *Am J Ophthalmol* 80:553, 1975.
47. Bokosky JE, Meyer RF, Sugar A: Surgical treatment of calcific band keratopathy. *Ophthalmic Surg* 16:645–647, 1985.
48. Chamon W, Azar DT, Rencs E, et al: A new model to test excimer laser ablations on spherical surfaces. *Invest Ophthalmol Vis Sci,* 33:765(suppl), 1992.

CHAPTER 9

Therapeutic Keratectomy: Corneal Smoothing

ROGER F. STEINERT

The argon fluoride excimer laser, emitting ultrashort pulses at 193 nm, precisely etches the cornea with only submicrometer damage to the adjacent nonablated stroma. The freshly ablated surface supports rapid and stable reepithelialization in advance of reformation of normal basal lamina complexes. Although the dominant interest in this laser has been for refractive applications, corneal surgeons have rapidly recognized the potential for treating corneal pathologic lesions.

The types of pathologic lesions under investigation for treatment with the excimer laser can be categorized into the following classification: (1) smoothing of an irregular surface, (2) removal of superficial opacities, (3) treatment of recurrent erosions due to epithelial basement membrane abnormalities, and (4) eradication of infectious keratitis. Each of these applications is under active investigation in the United States under the auspices of FDA investigational device exemptions, and many innovative applications have been pursued internationally. This chapter will illustrate applications in each of these categories of phototherapeutic keratectomy (PTK).

IRREGULAR SURFACE

The excimer laser can reduce, and in some cases eliminate, fine surface irregularities that often severely disrupt the optical performance of the anterior cornea. These fine irregularities must be distinguished from broad surface variations resulting in regular and irregular astigmatism. Techniques to deal with broadly varying surface contour are only in the conceptual stage at the current time.

Fine irregularities are not intrinsically removed by exposure to repeated pulses of the broad excimer beam. As shown in Figure 9.1, photons encountering the irregular surface will not discriminate between elevations and depressions. Tissue removed will largely replicate the original irregularity. Strategies must be devised, therefore, to protect deeper tissues (''valleys''), while exposing elevated pathologic iesions (''peaks'') to the ablating photons. Several factors complicate this problem. Some types of pathologic lesions ablate more readily than the surrounding tissue. This is generally observed with calcium, for example. On the other hand, clinical observations indicate that other types of opacity, such as the hyaline material in granular dystrophy, may ablate more slowly.

Epithelial hypertrophy commonly occurs in ar-

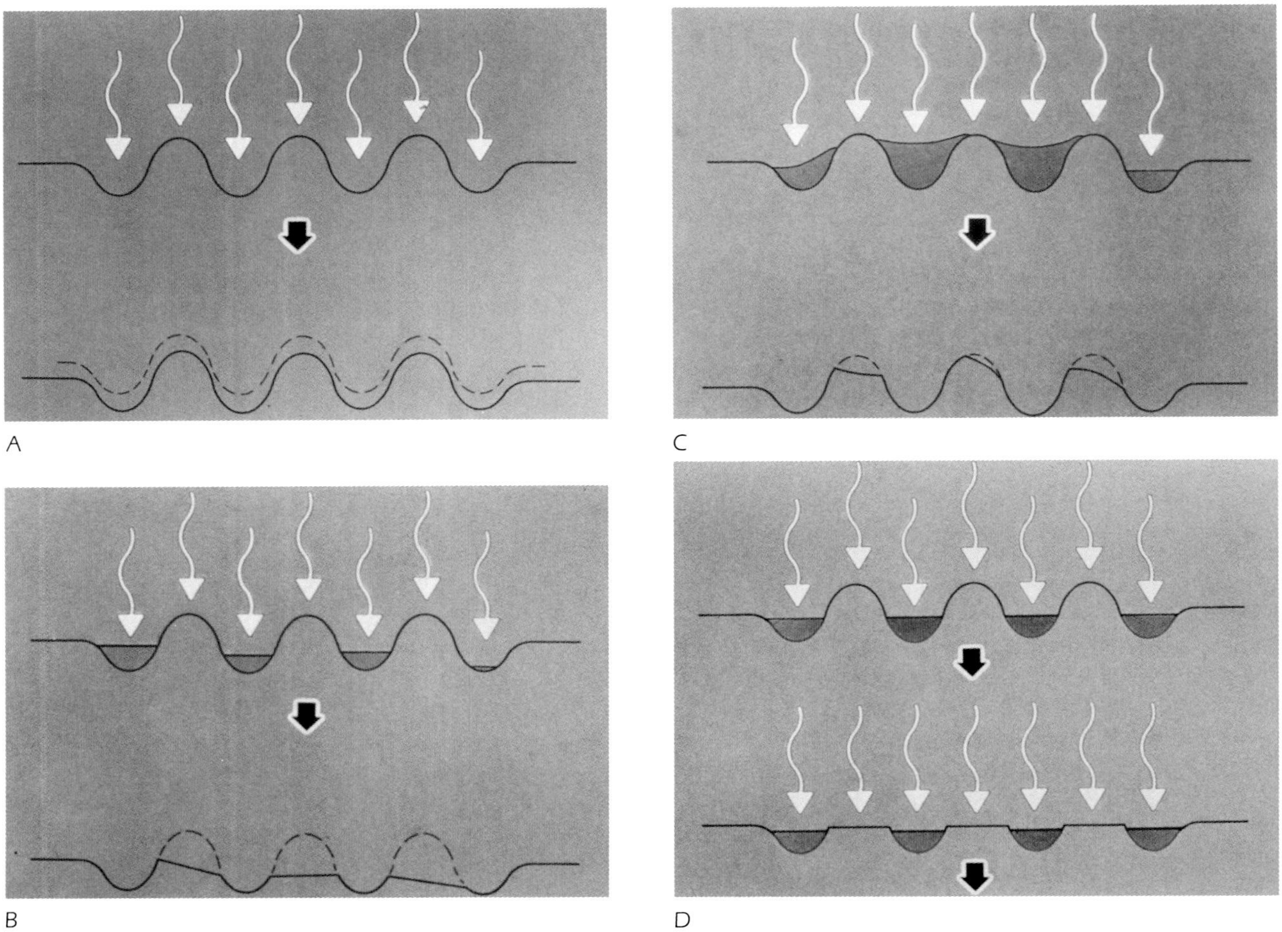

FIGURE 9.1. (A) Ablation by excimer laser photons will simply replicate any irregularity in the surface. (B) A low-viscosity fluid will protect some of the lower valleys but run off unevenly, resulting in irregularity of the surface. (C) A high-viscosity fluid will be retained and protect some of the peaks as well as the valleys, also resulting in irregularity. (D) An ideally viscous fluid will be retained evenly in the valleys while exposing the peaks. Through repeated applications of the fluid during the ablation, a smooth surface will ultimately be achieved.

eas of corneal depression. Leaving the epithelium to protect valleys, while exposing peaks through selective deepithelialization with a blade, can take advantage of the masking effect of epithelium. As an example, one strategy for removing the irregularities of Reis-Buckler's dystrophy involves ablating through the epithelium that is intermixed with the abnormal substance until epithelium is largely absent, as judged by the disappearance of the spontaneous fluorescence that occurs during epithelial ablation.

Bulk removal of a large irregularity such as a Salzmann nodule or elevated scar is most effectively performed first with a blade, reserving the excimer for improving the regularity of the surface after the blade excision.

Beyond taking advantage of the epithelium, masking fluids are often critical in protecting the valleys while continuing to allow ablation of elevated peaks. At the current time the most common masking fluids are artificial tear substances. These are readily available in various viscosities. In a study in our laboratory, Kornmehl et al.[1] compared several different artificial tear substances of differing viscosity to saline and a nonfluid control in an experimental model of surface irregularity. In this model, where the corneal surface was initially roughened with sandpaper, solutions of moderate viscosity yielded a smoother surface than more viscous artificial tears or the nonviscous saline solution. All these fluids outperformed a nonfluid control. Figure 9.2 shows the scanning electron micrographic changes demonstrated in this study, with the smoothest result obtained by the interme-

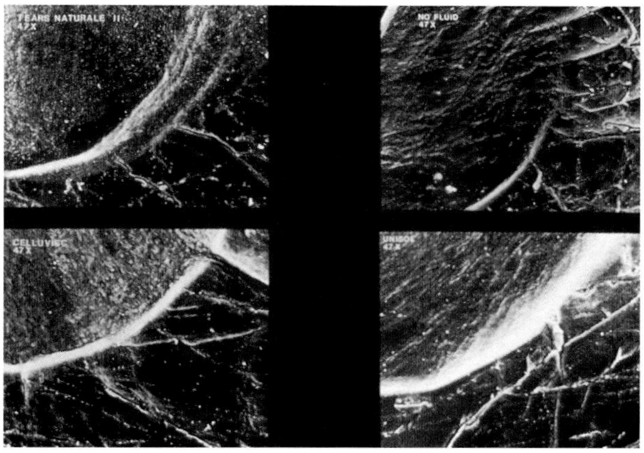

A

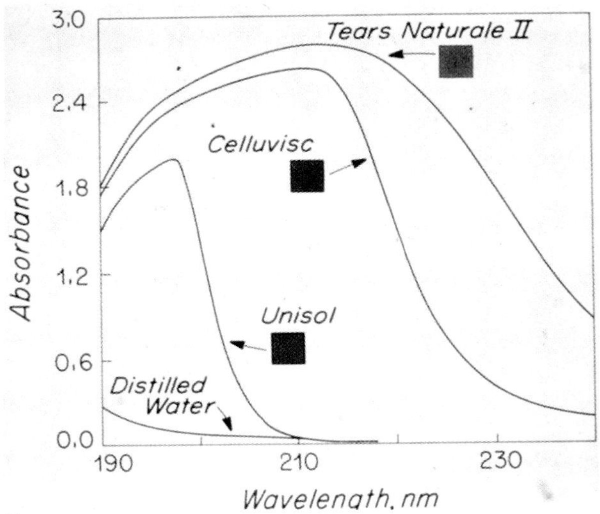

B

FIGURE 9.2. (A) Scanning electron micrographs comparing the smoothing achieved by different fluids. The smoothest surface was obtained with the intermediate-viscosity Tears Naturale II® (upper left). The high-viscosity Celluvisc solution was almost as good as Tears Naturale II® (lower left). The worst result was obtained in the control application of no fluid (upper right). The low-viscosity normal saline solution (Unisol®) was distinctly less smooth than the artificial tear solutions (lower right). (B) At 193 nm the absorption of artificial tears or saline solutions is higher than that of distilled water.

diate-viscosity substance. Figure 9.1 demonstrates the theoretical concept that a fluid with inadequate viscosity will tend to run off, inadequately protecting the valleys, while a too-viscous substance will drape over the peaks, giving some undesirable protection to the elevations where ablation is desired.

In addition to the viscosity effect, different solutions may have differing effectiveness in absorption of 193 nm photons down to a level adequate to prevent ablation of the underlying tissue by a thin film of the fluid. Enhancing absorption at 193 nm may be one step toward identifying a more effective masking fluid for phototherapeutic keratectomy of an irregular surface. Even better, one can hypothesize a substance such as a gel that would be uniformly applied over the cornea and molded into a new smooth anterior surface. This gel would then be ablated and, as ablation progressed, would first expose the peaks while protecting the valleys without the need for repeated artful application of viscous fluids. For this gel to be fully effective, the ablation rate of the gel would have to match that of the pathologic tissue. Such a gel has yet to be identified.

Figure 9.3 shows the ablation of an apical nodule from a patient with keratoconus.[2] The nodule was optically insignificant but caused reduction in contact lens tolerance from 8 to 2 hours daily. The nodule had been surgically excised once and rapidly recurred. After the excimer laser ablation down to a level slightly below the adjacent Bowman's layer, the nodule has not recurred in 2 years of follow-up. Figure 9.4 illustrates a patient with improved although still imperfect anterior corneal contour following excimer laser ablation of scarring that occurred postoperatively following surgical excision of a pterygium through the visual axis. Other suitable candidates are patients with Salzmann's nodular degeneration in the visual axis. Excision of the nodules with a blade followed by excimer PTK smoothing yields an intermediate improvement in acuity, but some degree of irregularity frequently persists. Sher and coworkers[3] reported some improvement in visual acuity in 80% of patients with Salzmann's nodular degeneration.

SUPERFICIAL CORNEAL OPACITIES

Considerable overlap exists between the categories of surface irregularity and superficial corneal opacities. Whether the superficial opacity is due to trauma, prior keratitis, or anterior dystrophy, visual impairment is often due to a combination of the opacity itself and accompanying irregularity. A hard contact lens refraction is the best way to evaluate the relative contribution of each of these components to the visual loss.

Common examples of superficial opacities include Reis-Buckler's dystrophy, early relatively anterior granular and lattice stromal dystrophies, scars after herpetic keratitis, and degenerations including nodule formation and band keratopathy.

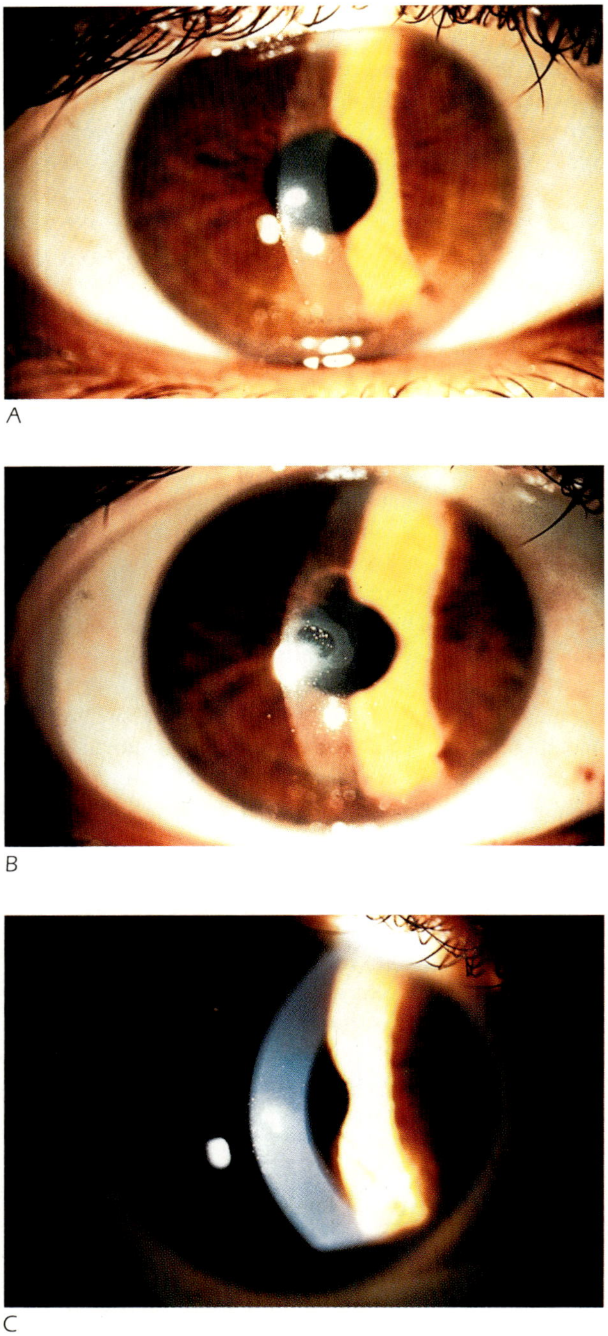

FIGURE 9.3. (A) A patient with keratoconus and an apical nodule leading to decreased contact lens tolerance. (B) Immediately after excimer ablation the opacity has been reduced. This is partially obscured by the adjacent light reflex. Partial ablation of the adjacent epithelium can be seen as a gray ring. (C) One year postoperatively the opacity partially remains as a subepithelial haze, but the surface is smooth and contact lens tolerance improved.

In the evaluation of a potential candidate for PTK, it is critical to assess the depth of the opacity. In some conditions, such as Reis-Buckler's dystrophy, the location of the pathologic lesion is known to be limited to the anterior stroma. In lattice or granular dystrophy, the surgeon must carefully examine the optically significant opacities in the visual zone and assess their depth. Postinflammatory scarring is more difficult to assess, because the posterior extent of the opacity is typically ill-defined and often deeper than initially appreciated at slit lamp examination. On the other hand, partial removal of the opacity may be adequate for the patient's visual needs. The use of an optical pachymeter (Haag-Streit, Bern, Switzerland) can be a useful adjunct in measuring the depth of the opacity, although the opacity itself may preclude accurate use of this device.[4]

Depending upon the excimer laser employed and the surgeon's preference, the ablations are performed as a planar disc or with a combination of a myopic followed by a hyperopic ablation. These approaches are intended to reduce the inevitable induced hyperopic shift.[3,5] Although the initial ablation may be planar and retain the original anterior corneal curvature, postlaser remodeling with new collagen formation and epithelial hyperplasia at the periphery of the treatment zone results in net flattening and a hyperopic shift. In assessing the suitability of a candidate for PTK, therefore, it is important to evaluate the patient's optical status. Unless the patient is moderately myopic preoperatively and either has bilateral disease or readily accepts contact lens correction in the fellow eye, the potential for unacceptable anisometropia is high. In most cases we carefully review with the patient the potential for postoperative hyperopia and the need for postoperative contact lens use in order to rehabilitate the eye after the opacity and/or irregularity has been eliminated. Postoperative use of a hard contact lens will often be of additional benefit to the patient by optically eliminating residual irregular and regular astigmatism.

In addition to the hyperopic shift, deeper ablation, particularly exceeding 50 μm, is usually accompanied by haze that can become visually significant at its extreme. It is unclear whether intensive postlaser steroid treatment will significantly retard scarring, or to what extent intensive steroid treatment will lead to a more pronounced permanent hyperopic shift by retarding wound healing.

Figures 9.5 to 9.8 illustrate patients who underwent PTK for an anterior herpetic scar, granular

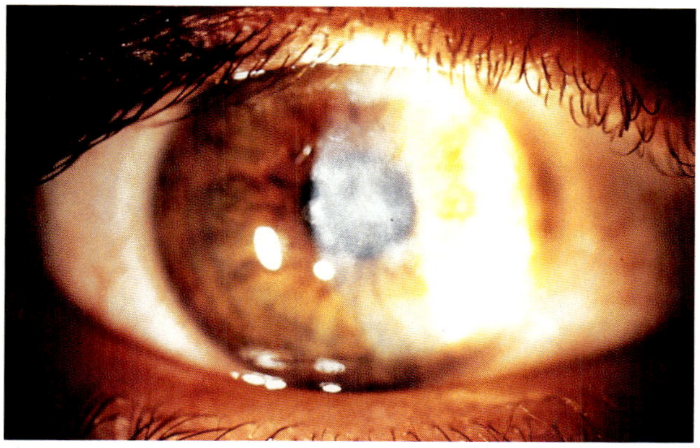

A

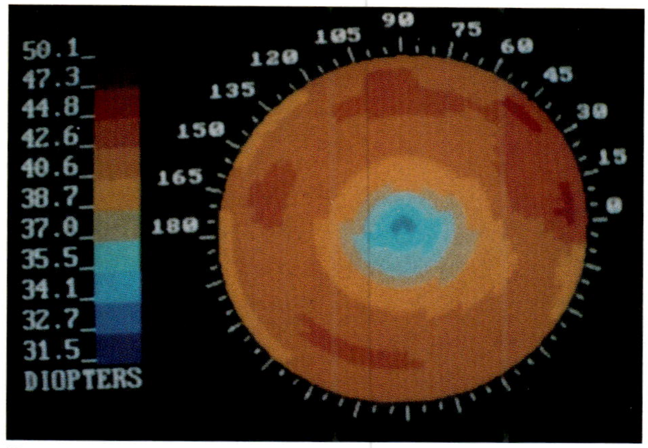

D

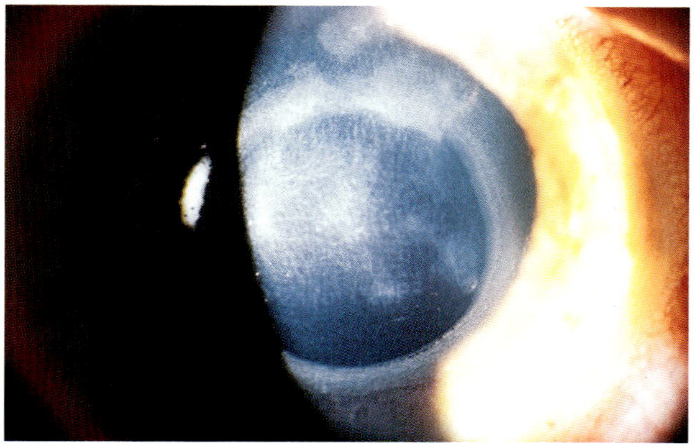

B

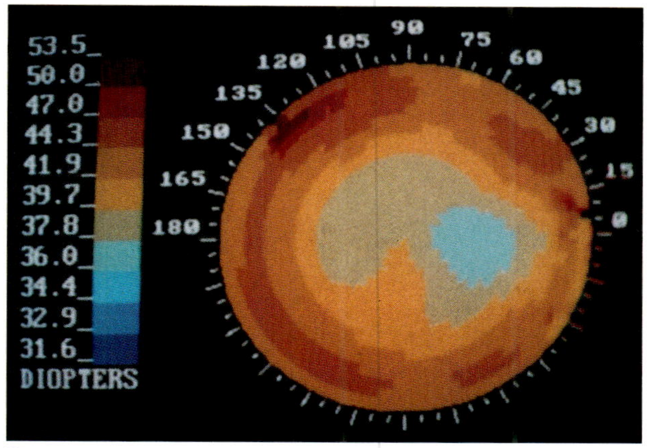

E

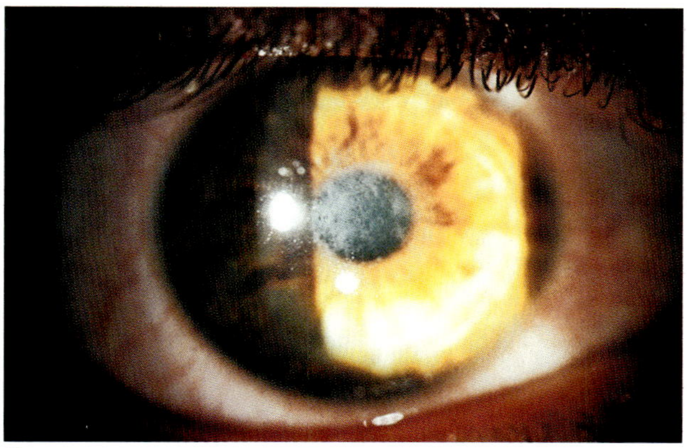

C

FIGURE 9.4. (A) After excision of a pterygium that extended through the pupillary zone, there is moderate residual scar formation partway through the pupil and irregular optics throughout the pupillary zone. One week after excimer ablation, marked improvement in the central opacity can be appreciated. (B) Four months postoperatively, a partial return of the haze can be seen in the superior pupil. (C) One year postoperatively, essentially complete return of the corneal scar has occurred. The adjacent clear cornea is smoother than preoperatively, however, resulting in persistent improved visual acuity. (D) Preoperative photokeratoscopy demonstrates the irregular corneal optics extending beyond the area of the opacity itself. (E) Marked improvement in the quality of the mires has occurred postoperatively, although irregular astigmatism persists.

dystrophy, the Avellino variant of lattice dystrophy, and Reis-Buckler's dystrophy.

RECURRENT CORNEAL EROSIONS

Painful recurrent erosion syndrome, whether due to trauma or anterior membrane dystrophy (Cogan's dystrophy or map-dot-fingerprint dystrophy), is due to abnormalities in the epithelial basement membrane complex. The vast majority of these cases will respond to topical lubrication therapy, bandage soft contact lenses, debridement of the epithelium and basement membrane, or anterior stromal micropuncture. An occasional patient will continue to suffer painful recurrent erosions despite all of these

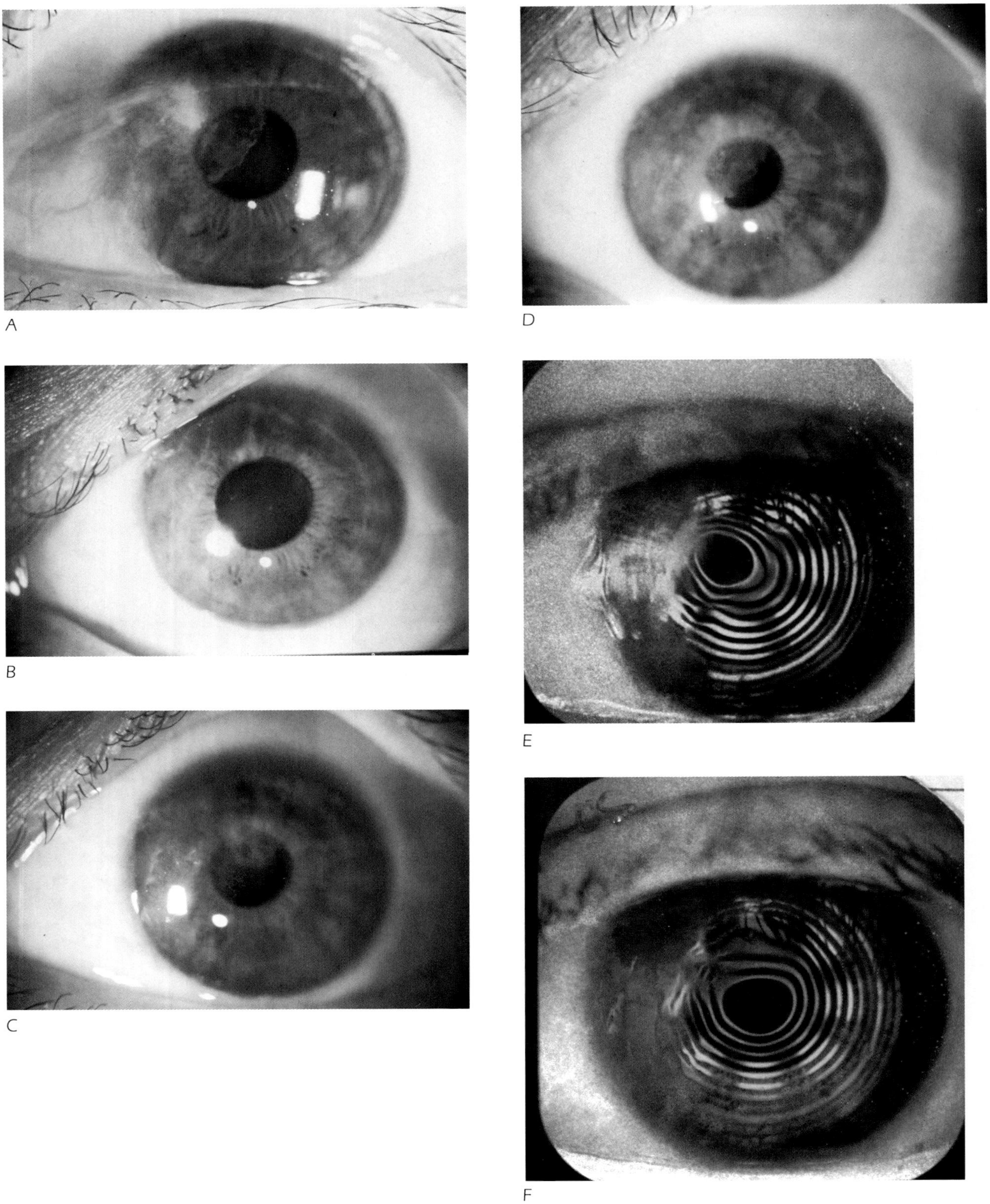

FIGURE 9.5. (A) A patient with superficial anterior stromal haze due to several episodes of herpetic keratitis. (B) Immediately after excimer ablation with a 5 mm disc, marked improvement in the haze can be seen. Some deeper haze remains. (C) Three months postoperatively, improvement in the opacity is appreciated although some opacity remains. (D) Preoperative topography demonstrates a marked central flattening in addition to the scar. (E) Postoperatively, the topography demonstrates persistent flattening but a much larger uniform central optical zone.

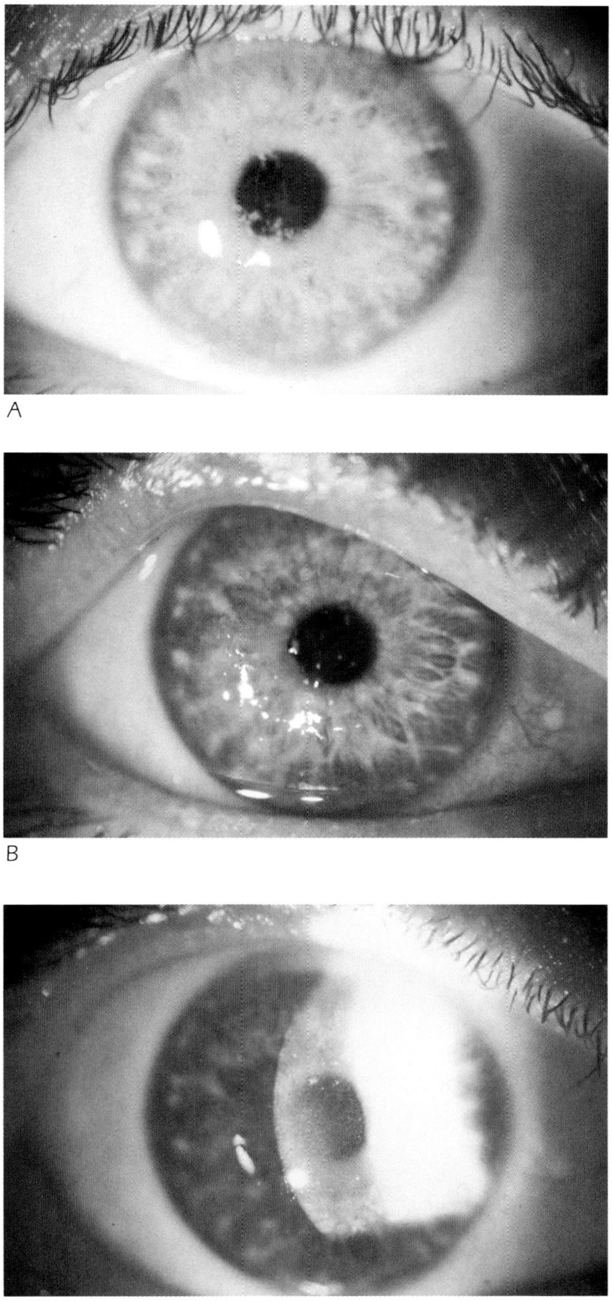

A

B

C

FIGURE 9.6. (A) A patient with granular corneal dystrophy preoperatively. (B) Immediately postoperatively, improvement has occurred in the residual granules. Before reepithelialization occurs, the elevation of the residual granules can be seen. (C) Three months postoperatively, the slit beam illumination distinctly shows the improved clarity in the area of ablation. A fine reticular haze is present in the ablation zone, although most of the granular opacities have been eliminated.

measures, however. Superficial PTK can be curative in that setting. The ablated anterior corneal stromal surface appears to be highly supportive of stable reepithelialization. Although completely normal reformation of the basal lamina complex including normal density of hemidesmosomes and anchoring fibrils may take months to years, most investigators of photorefractive keratectomy have been impressed at the rapid and stable reepithelialization that occurs after ablation, with absence of punctate keratitis, staining defects, or symptoms of recurrent erosion.

The objective of PTK in this setting is simply to remove enough of the superficial Bowman's layer to permit formation of a new basement membrane with adhesion structures. The technique is, therefore, the most superficial of the PTK procedures. Our current technique is to debride the epithelium in the involved area and, using a large spot size such as 5 mm, apply 16 pulses. On the average this will remove no more than 4 μm of Bowman's layer. No optical effect is seen with such a superficial ablation, and therefore the treatment may be applied centrally or eccentrically. Figure 9.9 shows the appearance of one such cornea in a patient who had painful recurrent erosions despite all conventional treatment including aggressive anterior stromal micropuncture. She has been symptom-free for over 6 months since the treatment, whereas previous erosions had occurred at least every 2 weeks for several years. Because these cases are rare, caution should be exercised in aggressive application of this technique until adequate experience is gained with the long-term success rate.

INFECTIOUS KERATITIS

The first therapeutic application proposed for the excimer laser was the eradication of infectious keratitis. In a rabbit model, Serdarevic and coworkers[6] demonstrated ablation of superficial fungal keratitis. An initial expectation of the excimer laser was for sterilization of the organisms by the ultraviolet radiation in addition to the bulk removal of infected tissue.

With improved understanding of the mechanisms of excimer laser ablation, however, workers in the field rapidly appreciated that 193 nm wavelengths are heavily absorbed by corneal tissue and largely extinguished within 1 μm. Sterilization of organisms remote from the ablation zone cannot occur at this wavelength.[7] Longer wavelengths with deeper

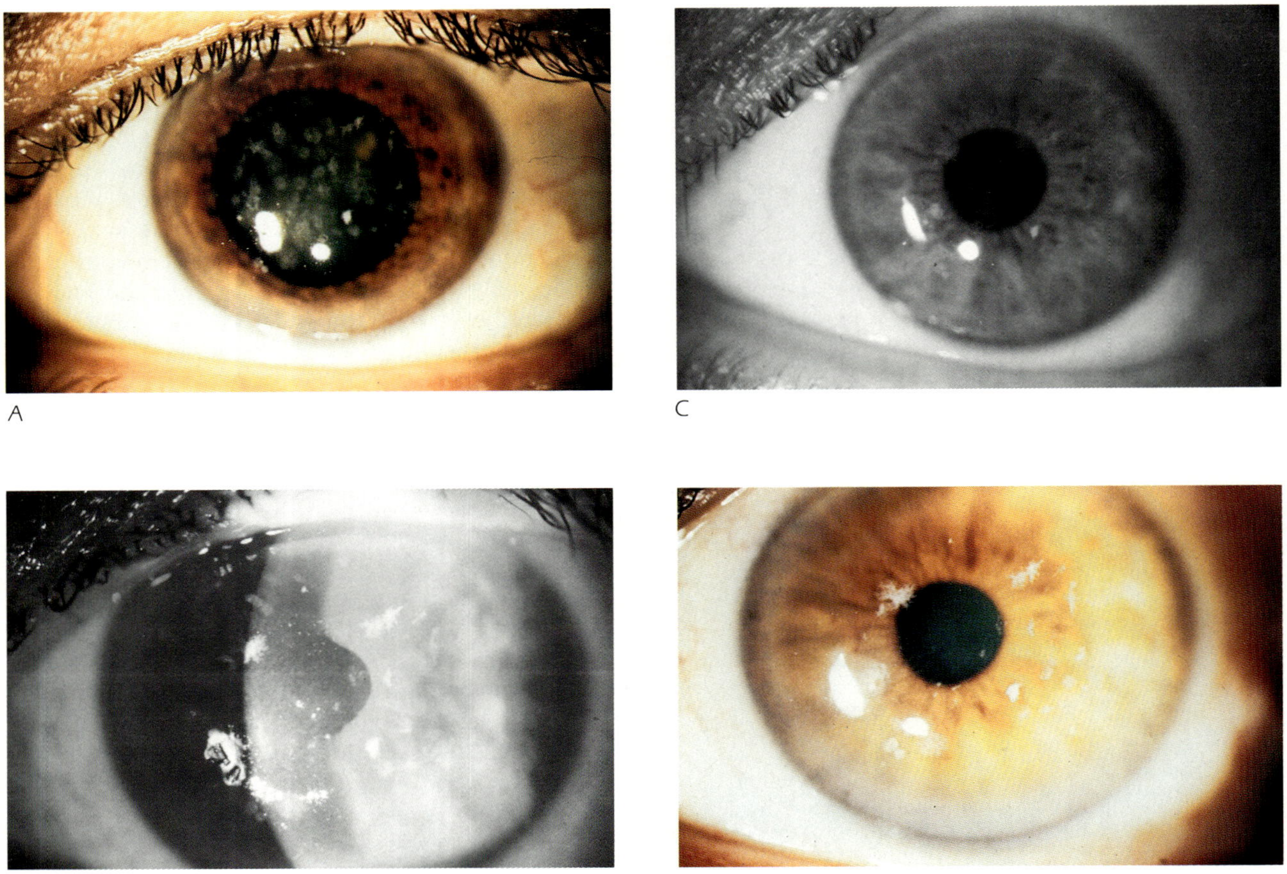

FIGURE 9.7. (A) The preoperative appearance of a patient with the granular appearance of the Avellino variant of lattice dystrophy. Most of the opacities are quite superficial. (B) Four days after excimer ablation, reepithelialization has occurred and most of the opacities are eliminated from the pupillary zone. (C) One month postoperatively, dramatic improvement in the granular opacities has been achieved. (D) Four months postoperatively, the central zone remains free of granular opacities. A trace reticular haze is present.

penetration, such as 248 nm, might possibly have a better germicidal effect. This wavelength is close to that used by germicidal ultraviolet lamps. These longer wavelengths are also generally believed to be significantly more mutagenic, however.

An additional limitation to effective treatment of infectious keratitis with the excimer laser is the deep stromal involvement by most organisms, exceeding the area of clinically observable infiltrate. Fungal keratitis is the most prominent of these examples; the fungal organisms typically penetrate into deep stroma down to the level of Descemet's membrane within the first few days of infection. Perhaps the most superficial of infections is herpetic epithelial keratitis. In disease limited to the epithelium, however, no investigators have yet reported any advantage of the excimer laser compared with antiviral medication and/or simple debridement of the epithelium with a cotton tip applicator.

Recently Eiferman and colleagues[8] reported the successful treatment of infectious crystalline keratopathy with the excimer laser. This infection is highly resistant to antibiotics. Most cases of an infectious crystalline keratopathy involve at least the midstroma and, therefore, would not be amenable to excimer laser ablation. For highly superficial infectious crystalline keratopathy, however, ablation by the excimer laser may be attempted. Because the alternative treatment is usually penetrating keratoplasty, initial treatment with the excimer laser may be a reasonable first effort as long as it does not result in undue delay of keratoplasty while infection spreads. Suitable candidate patients are expected to be quite rare.

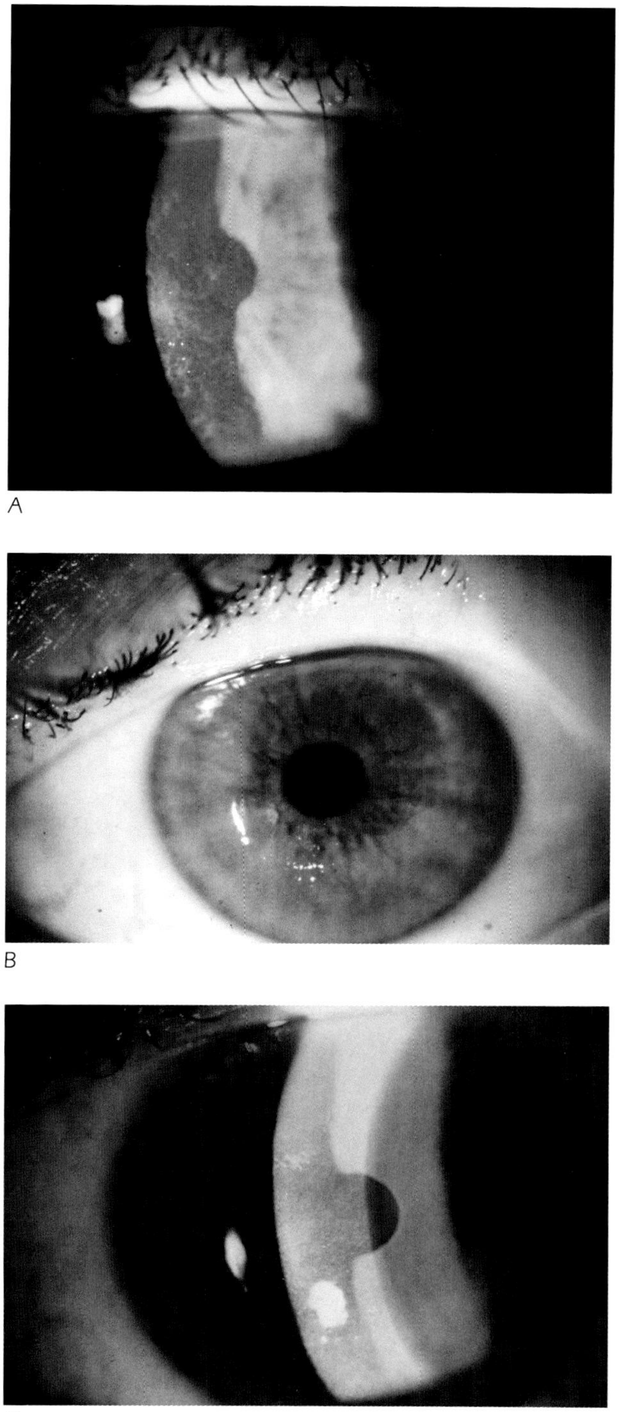

A

B

C

FIGURE 9.8. (A) The preoperative appearance of a patient with Reis-Buckler's dystrophy. (B) Four days after PTK, marked clearing of the pupillary zone is seen. (C) Four months postoperatively, central clarity remains improved but with a fine superficial reticular haze.

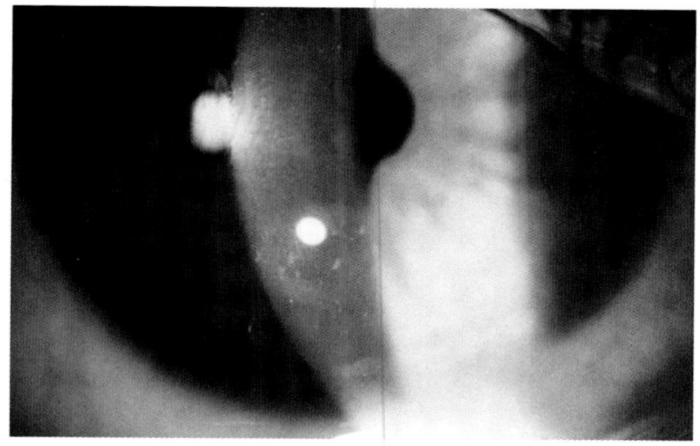

FIGURE 9.9. A patient with painful recurrent erosions despite previous anterior stromal micropuncture. The pinpoint scars from the anterior stromal micropuncture can still be seen. Stable reepithelialization has occurred without any opacification.

REFERENCES

1. Kornmehl EW, Steinert RF, Puliafito CA: A comparison study of masking fluids for excimer laser phototherapeutic keratectomy. *Arch Ophthalmol* 109:860–863, 1991.
2. Steinert RF, Puliafito CA: Excimer laser phototherapeutic keratectomy for a corneal nodule. *Refract Corneal Surg* 6:352, 1990.
3. Sher NA, Bowers RA, Zabel RW, et al: Clinical use of the 193 nm excimer laser in the treatment of corneal scars. *Arch Ophthalmol* 109:491–498, 1991.
4. Stark WJ, Gilbert ML, Gottsch JD, Munnerlyn C: Optical pachymetry in the measurement of anterior corneal disease: An evaluative tool for phototherapeutic keratectomy. *Arch Ophthalmol* 108:12–13, 1990.
5. Stark WJ, Chamon W, Kamp MT, Enger CL, Rencs EV, Gottsch JD: Clinical follow-up of 193 nm ArF excimer laser photokeratectomy. *Arch Ophthalmol* 1992, in press.
6. Sedaravec O, Darrell RW, Krieger RR, Trokel SL: Excimer laser therapy for experimental *Candida* keratitis. *Am J Ophthalmol* 99:534–538, 1985.
7. Gottsch JS, Gilbert ML, Goodman DF, Sulewski ME, Dick JD, Stark WJ: Excimer laser ablative treatment of microbial keratitis. *Ophthalmology* 98:146–149, 1991.
8. Eiferman RA, Forgery DR, Cook YD: Excimer laser ablation of infectious crystalline keratopathy. *Arch Ophthalmol* 110:18, 1992.

CHAPTER 10

Corneal Trephination With the Excimer Laser for Penetrating Keratoplasty

GERHARD K. LANG

GOTTFRIED O. H. NAUMANN

Current standard corneal transplantation techniques use circular, round, mechanical trephines, either operated by hand or motor-driven, under visual control through the operating microscope. The anatomic and functional results of this sight-improving procedure are acceptable. The two major problems of the procedure are excessive astigmatism and immunologic graft rejections. Excessive corneal astigmatism and optical irregularities can result from incongruent cut surfaces of donor and patient corneas and disparities in corneal thickness, which were evident in a histopathologic study.[1] Immunologic graft rejection occurs in 10% of avascular corneas and increases in frequency in vascularized corneas and as the diameter of corneal graft increases. Although for optical purposes it is desirable to have the corneal graft as large as possible, immunologic requirements aim for the smallest possible graft.[2] Our hypothesis has been that the excimer laser could prove useful in keratoplasty surgery, both as a means of minimizing wound irregularities (and thereby limiting postoperative astigmatism) and as a means of allowing noncircular trephinations.

TECHNIQUE

The ultraviolet excimer laser technique enables us to overcome the mechanical limitations of the trephination procedure and to produce trephination of any desired pattern (elliptic, circular with notches, etc.) (Fig. 10.1). We have introduced a new elliptic incision for corneal transplantation using an excimer laser with wavelength of 193 nm (Figs. 10.2 and 10.3).[3] An elliptic excision is created in the recipient and in the donor corneas. For this purpose, it is necessary to obtain an intact donor globe, rather than simply a corneoscleral rim. Ablation is performed by moving the laser slit around the edge of the mask and continuing until Descemet's membrane is reached and a perforation occurs. At that point, fluid loss prevents further tissue excision, and the button is removed using corneal scissors to cut the remaining Descemet's membrane. This new approach has several theoretical advantages. First, experimental studies have shown that noncontact, nonthermal excimer laser trephination produces congruent, parallel, and smooth-cut margins and avoids deviations in cutting direction known to result from mechanical trephination (Fig. 10.4).[3,4] Second, because the outline of the

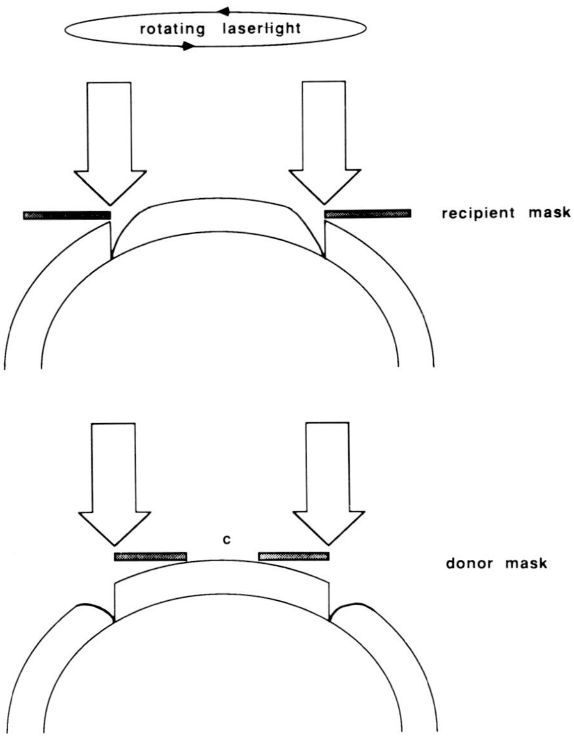

FIGURE 10.1. Open mask system. Schematic cross-section of recipient mask device (top) and donor mask (bottom). Note the wide triangular wound cleft with unbeveled edges at the outside (top) and inside (bottom) of the excimer laser cut.

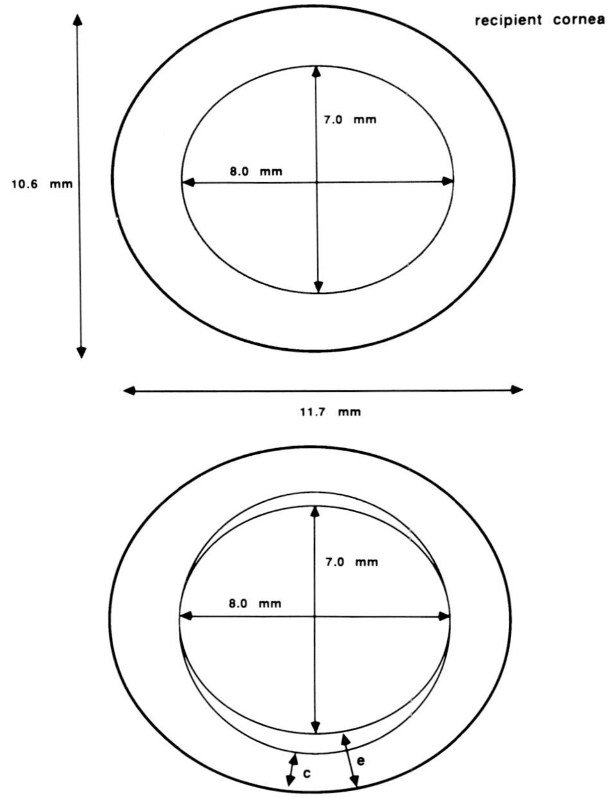

FIGURE 10.2. Elliptic trephination (7.0/8.0 mm) and elliptic outline of the human cornea (top). Compared with a circular 8.0 mm trephination (c) an elliptic 7.0/8.0 mm transplantation (e) provides a wider distance to the limbus in the critical superior and inferior area with more safety for suture placement (bottom). From Lang et al: *Ophthalmic Surg* 20:342–346, 1989.

corneoscleral limbus is not circular but rather elliptic, an elliptic shape of the corneal graft intuitively makes sense.[5] The elliptic graft provides a uniform distance from the graft to conjunctival limbal vessels in every sector (Fig. 10.2). A larger-diameter circular graft would result in closer approximation of the graft–host junction to limbal vessels superiorly and inferiorly, possibly increasing the risk of allograft reaction. This allows larger graft diameters in the horizontal plane and still permits the placement of sutures in an area with intact Bowman's layer, reducing the risk of suture loosening. Third, an elliptic donor button fits snugly into the elliptic recipient cornea opening and appears resistant to torsion, in comparison with a round button in a circular opening. Thus placement of the four cardinal sutures by the surgeon is simplified. Finally, the elliptic button is smaller and weighs about 12% less than a circular transplant that has the maximal diameter of the ellipse. Thus, the elliptic dimensions combine to minimize the disadvantages and maximize the advantages as far as immunologic or optical astigmatic requirements are concerned. Before clinical application of this technique, the Erlangen Excimer Laser Study Group ruled out concerns in terms of laser mutagenicity and healing by experimental studies.[5,6]

RESULTS

To date, we have performed 40 excimer laser penetrating keratoplasties, but not all patients have had their sutures removed. We have reported our early experience in the first patients with excimer laser elliptic penetrating keratoplasty (Figs. 10.5 and 10.6).[3] However, these are only patients with a short follow-up, and we hesitate to make definitive statements in the absence of longer-term results. Our clinical impression is that these corneas exhibit

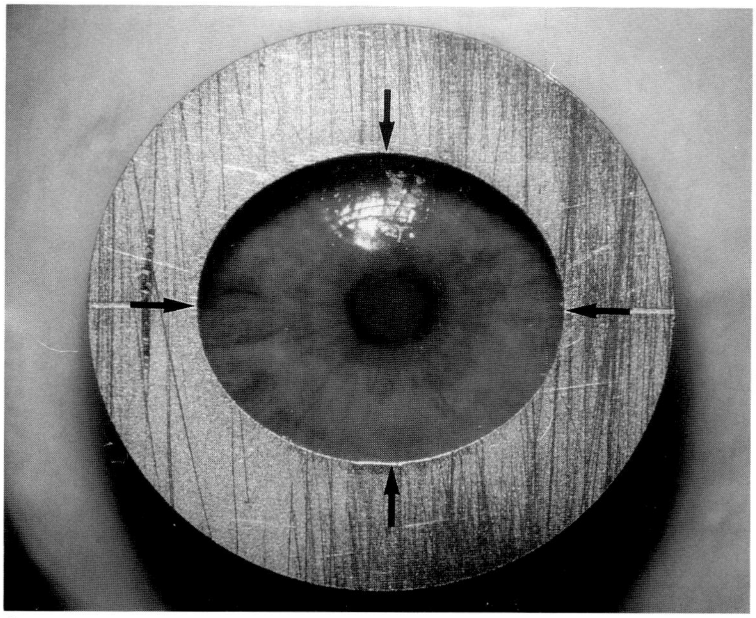

A

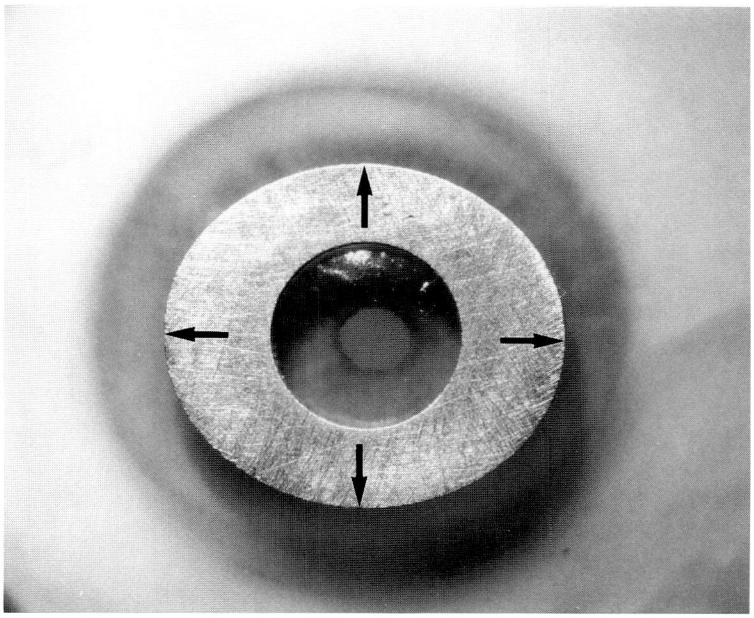

B

Figure 10.3. An elliptic recipient mask (A) and an elliptic donor mask (B) placed on human eyes for demonstration. The elliptic margins of the mask where the laser beam is scanned around are marked by arrows.

excellent postoperative clarity with extremely vertical graft–host junctions.

DISCUSSION

Because excimer laser technology allows the corneal surgeon to produce any trephination shape desired, the outline of the graft was adjusted to the physiologic outline of the cornea. This development led, to the best of our knowledge, to the first elliptic corneal transplantations in humans. Use of the excimer laser for this purpose is, of course, quite expensive compared with conventional mechanical, especially hand-held, trephines, and it would therefore be incumbent upon us to prove that the use of the new technology substantially improves clinical outcome. Also, the time required to complete the laser

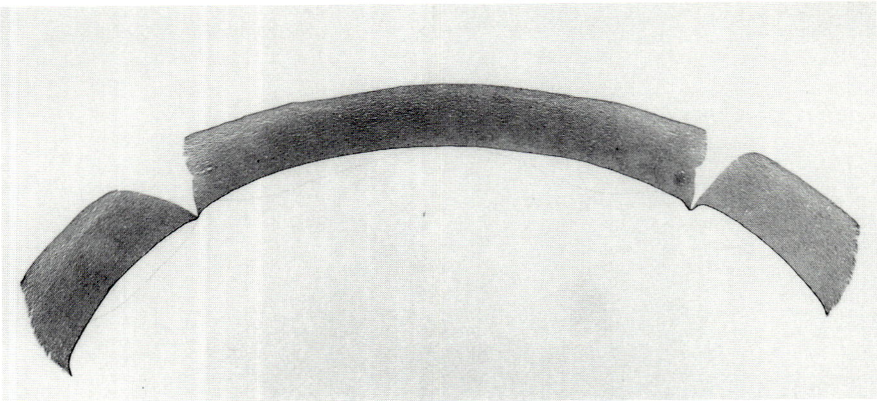

A

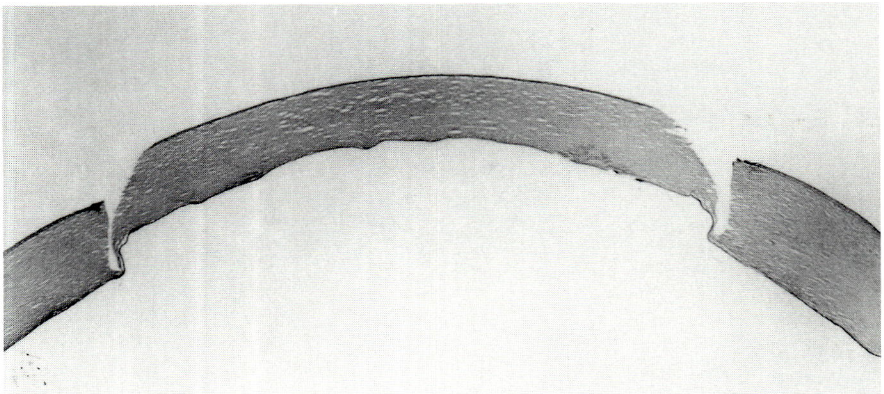

B

FIGURE 10.4. Light micrograph of a human autopsy cornea after excimer laser trephination using the recipient mask (A) and the donor mask (B). Note the wide open triangular wound cleft and the straight and smooth outer (recipient) and inner (donor) cut edge. From Lang et al: *Ophthalmic Surg* 20:262–267, 1989.

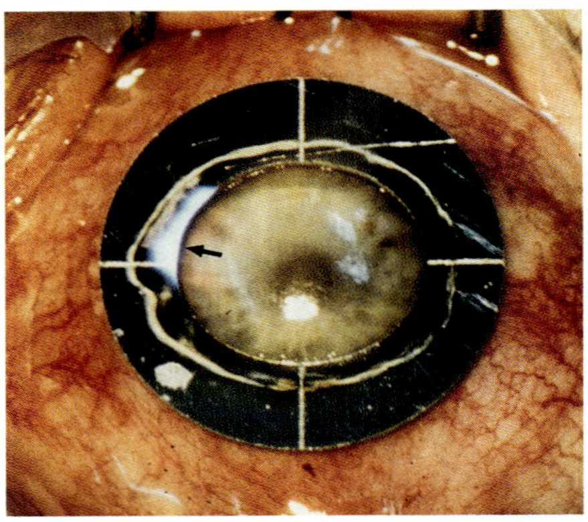

Figure 10.5. Intraoperative status. The open mask for the recipient trephination is well centered on the pupil. The excimer laser beam (arrow) is positioned half on the mask and half on the cornea and is directed by hand along the mask until perforation occurs. From Lang et al: *Arch Ophthalmol:* 108, 914–915, 1990.

excisions and the need for intact donor globes are relative deficits of this laser trephination procedure.

Is the excimer laser the corneal trephine of the future? To make this claim, we believe the cost of the laser mandates that it be proved to be dramatically better (statistically and clinically) than conventional trephination techniques in minimizing postoperative astigmatism. Other factors beside wound edge morphology are undoubtedly important in determining postoperative astigmatism, however, including interindividual variability in wound healing, anterior–posterior displacement of the graft–host junction due to faulty suture placement, and so forth. It may be overly simplistic to expect that improved corneal trephination alone will eliminate postkeratoplasty astigmatism. While our work to date is promising, it is simply too early for us to advocate replacement of mechanical trephines with the laser. We plan to continue our work in this area over the next several years, until we can convincingly demonstrate the relative merits of mechanical and laser trephination.

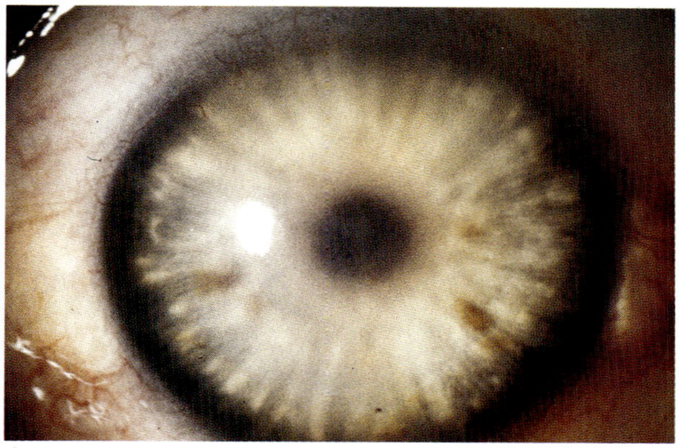

A

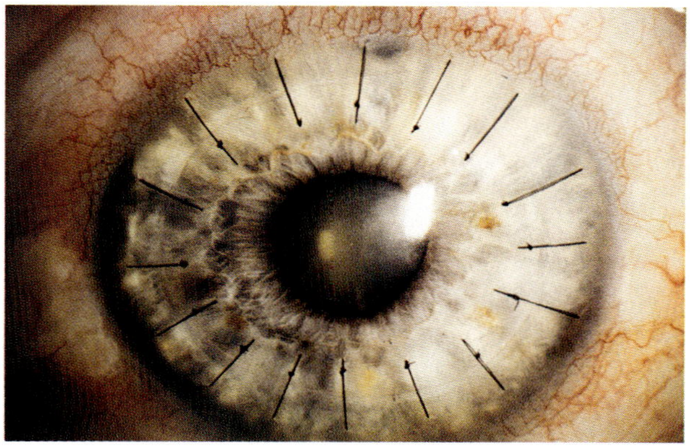

B

FIGURE 10.6. (A) Preoperative status. Posttraumatic bullous keratopathy with diffuse corneal scarring in a 63 year-old white man. (B) One year after elliptic excimer laser keratoplasty (7.0/8.0 mm for the recipient bed and 7.1/8.1 mm for the corneal graft). Sixteen interrupted 10-0 nylon sutures in place with knots buried in the crystal clear graft. Best-corrected visual acuity was 20/30. From Lang et al: *Arch Ophthalmol* 108:914–915, 1990.

REFERENCES

1. Lang GK, Green WR, Maumenee AE: Clinicopathological studies in keratoplasty eyes obtained postmortem. *Am J Ophthalmol* 101:28–40, 1986.
2. Naumann GOH, Sautter H: Surgery of the cornea. In Mackensen G, Neubauer H (eds): *Augenarzliche Operationen,* vol 1. Springer-Verlag, 1988, pp 491–566.
3. Lang GK, Naumann GOH, Koch JW: A new elliptical excision for corneal transplantation using an excimer laser. *Arch Ophthalmol* 108:914–915, 1990.
4. Lang GK, Schroder E, Koch JW, Yanoff M, Naumann GOH: Excimer laser keratoplasty. I: Basic concepts. *Ophthalmic Surg* 20:262–267, 1989.
5. Lang GK, Schroder E, Koch JW, Yanoff M, Naumann GOH: Excimer laser keratoplasty. II: Elliptical keratoplasty. *Ophthalmic Surg* 20:342–346, 1989.
6. Gebhart E, Lang GK, Tittelbach H, Rau D, Naumann GOH: Untersuchungen für Chromosomenmutagenität eines 193 nm Excimer Lasers. *Fortschr Ophthalmol* 87:229–233, 1990.
7. Koch JW, Lang GK, Kolkmeier J, Naumann GOH: Rorneale Wundheilung nach perforierender und nichtperforierender Excimer Laser Keratektomie. *Fortschr Ophthalmol* 87:615–622, 1990.

CHAPTER 11

New Directions in Excimer Laser Surgery

RONALD R. KRUEGER

PETER J. McDONNELL

Refractive surgery in general, and corneal laser surgery in particular, can be characterized as an area of intense basic research and rapid clinical development. How many ophthalmologists, 10 years ago, would have anticipated the ability to alter the anterior corneal curvature with shallow superficial ablations to correct myopia? Who would have believed that it would be feasible to excise Bowman's membrane without inducing corneal scarring sufficient to permanently reduce visual acuity? Given the inherent delay between writing a book chapter and having it available in print, can any book devoted to such a rapidly evolving field as excimer laser surgery avoid failing to address some of the topics that are new and exciting by the time it is published? To address this problem, this chapter will briefly describe some of the new directions of research in this field, directions that as of this writing are incompletely evaluated, in the expectation that some may prove clinically useful.

MODULATORS OF CORNEAL WOUND HEALING

All keratorefractive procedures are influenced by the effects of corneal wound healing, a phenomenon that exhibits inter-individual variability and that cannot be adequately predicted in laboratory studies. The use of relaxing incisions to correct postkeratoplasty astigmatism is one such situation; a cornea left spherical intraoperatively will likely be found to be substantially undercorrected shortly after surgery.[1] Wound healing after radial keratotomy accounts for some loss of effect during the early postoperative period, and despite research on use of some modulators of wound healing (corticosteroids, inhibitors of collagen cross-linkage, etc.), no effective pharmacologic means of controlling this wound healing has gained acceptance. Excimer laser superficial ablation (photorefractive keratectomy, PRK) is another excellent example of the importance of wound healing to the ultimate outcome of refractive surgery. When ablations are performed in polymethyl methacrylate (PMMA) as part of the instrument calibration, excellent reproducibility (± 0.25 D) is obtained from one ablation to the next.[2] In contrast, the results in experimental animals and in humans show substantial variability. Clinical trials to date demonstrate that an initial overcorrection is common after PRK, followed by a time-dependent loss of effect, with a stable end point achieved within 6 to 12 months.[3] Undercorrections are common, particularly as the intended myopic correction increases beyond 5 to 6 D. Suggested explanations for the variable end result of surgery include changes in epithelial thickness[4] and ingrowth of keratocytes into the area of ablation, with synthesis of new collagen,[5] thereby reducing the amount of stroma effectively removed by the ablation.

The latter change is worsened by the fact that the new collagen arrays are random, less organized, and composed of fibers of greater thickness and interfibrillar spacing.[6] This alters the corneal light scattering and produces a subepithelial haze. Immunohistochemical studies show this collagen to be type III in origin, not seen in normal corneas. In addition, there is an initial absence of sulfated keratan sulfate, which is thought to maintain precise spacing of collagen fibers.[7,8] The absence of sulfated keratan sulfate associated with corneal opacity is seen congenitally in macular corneal dystrophy. Immunofluorescence following excimer laser corneal ablation shows the absence of sulfated keratan sulfate in new collagen for up to 1 month,[7] but its gradual appearance in increasing amounts beyond 6 weeks as corneal haze begins to dissipate.[8]

The presence and deposition of new collagen produces subepithelial haze and reduces refractive predictability and stability. It is logical to expect that pharmacologic control and manipulation of the wound-healing response after PRK would improve the predictability of the results. The use of 5-fluorouracil and mitomycin C in trabeculectomy, and of mitomycin C in pterygium surgery, shows that results with some types of anterior segment surgery can be improved with adjunctive use of agents that suppress wound healing.

Corticosteroids have been widely used as part of the postoperative routine following PRK, but the clinical value of the corticosteroids remains to be convincingly demonstrated. It has been common among investigators performing clinical trials with the excimer laser to observe the occasional patient who, upon discontinuing corticosteroids, has a substantial loss of effect, with return of myopia. Some investigators, however, have not used corticosteroids in small groups of patients, without discernible effect on ultimate outcome. Tuft and colleagues[6] have examined the effect of corticosteroids on epithelial hyperplasia and new collagen production in rabbits and concluded that local steroids reduced collagen synthesis but did not affect the epithelium. A randomized clinical trial recently performed in London, England, addresses this issue of the efficacy of steroids following PRK and concludes that tropical corticosteroids given over 3 months do not significantly influence the ultimate refractive correction. Whether this indicates that corticosteroids should not be used at all, or that more frequent or longer-duration treatment should be considered, is unclear. Even if corticosteroids are not to be used, significant refractive regression is still a concern following PRK, and other stronger, more specific agents need to be investigated.

Talamo and colleagues[9] compared rabbit eyes treated with erythromycin alone, erythromycin-dexamethasone combination ointment, and erythromycin-dexamethasone combination ointment plus mitomycin C (0.5 mg/ml). They concluded that eyes receiving both dexamethasone and mitomycin C had much less new collagen formation and exhibited less anterior stromal opacity than did the other two groups. This work remains to be confirmed by others in animals or validated in human clinical trials.

The use of wound-healing inhibitors after excimer laser surgery has potential risks. The risk of marked pressure rises with corticosteroids is well appreciated, and the increased possibility of cataract formation as a consequence of 3 to 6 months of topical corticosteroid use cannot be discounted. Presumably, the ideal corticosteroid for this purpose would be one that achieves reasonable levels in the superficial stroma but that penetrates very poorly into the aqueous humor. At the same time that undesired processes of keratocyte migration and new collagen synthesis are underway in the first 6 weeks after surgery, important and highly desirable processes such as synthesis of new hemidesmosomes by the basal epithelium are underway. Inhibition of hemidesmosome formation might lead to faulty epithelial adhesion to the anterior stroma, resulting in problems of recurrent epithelial erosions and possibly delayed infectious keratitis.

The search for pharmacologic agents that control wound healing without the risk of acute or delayed ocular complications will undoubtedly continue as a major emphasis through this decade.

CONTROL OF ABLATION ENVIRONMENT

PARTICULATE EJECTION

The gaseous and particulate by-products of corneal ablation, first examined by Puliafito and colleagues[10] in 1987, demonstrate a mushroom cloud–like ejection of debris emanating from the surface of the cornea immediately following impact with the excimer laser pulse. This finding suggested the need to remove these by-products so that they would not interfere with the subsequent pulses of the laser

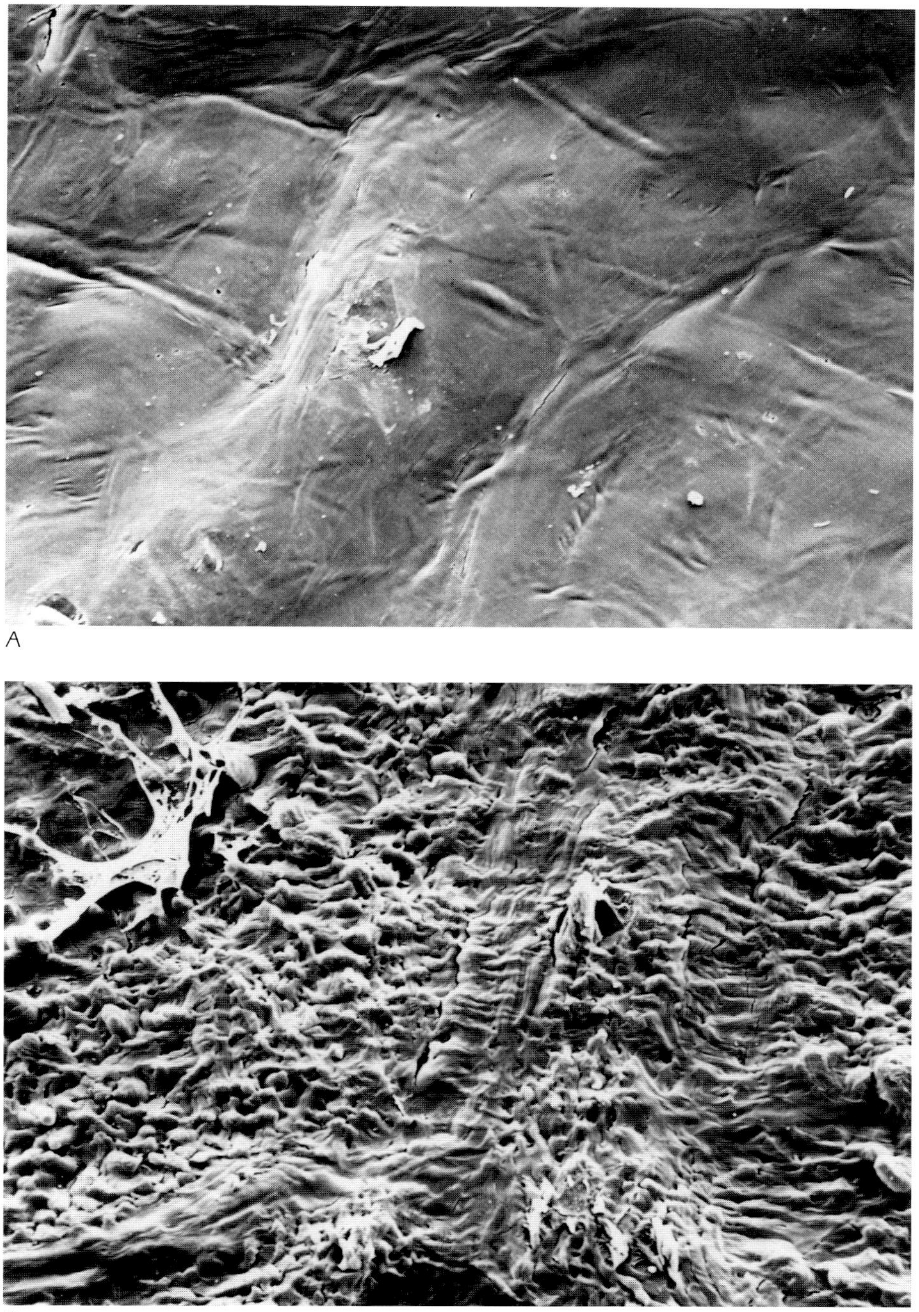

A

B

FIGURE 11.1. Scanning electron micrographs of the surface of ablated rabbit corneas immediately after ablation. (A) Surface of cornea treated without nitrogen gas blowing during ablation is smoother than (B) that of cornea treated with brisk nitrogen gas flow (5 standard ft^3/h. Both figures are taken at 500 × magnification.

beam. One manufacturer designed an effluent remover and a fixation ring with nitrogen blower to eliminate the gaseous and particulate debris so as to facilitate a smooth ablation pattern. The effluent remover not only aids in removing the ablation byproducts but also removes toxic ozone produced when the excimer laser reacts with oxygen. The nitrogen blower, although used in early investigational trials of myopic PRK, has been recently discontinued from use. The nitrogen gas blown across the surface of the cornea was noted to produce an undesirable effect, creating intraoperative loss of corneal transparency and histopathologically apparent corneal surface irregularities.[11] Scanning electron microscopy demonstrates greater surface roughening when nitrogen is blown across the ablating surface at high speeds, compared with the surface of excimer ablation in air with no blowing (Fig. 11.1). This effect is presumably from an uneven distribution of corneal dehydration created by the drying effect of blown gas. The net effect is that the nitrogen blower appears to roughen the surface rather than smooth it. With the nitrogen blower no longer in use, the question to be answered is whether the ablation by-products are adequately evacuated between laser pulses so as not to interfere with the beam homogeneity. Thus far, clinical experience suggests that this does not represent a problem. Other excimer laser manufacturers have not used the nitrogen blower in their clinical trials and seem unconcerned with the potential interference caused by particulate debris.

SURFACE HEATING

Although excimer laser photoablation is a predominantly nonthermal process, the release of energy as molecular bonds break does give rise to temperature changes on the surface. In 1988, Bende and colleagues[12] showed temperature increases of approximately 10 or 20°C in the stromal tissue adjacent to the excimer laser–ablated area. Other studies with excimer ablation of polymers show that high-temperature gases are created during the ablation process. These temperature increases may affect keratocyte activation and corneal wound healing.

Recently, we have shown that the shock waves created during excimer laser ablation travel twice as fast in helium as they do in either nitrogen or air (Fig. 11.2).[13] The more rapid dissipation of high-temperature and high-pressure wavefronts means that the corneal surface endures less exposure to hot gases created during the ablation process. An environment of cooled helium gas may be more favorable in reducing the corneal temperature than operating the laser under ambient conditions.

Another way corneal surface heating may be minimized is by reducing the excimer laser pulsewidth. Early studies by Krasinski and colleagues[14] have demonstrated the presence of a plasma created by the leading edge of the excimer pulse. This plasma shields the transmission of laser light at the end of the pulse and sequesters energy at the surface. By shortening the excimer laser pulse, one might eliminate the shielding effect and minimize the exposure of sequestered energy to the corneal surface. Although this and other methods of reducing surface temperatures are clinically and histologically unsubstantiated, they are being investigated and deserve mention.

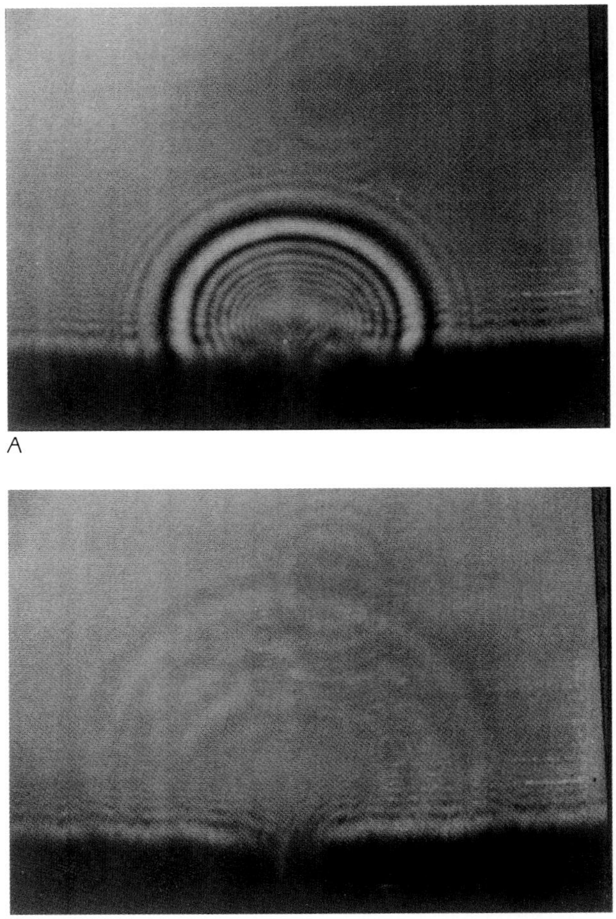
A

B

FIGURE 11.2. Shock wave of excimer laser ablation of a rubber stopper at 1000 mJ/cm^2 and 190 nm time delay in air (A) and helium (B). The velocity and distance traveled in helium is nearly twice that in air, suggesting more rapid dissipation of thermal gases from the surface. Similar findings are seen in ablation of corneal tissue.

TISSUE HYDRATION

Perhaps the most important environmental factor in excimer laser ablation is tissue hydration. Upon removal of the corneal epithelium, the corneal stroma can swell, while at the same time the light of an operating microscope can promote superficial dehydration. It has been shown that the pulse depth of excimer laser ablation depends strongly on the level of tissue hydration. Aside from nitrogen blown across the surface, causing a drying effect, most investigators operate under ambient conditions, attempting to begin the ablation process shortly after removal of the epithelium so as to minimize hydration changes. Some investigators have advocated blowing humidified nitrogen across the surface to maintain a constant level of hydration.[15] Although this has not been adopted into clinical practice, it does appear to eliminate the problem of surface drying associated with nitrogen. Studies are currently underway to determine the efficacy of using humidified gases during corneal ablation.

ABLATABLE MASKS

The interposition of an erodible disc-shaped mask between the laser and the cornea offers a potential means of altering anterior corneal contour. This technique involves placing over the cornea a mask composed of a material that is to be ablated by the laser. The thickness of the mask can be varied, so that the laser beam will perforate first in one region and begin ablating the underlying corneal tissue before the mask is perforated elsewhere (Fig. 11.3). A mask that is thinnest centrally would be appropriate for a myopic correction, a mask thickest centrally would be used for hyperopia, and a toric mask, properly aligned above the treated cornea, would be used for the correction of astigmatism.

In a report by Gordon and colleagues,[16] PRK using the erodible mask was performed on a limited number of patients with both myopia and astigmatism. PMMA masks, resting on a thin quartz substrate and fixed within a specialized eye cup, were used in both animal and human trials. The shapes of the masks were predetermined by shape transfer functions correlating the radius of curvature of the mask with the radius of curvature of a plastic target eye, and ultimately with the desired dioptric correction. The early clinical results on five patients undergoing PRK with the erodible mask suggest a final spherical overcorrection and cylindrical undercorrection in manifest refraction. These preliminary results are in agreement with early European trials, and future masks may require a greater cylindrical and lesser spherical component.

Although this is a promising technique, the successful use of erodible masks will require that their shape be accurately correlated with the desired dioptric correction. In addition, they must be made with great precision and reproducibility, be correctly centered, and, in the case of astigmatism treatment, correctly oriented with respect to the major and minor axes of curvature of the underlying cornea.

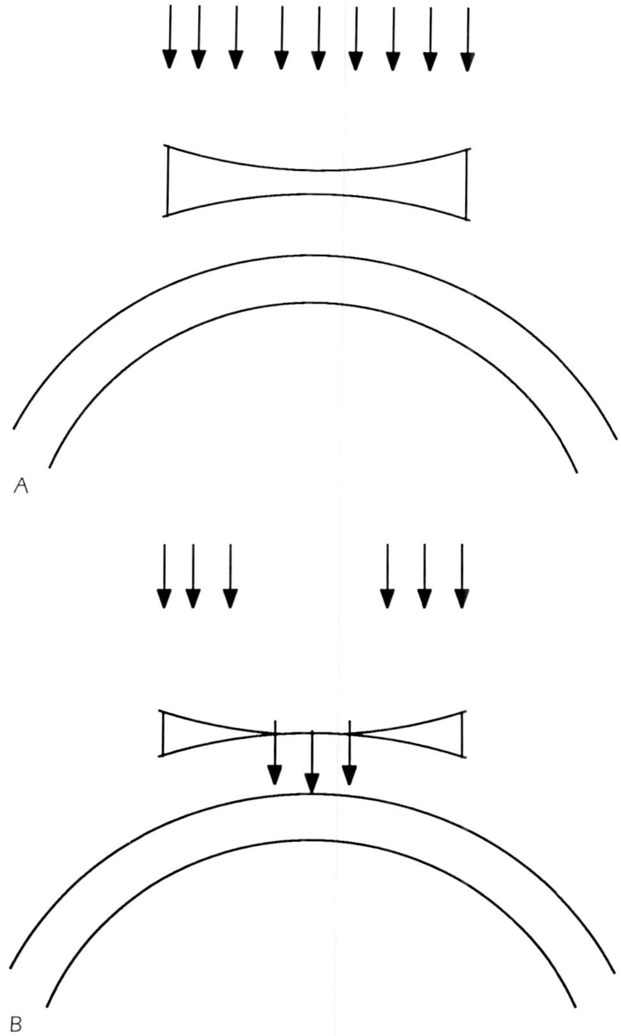

FIGURE 11.3. (A) Schematic illustration of broad-diameter excimer laser beam impinging on and ablating concave mask interposed between laser and cornea in procedure designed to correct myopia. (B) The thinnest central portion of the mask is perforated first, such that photons reach the underlying central cornea initially. When the task is completely eroded, the greatest amount of tissue will have been ablated centrally, with progressively less tissue removed toward the periphery of the ablation zone.

MOLDABLE COLLAGEN GEL

One approach to the problem of smoothing the irregularly shaped cornea, and of altering anterior corneal curvature for refractive purposes is the use of a gel placed on the corneal surface and molded to the desired curvature. We have used a suspension of collagen that becomes firm after application to the cornea to create a smooth temporary anterior surface, using a rigid contact lens as a mold.[17] The resulting surface is optically and ultrastructurally smooth, and the collagen gel ablates at the same rate as does corneal stroma (Fig. 11.4). The laser is then used to ablate through the gel and into the superficial corneal stroma with a uniform profile of ablation.

To correct hyperopia, the gel is molded using a

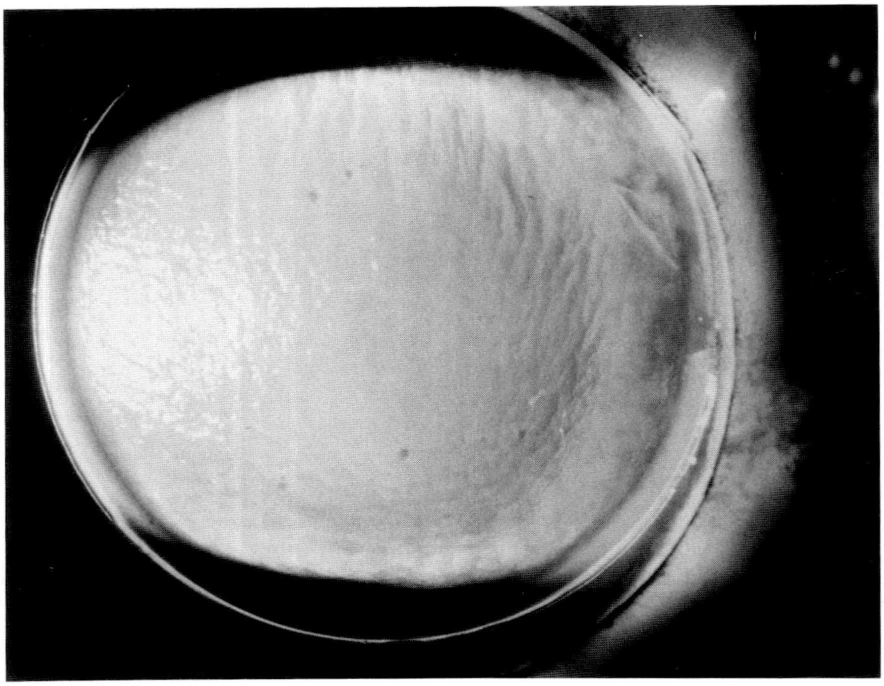

A

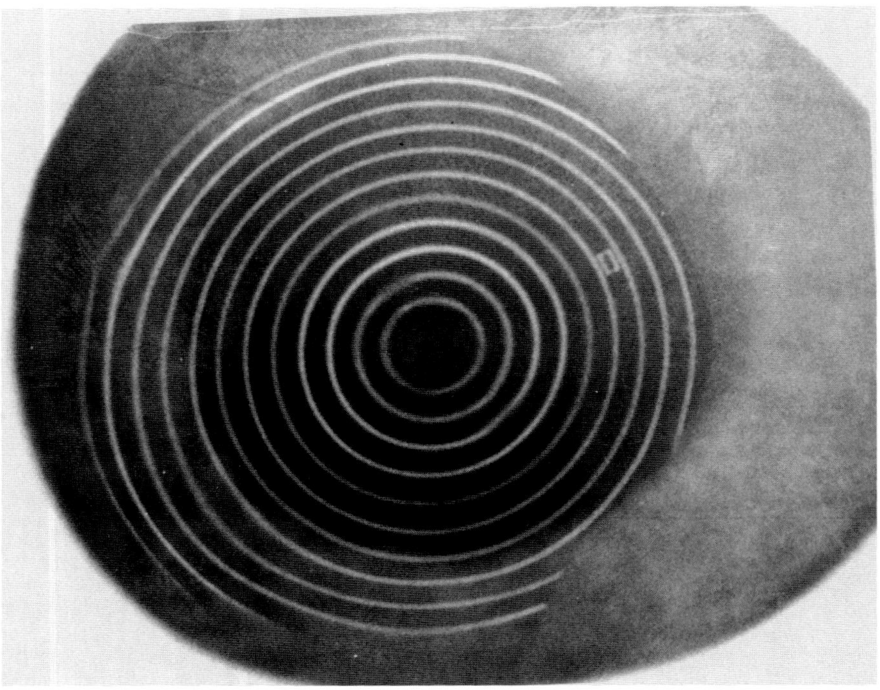

B

FIGURE 11.4. (A) Collagen gel solidified on surface of animal cornea. (B) Photokeratoscope image of spherical surface of collagen gel. Reprinted with permission from Englanoff JS, Kolahdouz-Isfahani AH, Moreira H, et al: In situ collagen gel mold as an aid in excimer laser superficial keratectomy. *Ophthalmology* (in press).

contact lens having a steep base curve equal to the desired postoperative corneal curvature, while myopia is corrected using a contact lens with a flat base curve. Corneal astigmatism, regular and irregular, is improved because the gel creates a smooth spherical or aspherical surface identical to the base curvature of the contact lens used as a mold. Using this technique, we have been able to achieve both flattening and steepening of the corneas of animals and have also demonstrated that preexisting keratometric cylinder can be eliminated.[17]

MULTIFOCAL CORNEAL ABLATIONS

Quantitative analysis of the results of refractive surgical procedures such as radial keratotomy have documented the lack of direct correlation between changes in visual acuity, cycloplegic refraction, and keratometric measurement.[18] Using computer-assisted analysis of corneal topography, we observed regional variation in corneal curvature in eyes of patients of the age at which presbyopia would be anticipated but who had excellent uncorrected distance and near acuities.[19,20] The regional variation in corneal power appeared to explain how a multifocal lens effect could be achieved. By contrast, patients with large homogeneous (in terms of corneal power) central corneas did not exhibit this multifocal effect. This observation has been confirmed by others.[21] Unfortunately, these inadvertently created multifocal lens effects in corneas after radial keratotomy may, at least in some patients, produce symptoms of visual distortion or monocular diplopia.[19-21]

We were intrigued by the possibility that multifocal corneas could be purposefully created with superficial ablations using the excimer laser. As PRK is currently performed for myopia, the surgeon attempts to create relatively large homogeneous zones of central flattening, and topographic analysis suggests that this is generally achieved.[22,23] Theoretically, if completely successful, such an approach would result, eventually, in 100% of corrected myopic patients experiencing presbyopia. To avoid this limitation, we have achieved experimental creation of multifocal ablations designed to allow correction of myopic refractive errors while allowing good uncorrected near vision.[24] To perform multifocal ablations, we used three strategies: (1) two concentric ablations, one of larger diameter (6 mm) and a second of smaller diameter (3 mm) (Fig. 11.5); (2) two ablations of 6 and 3 mm, with the 3 mm ablation decentered inferiorly by 2 mm; and (3) one single ablation in which the computer-controlled iris diaphragm is initially fully open to 6 mm and progressively closes until two-thirds of the pulses have been delivered, leaving the periphery of the ablation zone flattened, but the central area of approximately 3 mm diameter with no intended refractive change (Fig. 11.6). Computer-assisted topographic studies of plastic hemispheres and rabbit corneas suggest that we can, in fact, produce a bimodal distribution of corneal powers, such that good distance and near acuity might be achieved.

Of the strategies employed in this study to create a bifocal effect, we believe one (technique 3) appears most promising: performing an ablation with the diaphragm initially maximally opened and then interrupting the treatment so as to leave the central 3 mm of the ablation zone with a curvature unchanged from preoperatively. In this fashion, we can take advantage of pupillary miosis during accommodation decreasing the percentage of light rays reaching the retina that have traversed the flattened region of the cornea. Supporting this conclusion, we have demonstrated a shift to steeper values when we compare the central 3 mm to the central 6 mm of cornea using this strategy. In addition, if the patient is unhappy with the refractive outcome of this multifocal procedure because of monocular diplopia or a similar problem, this could be converted to a monofocal ablation by completing the treatment of the central 3 mm of the cornea.

Providing patients in the presbyopic age range with satisfactory uncorrected distance and near acuity is an exciting prospect. On the other hand, there are likely to be undesired consequences of such attempts. Multifocal contact and intraocular lenses have been developed and clinically tested as a response to the loss of accommodation with presbyopia or aphakia. While increasing depth of field, such devices can decrease contrast of the retinal image by at least 50% and decrease the limit of resolution by one or two lines.[25] Thus, there may be clinical settings in which these devices cause patients to experience negative effects from multifocal lenses or to be dissatisfied with their vision. We believe that the questions that are as yet unanswered about the optical performance of multifocal intraocular lenses and multifocal corneas argue for a conservative approach to human clinical trials of excimer laser ablation for creation of multifocal corneas.

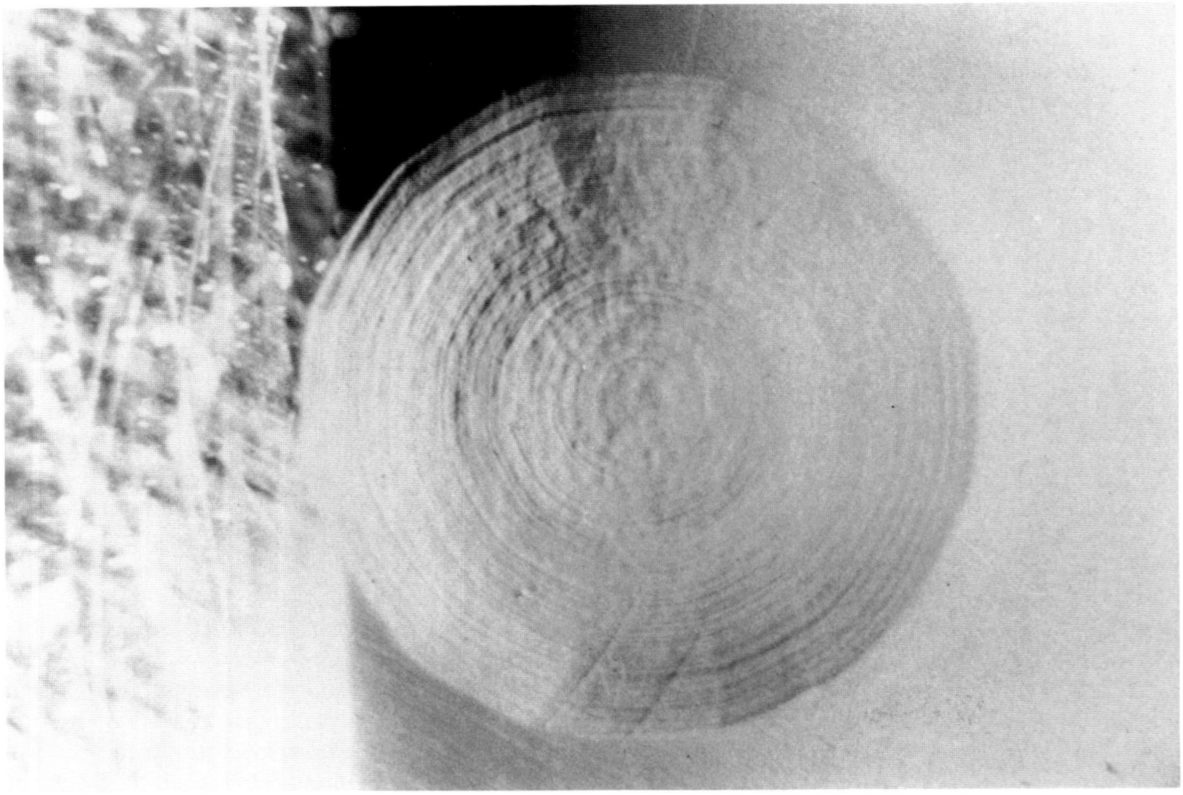

A

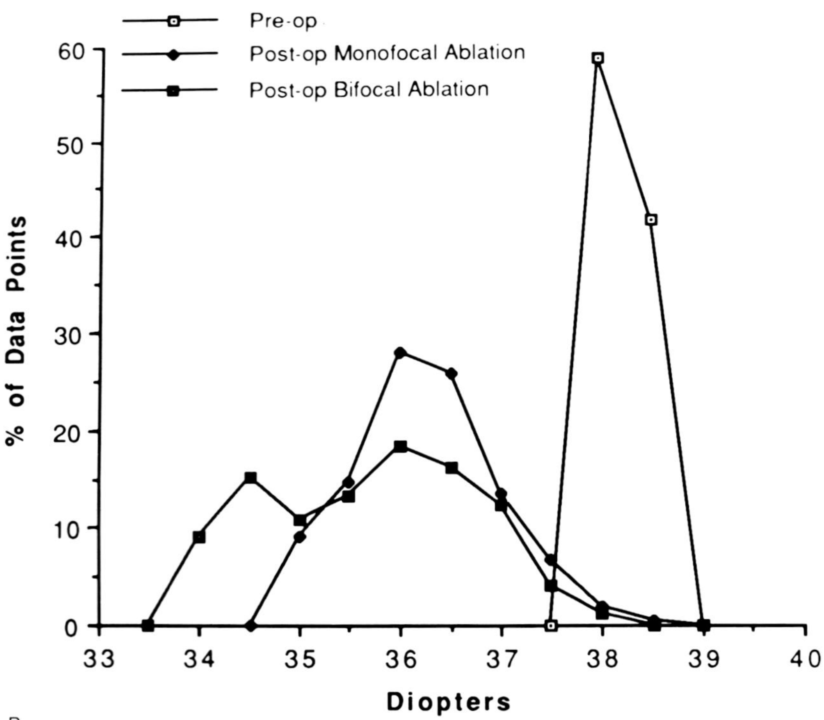

B

FIGURE 11.5. (A) Photograph of concentric bifocal ablation in plastic hemisphere. Outer myopic (4 D) ablation zone diameter is 6 mm, and inner myopic (additional 2 D) ablation zone diameter is 3 mm. (B) Distribution of surface powers of the central 6 mm of the hemisphere preoperatively, after single 4 D ablation (6 mm diameter), and after second 2 D ablation (3 mm diameter).

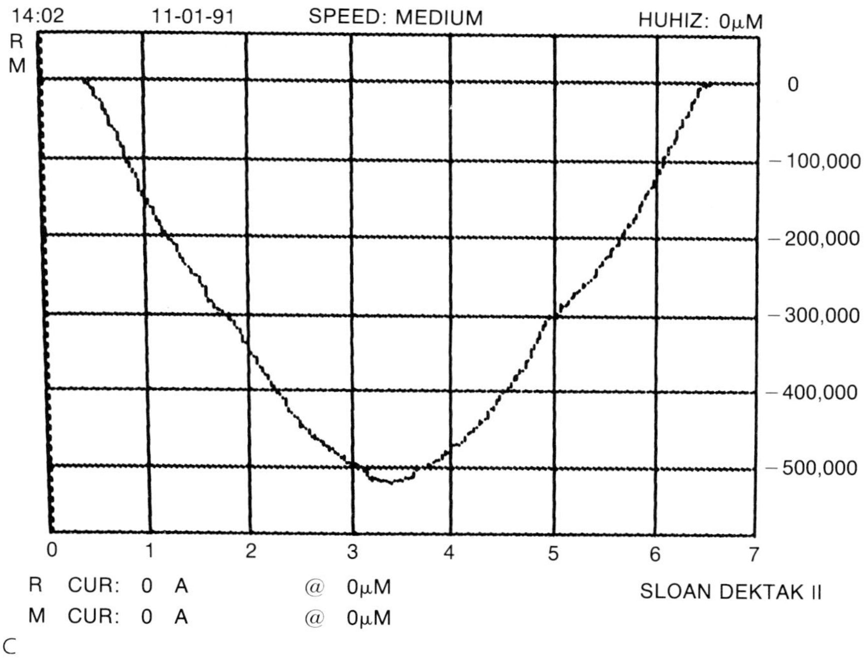

Continued (C) Profile scan through the center of a flat PMMA plastic block after both myopic ablations (6 mm, −4.00 D; 3 mm, −2.00 D) using technique 1. Reprinted with permission from Moreira H, Garbus J, Fascino A, et al: Multifocal corneal topographic changes with excimer laser photorefractive keratectomy. *Arch Ophthalmol* (in press).

LASER ADJUSTABLE SYNTHETIC EPIKERATOPLASTY

Although excimer laser PRK holds promise as a simple technique for inducing refractive change, the precision and stability of correction may vary between patients and in some cases may produce a less-than-optimal visual result. This lack of predictability in some patients is due mainly to the corneal wound-healing response, but also to differences in structural integrity between corneas, and variability of laser output. One way to overcome this problem would be to design a procedure that eliminates the variability of the wound-healing response and is adjustable and reversible to correct for variability and error during laser ablation. Laser adjustable synthetic epikeratoplasty (LASE), proposed by Thompson, Hanna, and Waring,[26] is a procedure in which excimer laser photoablation is used to sculpt a synthetic epikeratoplasty lenticule placed on the corneal surface. The lenticule, made of a synthetic polymer, would provide an acellular substrate that could be modified repeatedly to change the cornea's refractive power without disrupting the underlying corneal stroma or inciting a wound-healing response. The initial shape of the lenticule would be defined by the desired correction, as in conventional epikeratoplasty. The laser would then be used to resurface the lenticule to adjust for any inaccuracies in the initial result. Changes in the lenticule or in the refractive state of the eye could also be adjusted for at a later date, as needed. Should a new lenticule be needed, the old one could simply be removed and replaced, making the procedure reversible.

At present LASE is experimental and in the early research phase, and several concerns must be addressed before the concept can be clinically tested. The most important of these is the stability and biocompatibility of the material with human corneal collagen. For a material to be acceptable, it must be optically clear, support epithelial spreading and attachment, be permeable to nutrients and metabolites, and resist enzymatic degradation.[27] The lenticule must also be securely attached, but for the procedure to be reversible, it must not modify the shape of the underlying cornea.[26]

Investigators at the Yerkes Regional Primate Research Center of Emory University have been addressing these concerns and have tested various cross-linked collagen polymers and copolymers. One of the most promising is type IV collagen, a copolymer, which has been successfully secured on primate eyes.[27] Figure 11.7 shows such a collagen lenticule being secured within the corneal stroma. After partial-thickness trephination, a peripheral annular dissection into the corneal stroma is made, epithelium removed, and the lenticule inserted into the stromal pocket, conforming nicely to the contour of the cornea. Figure 11.8 shows the cornea

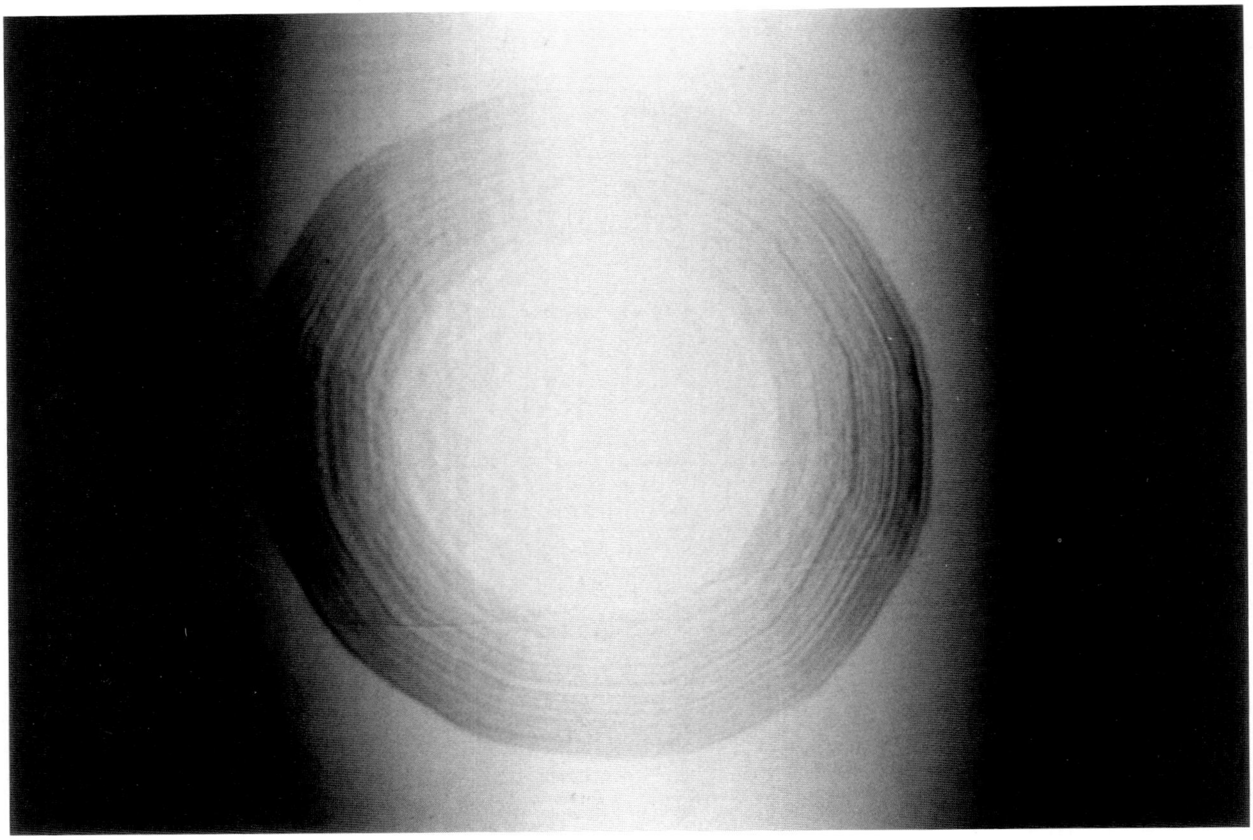

A

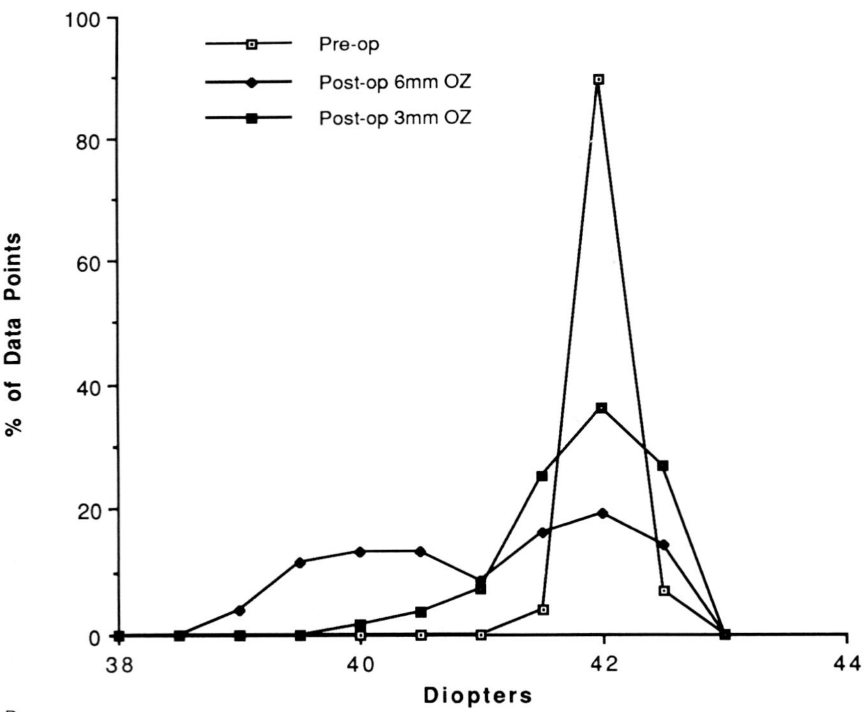

B

FIGURE 11.6. (A) Photograph of annual bifocal ablation in plastic hemisphere. Annular zone of stepped ablation surrounds central region of cornea, in which curvature is unchanged from preoperatively. (B) Distribution of surface powers of the central 6 mm of the hemisphere preoperatively, after single 4 D ablation (6 mm diameter), and after second 2 D ablation (3 mm diameter).

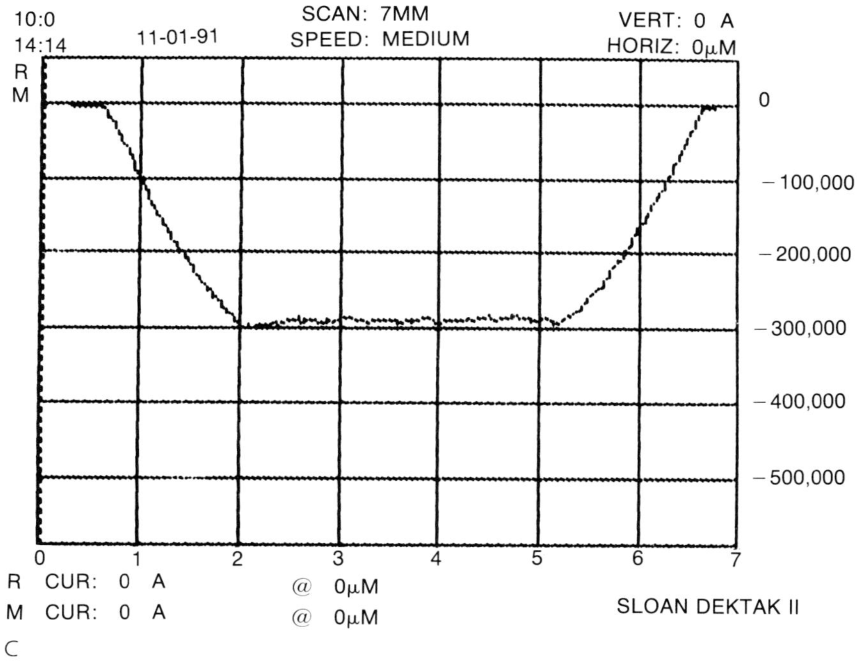

Continued (C) Profile scan through the center of a PMMA plastic block after myopic ablation using technique 3. Reprinted with permission for Moreira H, Garbus J, Fasano A, et al: Multifocal corneal topographic changes with laser photorefractive keratectomy. Published courtesy of *Ophthalmology,* in press, 1992.

of a rhesus monkey 20 days postinsertion of the synthetic type IV collagen lenticule. There is complete reepithelialization of the new corneal surface, and one can see the clarity of the lenticule sandwiched between the brightly reflective narrow band of epithelium and the underlying broad reflective corneal stroma. At present, the lenticule in this rhesus monkey cornea has remained stable and unaltered as a synthetic epikeratoplasty for over 3 years (Dale E. Reddick, M.S., personal communication, April 27, 1992). Although it has remained intact for such a long period, it is still composed of a material that is prone to enzymatic degradation and may not be optimal in its present form.

Once a suitable synthetic material is found, excimer laser sculpting of the lenticule is performed to achieve the desired correction without the influence of wound healing. Figure 11.9 shows a schematic representation of the excimer laser sculpting of a synthetic epikeratoplasty lenticule. The excimer light is focused through the appropriate optical system and projected onto the new corneal surface.

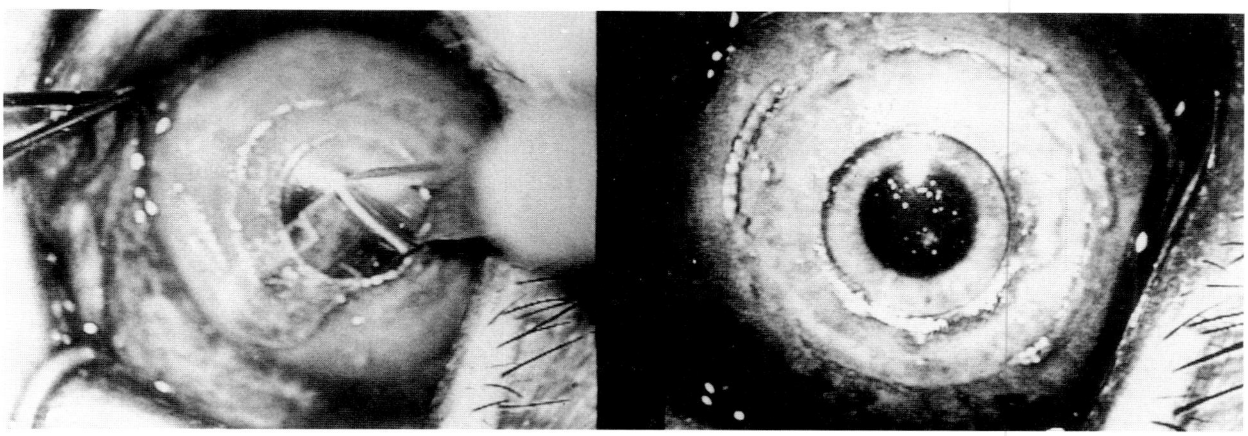

FIGURE 11.7. Technique used to secure a type 4 collagen synthetic lenticule onto the host cornea. As in epikeratoplasty, a peripheral stromal pocket is dissected (left), and the synthetic lenticule of desired shape is inserted to conform nicely with the underlying cornea (right). Photograph from Keith Thompson, M.D.

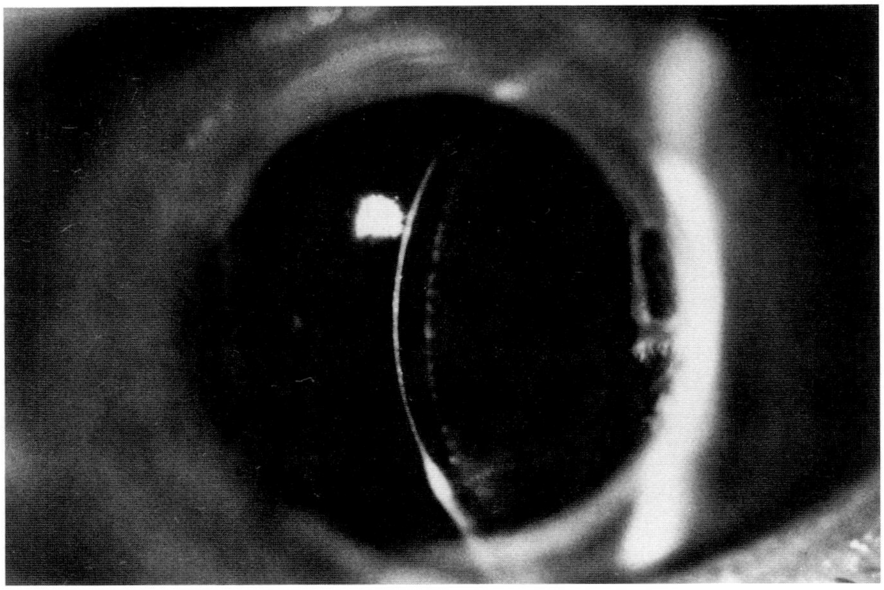

FIGURE 11.8. Reepithelialized cornea of a rhesus monkey 20 days postinsertion of a synthetic type 4 collagen lenticule. Not the brightly reflective narrow band of epithelium anterior to the nonreflective collagen lenticule and the underlying broad reflective corneal stroma. Photograph from Keith Thompson, M.D.

Once the surface is modified, reepithelialization should again occur and the lenticule remain stable, as before, but with a new refractive surface.

LASER IN SITU KERATOMILEUSIS

Earlier in this book, we discussed excimer laser PRK for high myopia (principally, −10 to −20 D). In this technique, three ablations are performed at gradually increasing ablation diameters, 4, 5, and 6 mm, the net effect being a graded ablation of less total depth than an equivalent one-stage ablation. A smaller total depth of ablation may lead to less postoperative haze and refractive regression.

Another approach to correcting high myopia with the excimer laser is that of laser in situ keratomileusis (LASIK). Keratomileusis, first described by Barraquer in 1961,[28] is a procedure whereby a partial-thickness corneal cap is excised using a microkeratome and then reshaped prior to suturing it back onto the cornea. Conventional keratomileusis as described by Barraquer reshapes the lenticule with a cryolathe; the corneal cap is frozen, lathed, and then thawed in glycerol prior to resuturing to the cornea. This procedure was modified by Ruiz and Rowsey in 1987[29] so that two microkeratome sections are made, thereby avoiding the need for the cryolathe. The procedure, termed *in situ keratomileusis,* reshapes the corneal stroma by removing a convex meniscus of tissue with the second pass of the instrument. The second pass or cut is performed on the underlying exposed stroma, rather than the corneal cap, making it fundamentally different from keratomileusis using a cryolathe. LASIK goes one step further and uses an excimer laser rather than the second pass of the microkeratome to ablate the underlying corneal stroma to the desired correction. LASIK offers a unique refinement to keratomileusis by introducing the excimer laser and broadens the scope of myopic PRK by allowing the correction of high myopia without disrupting Bowman's membrane centrally.

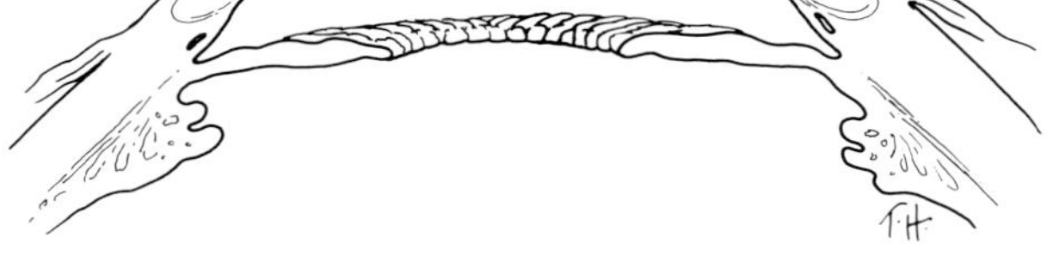

FIGURE 11.9. Schematic representation of excimer laser sculpting of a synthetic epikeratoplasty lenticule.

Why use both an expensive and complex laser and a microkeratome to reshape the cornea when either one could be used independently? The answer lies in the difficulties encountered with using either instrument alone for correcting high myopia. As mentioned in the previous paragraph, excimer laser PRK, whether for high or low myopia, requires ablation of the central few millimeters of Bowman's membrane. For low myopia, this seems to be associated with relatively small amounts of scar formation and refractive regression, but for high myopia, these problems are more prominent. With in situ keratomileusis, most microkeratome instruments can remove the corneal cap with fair predictability. The second pass of the instrument, however, is often associated with variability of smoothness, due to the change in resistance of a thinner cornea. This can result in irregular astigmatism and monocular diplopia in up to 25% of patients undergoing the procedure.[30] LASIK combines the precise sculpting of the excimer laser with the relative predictability of the initial cut of the microkeratome to reshape the midcorneal stroma without the negative effects of using either instrument independently.

LASIK, although not clinically investigated in this country, has been tested abroad with promising results. The first published article on this subject was by Pallikaris and colleagues in 1990;[31] he described the procedure as performed in a rabbit model. They used the ArF excimer laser to produce a 3 mm circular ablation on the central part of the exposed corneal stroma, after creating a central corneal flap with a modified microkeratome. Fifteen rabbit corneas underwent the procedure and were examined biomicroscopically and histopathologically at various time intervals and found to have good results. A mild haze was seen at 3 days postoperatively, with progressive improvement over a month, and electron and light microscopy showed an initially smooth surface in both the dissected and ablated areas, with only increased numbers of keratocytes along the ablation interface at 4 weeks. The unique feature of this procedure was that the corneal cap was not completely removed but was developed as a 200 μm nasally based flap that could be reapposed without sutures. Human studies on six blind eyes[32] verify the utility of the corneal flap technique by creating nasally based flaps of 300 μm depth and allowing them to heal without further reshaping by the placement of a bandage soft contact lens. Good optical clarity was maintained, and minimal astigmatism was seen after 4 weeks, suggesting the importance of a flap in allowing the cornea to heal in its original position.

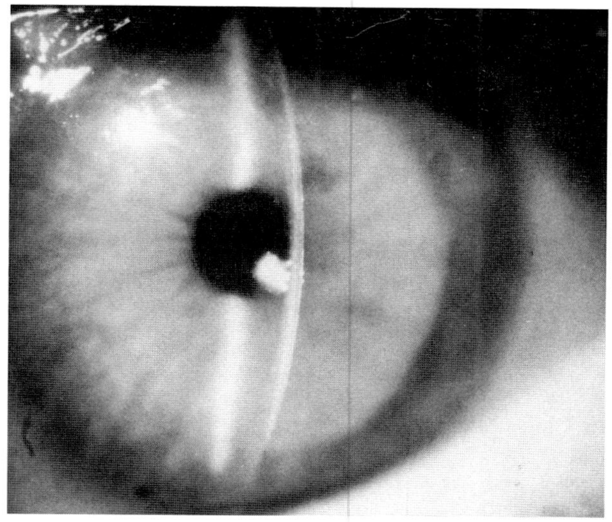

FIGURE 11.10. Slit lamp photograph of a human eye 2 days following LASIK. Note the prominent intrastromal interface and fine undulations of corneal stroma caused by the rotating microkeratome. Photograph from Ioannis Pallikaris, M.D.

Currently, Dr. Pallikaris and his colleagues at the University of Crete, Greece, are carrying out a study on 10 partially sighted human eyes with myopia of 12 to 20 D and best-corrected visual acuities of 20/50 or less (Ioannis Pallikaris, M.D., personal communication, April 27, 1992). Six of these patients have greater than 6 months follow-up and have stable refractions and less induced astigmatism than conventional myopic keratomileusis patients. The disadvantage with the technique, thus far, is the lower predictability of outcome compared with low myopic photorefractive corrections. Figure 11.10 shows a slit lamp photograph of a human eye 2 days following LASIK. The slit beam shows a prominent interface within the corneal stroma, and one can also see fine undulations produced by the rotating microkeratome, as noted against the iris detail. Figure 11.11 shows a similar patient with 17 D of correction 2 months following the procedure. One can note a fine interface within the slit beam and relatively good corneal clarity. In their series, the postoperative refractive corrections have all remained stable. They anticipate improvement in predictability in future series.

A new and competing approach to LASIK is that of excimer laser intrastromal keratomileusis, or intrastromal photokeratomileusis (PKM). This technique, introduced by Burrato and colleagues in March of 1992,[33] uses the excimer laser to reshape the undersurface of the corneal cap or lenticule

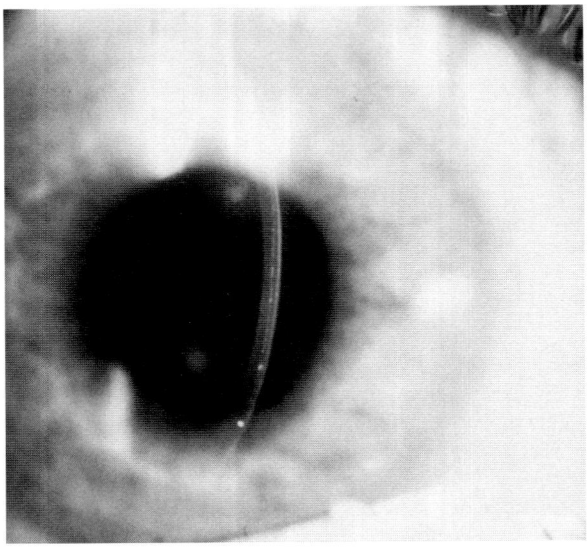

FIGURE 11.11. Slit lamp photograph of a human eye with 17 D correction 2 months following LASIK. Note the fine intrastromal interface and relatively good corneal clarity. Photograph from Ioannis Pallikaris, M.D.

rather than the exposed corneal stromal bed. In their procedure, a microkeratome is used to remove a 300 μm corneal cap that is marked along its optical axis. The lenticule is then inverted and placed on a hard rubber surface where a 3.5 to 4.5 mm diameter excimer laser myopic correction is performed for the desired refractive change. The lenticule is then sutured back onto the corneal bed with a single, running, antitorque 10.0 nylon suture. They report the results of this technique performed on 30 sighted human eyes of 22 myopic patients, with 6 months of follow-up. A marked refractive reduction from -17.875 ± -3.32 D to -2.125 ± -1.40 D was observed, with 80% having a final outcome within 1 D of the desired correction. Best-corrected visual acuities remained the same or better in 90% of patients. Uncorrected visual acuity improved from less than 20/200 preoperatively to 20/100 or better in 93% of eyes. Complications included irregular astigmatism (13%), poor night vision (3%), intrastromal haze (10%), and irregularities in Bowman's membrane (7%). The latter finding of wrinkles in Bowman's membrane, seen in two patients, was associated with a lenticular cap of less than 250 μm in depth. They recommend that whenever the thickness of the corneal cap is less than 250 μm, in situ photoablation be performed.

The relative safety and efficacy of LASIK and laser intrastromal keratomileusis remain to be determined. With LASIK, the ease and convenience of creating a flap that can be reapposed without the use of sutures certainly has its advantages. Likewise, the simplicity of laser intrastromal keratomileusis in ablating a lenticule along a premarked optical center suggests its advantage over in situ ablation. Only further controlled clinical studies and careful research will establish the qualities of these procedures and perhaps introduce a new and acceptable surgical alternative for correcting high myopia.

ON THE HORIZON

The proliferation of manuscripts, journals, and companies focusing on laser corneal surgery is almost overwhelming. While the excimer laser has seized the spotlight, other lasers are being intensively investigated. Lasers that are at various points along the time line from preliminary animal studies to human clinical trials include the holmium yag laser (for laser thermokeratoplasty), solid-state lasers that emit ultraviolet wavelengths close to that of the 193 nm excimer laser, and nanosecond, picosecond, and femtosecond yag lasers for intrastromal surgery. The next decade will witness competition among differing laser technologies. Very possibly, multiple lasers will prove clinically useful, with each "carving out" its own niche within the field of refractive surgery.

The use of these lasers will stimulate basic studies in corneal topography, corneal biomechanics, and pharmacologic modulation of corneal wound healing. As with intraocular lenses, we will see efforts to develop a satisfactory technique for creating multifocal corneas.

With the ultimate goal of these efforts being the creation of an emmetropic eye with a clear cornea (preferably such that no opacity is detectable), refractive surgery is the frontier within our specialty.

REFERENCES

1. Troutman RC, Swinger C: Relaxing incision for control of postoperative astigmatism following keratoplasty. *Ophthalmic Surg* 11:117–120, 1980.
2. McDonnell PJ, Moreira H, Garbus J, et al: Photorefractive keratectomy to create toric ablations for correction of astigmatism. *Arch Ophthalmol* 109:710–713, 1991.
3. Gartry DS, Kerr-Muir MG, Marshall J: Photorefractive keratectomy with an argon fluoride excimer laser: A clinical study. *Refrac Corneal Surg* 7:420–435, 1991.
4. Fantes FE, Hanna KD, Waring GO III, et al: Wound healing after excimer laser keratomileusis (photore-

fractive keratectomy) in monkeys. *Arch Ophthalmol* 108:665–675, 1990.

5. Goodman GL, Trokel SL, Stark WJ, et al: Corneal healing following laser refractive keratectomy. *Arch Ophthalmol* 107:1799–1803, 1989.
6. Tuft SJ, Zabel RW, Marshall J: Corneal repair following keratectomy: A comparison between conventional surgery and laser photoablation. *Invest Ophthalmol Vis Sci* 30:1769–1777, 1989.
7. Malley DS, Steinert RF, Puliafito CA, et al: Immunofluorescence study of corneal wound healing after excimer laser anterior keratectomy in the monkey eye. *Arch Ophthalmol* 108:1316–1322, 1990.
8. SundarRaj N, Geiss MJ III, Fantes F, et al: Healing of excimer laser ablated monkey corneas: An immunohistochemical evaluation. *Arch Ophthalmol* 108: 1604–1610, 1990.
9. Talamo JH, Gollamudi S, Green WR, et al: Modulation of corneal wound healing after excimer laser keratomileusis using topical mitomycin C and steroids. *Arch Ophthalmol* 109:1141–1146, 1991.
10. Puliafito CA, Stern D, Krueger RR, et al: High speed photography of excimer laser ablation of the cornea. *Arch Ophthalmol* 105:1255–1259, 1987.
11. Campos M, Cuevas K, Garbus J, et al: Corneal wound healing after excimer ablation: Effects of nitrogen gas blower. *Ophthalmology* 99:893–897, 1992.
12. Bende T, Seiler T, Wollensak J: Side effects in excimer corneal surgery: Corneal thermal gradients. *Graefes Arch Clin Exp Ophthalmol* 226:277–280, 1988.
13. Krueger RR, Krasinski JS, Radzewicz C, et al: High speed shadowgraphy of excimer laser excited shock wave: The effect of helium on propagation [*sic*] velocity. *Invest Ophthalmol Vis Sci* 33:765, 1992.
14. Krasinski JS, Radzewicz C, Krueger RR: Experimental evidence of excimer laser plasma shielding and its dependence on pulsewidth. *Invest Ophthalmol Vis Sci* 33:1106, 1992.
15. Waring GO III: Development of a system for excimer laser corneal surgery. *Trans Am Ophthalmol Soc* 87:854–983, 1989.
16. Gordon M, Brint SF, Durrie DS, et al: Photorefractive keratectomy (PRK) at 193 nm using an erodible mask. *Ophthalmic Technol II* SPIE 1644, 1992 (in press).
17. Englanoff JS, Kolahdouz-Isfahani AH, Moreira H, et al. In situ collagen gel mold as an aid in excimer laser superficial keratectomy. *Ophthalmology* (in press).
18. Santos VR, Waring GO III, Lynn MJ, et al: Relationship between refractive error and visual acuity in the Prospective Evaluation of Radial Keratotomy (PERK) study. *Arch Ophthalmol* 105:86–92, 1987.
19. McDonnell PJ, Garbus J, Lopez PF: Topographic analysis and visual acuity after radial keratotomy. *Am J Ophthalmol* 106:692–695, 1988.
20. Moreira H, Garbus JJ, Lee M, et al: Multifocal corneal topographic changes after radial keratotomy. *Arch Ophthalmol* 110:994–999, 1992.
21. Maguire LJ, Bourne WM: A multifocal lens effect as a complication of radial keratotomy. *Refract Corneal Surg* 6:394–397, 1989.
22. McDonald MB, Frantz JM, Klyce SD, et al: One-year refractive results of central photorefractive keratectomy for myopia in the nonhuman primate cornea. *Arch Ophthalmol* 108:40–47, 1990.
23. McDonald MB, Frantz JM, Klyce SD, et al: Central photorefractive keratectomy for myopia: The blind eye study. *Arch Ophthalmol* 108:799–808, 1990.
24. Moreira H, Garbus J, Fasano A, et al: Multifocal corneal topographic changes with excimer laser photorefractive keratectomy. *Arch Ophthalmol* (in press).
25. Holladay JT, van Dijk H, Lang A, et al: Optical performance of multifocal intraocular lenses. *J Cataract Refract Surg* 16:413–422, 1990.
26. Thompson KP, Hanna K, Waring GO III: Emerging technologies for refractive surgery: Laser adjustable synthetic epikeratoplasty. *Refract Corneal Surg* 5:46–48, 1989.
27. Thompson KP, Hanna K, Waring GO III, et al: Current status of synthetic epikeratoplasty. *Refract Corneal Surg* 7:240–248, 1991.
28. Barraquer JI: Queratoplastia. *Arch Soc Am Oftal y Optom* 3:147–168, 1961.
29. Ruiz LA, Rowsey JJ: In situ keratomileusis. *Invest Ophthalmol Vis Sci* 29 (suppl): 392, 1988.
30. Bas AM, Nano HD: In situ myopic keratomileusis results in 30 eyes at 15 months. *Refract Corneal Surg* 7:223–231, 1991.
31. Pallikaris IG, Papatzanaki ME, Stathi EZ, et al: Laser in situ keratomileusis. *Lasers Surg Med* 10:463–468, 1990.
32. Pallikaris IG, Papatzanaki ME, Siganos DE, et al: A corneal flap technique for laser in situ keratomileusis: Human studies. *Arch Ophthalmol* 109:1699–1702, 1991.
33. Buratto L, Ferrari M, Rama P: Excimer laser intrastromal keratomileusis. *Am J. Ophthalmol* 113:291–295, 1992.

Index

A

Ablatable masks, for astigmatism, 102, *see also* Erodible mask
Ablation, corneal, *see* Cornea, ablation of
Acuity, visual, *see* Visual acuity
Adrenal cortex hormones, *see* Corticosteroids
Alignment subsystem, of excimer laser, 10–11
Animal studies, with excimer laser, 13–14
Argon fluoride excimer laser, 7–8
Astigmatism, *see also* Photorefractive keratectomy (PRK), for astigmatism
  beam delivery in, 9–10
  corneal topography in, 24, 98–99
  erodible masks for, 61
  irregular astigmatism, 102
  naturally occurring, 99
  postcataract extraction, 102
  postkeratoplasty, 99–101
  postulcer astigmatism, 101

B

Barraquer, S. I., on keratomileusis, 82, 148
Bates, W. H., on astigmatism, 94
Beam delivery, by excimer laser, 8
Bende, T., on surface heating, 140
Berlin, Michael, on excimer lasers, 63
Blind eye studies, of myopia, 28–30
Blum, S. E., on excimer laser, 3
Brau, Charles
  on excimer laser, 2
  on rare gas dimers, 2
Brint, Steven F., on keratomileusis, 90
Buratto, L., on keratomileusis, 90, 149–150

C

Case studies, in phototherapeutic keratectomy, 111–117
Cataract extraction, astigmatism following, 102
Center, Robert, on rare gas dimers, 2
Centration, in photorefractive keratectomy, 30–33
Clear lens extraction, for high myopia, 82
Collagen gel, moldable, in corneal smoothing, 142–143
Color-coded maps, in corneal topography, 24–28
Computers, in keratoscopy, 22–24
Consent, informed, *see* Informed consent
Contact lenses
  for high myopia, 80–81
  warpage of, keratoconus vs., 25–26
Contour maps, of corneal surface, 23
Cooper Laboratories, laser experimentation by, 6–7
Cornea
  ablation of
    algorithm of, 37
    double, 89–90
    elliptical, 102
    environment of, 138–141
    for high myopia, 86
    history of, 12–13, 20–24, 105
    masks in, 141
    multifocal, 143–144
    multizone, 89
    particulate ejection in, 138–140
    surface heating in, 140
    tissue hydration in, 140–141
    variable diameter, 86
  contour maps of, 28
  dystrophy of, 109–110
  erosions of, 111, 125–127
  flattening of, 110
  heating of, 140
  lasers interacting with, 12–13
  opacities of
    histopathologic studies in, 107–108
  postoperative care in, 107–108
  preoperative preparation in, 105–106
  scars of, 105
    superficial, 123–125
    surgery for, 106–107
  smoothing of
    collagen gel in, 142–143
    of irregular surfaces, 121–125
  topography of
    in astigmatism, 98–99
    color-coded maps of, 24–28
    in epikeratophakia, 26–27
    future of, 34
    in preoperative screening, 33–34
    trephination of, 12, 131–135
  wound healing in, 107, 137–138
Corticosteroids, postoperative use of, 138
Cotliar, A. M., on radial laser incisions, 13

Curtin, B. J., on myopia grading, 78
Crystalline keratopathy, infectious, 128

D

Damiano, R. E., on radial keratotomy, 70
Decomposition, photoablative, from argon fluoride laser, 3
Degenerative myopia, 77–79
Dehydration, tissue, in corneal ablation, 140–141
Deitz, Michael B.
  on photorefractive keratectomy, 49
  on radial keratotomy, 69–70
Del Pero, R. A., animal studies by, 14
Dimers, rare gas, 1–2
Dioptic stability, in myopic photorefractive keratectomy, 48
Double ablation, for high myopia, 89–90
Double yag laser, for high myopia, 90
Dystrophy, corneal, after phototherapeutic keratectomy, 109–110

E

Eiferman, R. A., on infectious crystalline keratopathy, 128
Ejection, particulate, in corneal ablation, 138–140
Elliptical ablation, in astigmatism, 102
Epikeratophakia
  corneal topography in, 26–27
  for high myopia, 81–82
Epikeratoplasty, laser adjustable synthetic, 145–148
Epithelial disorders, from large-area photorefractive keratectomy, 60
Epithelial hypertrophy, 121–122
Epithelial keratitis, herpetic, 128
Erodible mask photorefractive keratectomy, 60–62, 141
Erosions, corneal, 111, 125–127
Ewing, James, on rare gas dimers, 2
Excimer laser
  argon fluoride, 7–8
  for astigmatism, 96
  beam delivery by, 8
  in corneal ablation, 86
  defined, 1
  for high myopia, 83–86, 90
  history of, 1–7
  instrumental variations in, 11–12
  interaction with cornea, 12–13
  studies with
    animal, 13–14
    human, 14–16
  subsystems of
    alignment, 10–11
    laser, 8
    optical, 8–10
Extraction
  clear lens, for high myopia, 82
  cataract, astigmatism following, 102

F

Fibroblastic keratocytes, postoperative haze from, 50
Follow up, in astigmatism, 98
Food and Drug Administration (U.S.), on myopia, 37–39
Forstot, S. L., on radial keratotomy, 70
Fungal keratitis, 128
Fyodorov, Svyatoslav N.
  on intraocular implantation, 82–83
  on radial keratotomy, 81

G

Gartry, D., on photorefractive keratectomy, 60, 70–71
Gas dimers, rare, 1–2
Gel, moldable collagen, in corneal smoothing, 142–143
Golde, on rare gas dimers, 2
Goodman, G. L., animal studies by, 14
Gordon, Eugene, laser experimentation by, 4
Gordon, M., on erodible masks, 141
Gould, Gordon, on excimer laser, 1–2
Guyton, D.L., on astigmatism, 102

H

Haag-Streit optical pachometer, in corneal measurement, 106
Halo effect, after large-area photorefractive keratectomy, 59
Hanna, K., on laser adjustable synthetic epikeratoplasty, 145
Hao-Lin Chen, on rare gas dimers, 2
Haze
  after large-area photorefractive keratectomy, 57–58
  stromal, in myopic photorefractive keratectomy, 49–50
Healing, wound, *see* Wound healing
Heating, of corneal surfaces, 140
Herpetic epithelial keratitis, 128
High myopia, *see* Myopia, high
Histopathologic studies, in corneal opacities, 107–108
History
  of corneal opacities, 105
  of excimer laser, 1–7
  of photorefractive keratectomy, 53–54
Hofbauer, John, on excimer lasers, 63
Hogan, C., on excimer laser photorefractive keratectomy, 47–48
Holladay, on radial keratotomy, 64
Houtermans, F. G.
  on rare gas dimers, 1
  on rotating-slit system, 11
Huestis, D. L., on excimer laser, 2
Human studies, with excimer laser, 14–16
Hydration, tissue, in corneal ablation, 140–141
Hyperopia
  collagen gel in, 141–143
  after phototherapeutic keratectomy, 108–109
Hyperopic photorefractive keratectomy, 55
  erodible masks for, 61

Hyperplasia, epithelial, 110
Hypertrophy, epithelial, 121–122

I
Implantation, intraocular, for high myopia, 82–83
Interferometry, in keratoscopy, 21
Informed consent
  in astigmatism, 96
  in photorefractive keratectomy, 65–66
  in radial keratotomy, 65
In situ keratomileusis, 148–150
Instrumental variations, in excimer laser, 11–12
International standard scale, in corneal topography, 23
Intraocular lens implantation, for high myopia, 82–83
Intraocular pressure, from large-area photorefractive keratectomy, 60
Intraoperative care, in astigmatism, 98
Intrastromal keratomileusis, 149–150
Irregular astigmatism, 102

K
Kaufman, Herbert E.
  on epikeratophakia, 81
  on excimer lasers, 63
  on intraocular implantation, 82
Keck, James, on rare gas dimers, 1
Keratectomy, photorefractive, *see* Photorefractive keratectomy (PRK)
Keratitis, infectious, 127–129
Keratoconus
  corneal topography in, 24–26
  preoperative screening for, 33
Keratocytes, fibroblastic, postoperative haze from, 50
Keratomileusis
  for high myopia, 82, 90
  laser *in situ,* 148–150
Keratopathy
  infectious crystalline, 128
  primary band, 111
Keratoplasty
  astigmatism following, 99–101
  penetrating, 105, 131–135
Keratoscopy
  computerized, 22–24
  history of, 20–22
Keratotomy, radial, *see* Radial keratotomy (RK)
Klyce, S. D.
  on epikeratophakia, 81
  on topographic analysis, 33
Kornmehl, E. W., on corneal smoothing, 122
Krasinski, J. S., on surface heating, 140
Krueger, R. R., on laser corneal ablation, 13

L
Lambda Physik, laser delivery system of, 53
Lamellar keratectomy, in animals, 13
Lans, on radial keratotomy, 81
Large-area photorefractive keratectomy, 56–60
Laser adjustable synthetic epikeratoplasty (LASE), 145–148
Laser, excimer, *see* Excimer laser
Laser *in situ* keratomileusis (LASIK), 148–150
Lavery, Frank L., on double ablation, 89–90
Leach, David, on multizone ablation, 89
Lenses
  in beam delivery, 10
  clear, extraction of, 82
  contact
  for high myopia, 80–81
  warpage of, 25–26
L'Esperance, F. A.
  human studies by, 14
  keratectomies by, 37, 64
Linsker, R., on excimer laser, 3
Liu, J. C., on myopic photorefractive keratectomy, 47
Loertscher, H., on corneal trephination, 12
Louisiana State University (LSU), myopia studies at, 28–33

M
McDonald, Marguerite B.
  on epikeratophakia, 81–82
  on high myopia, 89
  on keratectomies, 37–38
  on multizone ablation, 89
  on photorefractive keratectomy, 14–16, 28, 63, 64, 70
  myopic, 38, 46–48, 49
  on topographic analysis, 33
McDonnell, P. J., on photorefractive keratectomy, 16
Macy, Jonathan, on excimer lasers, 63
Maguen, Ezra, on excimer lasers, 63
Malignant myopia, 77–79
Maps, color-coded, in corneal topography, 24–28
Marshall, John
  animal studies by, 13–14
  laser experimentation by, 6
Masks
  ablatable, for astigmatism, 102
  erodible, in photorefractive keratectomy, 60–62
Measurement
  in corneal opacities, 106
  in keratoscopy, 21
Meditec, laser delivery system of, 53
Modeling, topographic, 22–24
Moldable collagen gel, in corneal smoothing, 141–143
Muller, D., on erodible masks, 60
Multifocal corneal ablations, 143–144
Multistep variable diameter corneal ablation, 86
Munnerlyn, Charles
  ablation algorithm of, 37
  laser experimentation by, 6–7
Myopia
  degenerative, 77–79
  high
    clear lens extraction for, 82

Myopia (*contd.*)
clinical features of, 79–80
corneal ablation for, 86
double yag laser for, 90
epikeratophakia for, 81–82
excimer laser therapy for, 83–86, 90
intraocular lens implantation for, 82–83
keratomileusis for, 82, 90
nonsurgical treatment of, 80–81, 83
pathologic vs., 77–79
physiologic aspects of, 80
posttreatment management of, 85–86
preoperative evaluation in, 84
radial keratotomy for, 81
scleral reinforcement for, 91
sociological aspects of, 80
surgery for, 81–83
visual aspects of, 80
malignant, 77–79
pathologic, 77–79
photorefractive keratectomy for
complications of, 49–50
early studies in, 37–39
patient selection in, 39–40
postoperative evaluation in, 45–46
results of, 46–49
technique in, 41–45
topographic analysis of, 28–33
progressive, 77–79
radial keratotomy for, 27–28

N

Nesburn, Anthony, on excimer lasers, 63
Neuhann, Thomas, on excimer lasers, 63
Nonsurgical treatment, of high myopia, 80–81, 83

O

Opacities, corneal, *see* Cornea, opacities of
Optical measurement
in corneal opacities, 106
in keratoscopy, 21
Optical subsystem, of excimer laser, 8–10

P

Pallikaris, I. G., on keratomileusis, 149
Parker, P., on preoperative myopia, 48
Particulate, ejection, in corneal ablation, 138–140
Pathologic myopia, 77–79
Patient(s)
costs to, 73–74
experiences of
in photorefractive keratectomy, 66–69
preparation of, for excimer laser surgery, 97–98
in radial keratotomy, 66–69
selection of
for photorefractive keratectomy, 39–40, 65, 96
for radial keratotomy, 65
for therapeutic keratectomy, 105–106
Pellier de Quengsy, on artificial implants, 105
Penetrating keratoplasty, 105, 131–135
PERK (Prospective Evaluation of Radial Keratotomy)
for high myopia, 84
for photorefractive keratectomy, 47
Photoablative decomposition, from argon fluoride laser, 3
Photorefractive keratectomy (PRK), *see also* Myopia, photorefractive keratectomy for
in animals, 13–14
for astigmatism
history of, 94–96
intraoperative care in, 98
patient preparation for, 97–98
patient selection in, 96
postoperative care in, 98
procedures in, 96–98
results of, 99–101
centration of, 30–33
costs of, 73–74
in Europe, 53–62
history of, 53–54
hyperopic, 55
mechanisms of, 64–65
preoperative screening in, 33–34
radial keratotomy vs., 63–74
results of, 70–71
rotating-slit delivery system for, 11
side effects of, 71–72
techniques of
erodible mask, 60–62
large area, 56–60
scanning slit, 54–55
in U.S., 37–50
Phototherapeutic keratectomy (PTK)
for corneal opacities
case studies in, 111–117
complications of, 106–107
for corneal erosions, 111
histopathologic studies in, 107–108
history of, 105
hyperopic effect from, 110
patient selection in, 105–106
planning for, 106
postoperative care in, 107–108
results of, 108–109
techniques of, 106–107
for corneal smoothing
in infectious keratitis, 127–129
in irregular surfaces, 121–125
in recurrent erosions, 125–127
Physiologic aspects, of high myopia, 80
Piebenga, Larry W., on myopia, 38
Piovella, M., on high myopia, 88–89
Postcataract extraction astigmatism, 102
Postkeratoplasty astigmatism, 99–101
Postoperative care
in astigmatism, 98

in high myopia, 85–86
in photorefractive keratectomy, 45–46, 67
in therapeutic keratectomy, 107–108
in radial keratotomy, 66
Postulcer astigmatism, 101
PRK, *see* Photorefractive keratectomy
Preoperative evaluation
in corneal opacities, 105–106
in high myopia, 84
in photorefractive keratectomy, 33–34
Preparation of patient, for excimer laser surgery, 97–98
Pressure, intraocular, from large-area PRK, 60
Primary band keratopathy, 111
Progressive myopia, 77–79
Prospective Evaluation of Radial Keratotomy (PERK)
for high myopia, 84
for photorefractive keratectomy, 47
Pseudomonas aeruginosa, in astigmatism, 101
PTK, *see* Phototherapeutic keratectomy
Puliafito, C. A., on corneal ablation, 12–13, 138

R

Radial keratotomy (RK)
costs of, 73–74
for high myopia, 81
informed consent in, 65
mechanisms of, 64
in myopia, 27–28
patient selection in, 65
photorefractive keratectomy vs., 63–74
results of, 69–70
side effects of, 71–72
Rare gas dimers, 1–2
Rasterstereography, in keratoscopy, 21
Reddick, Dale E., on synthetic epikeratoplasty, 147
Refraction, after large-area PKR, 56–57
Refractive keratectomy, *see* Photorefractive keratectomy (PRK)
Reinforcement, scleral, for high myopia, 91
Rhodes, Charles
on excimer laser, 2
on rare gas dimers, 1–2
RK, *see* Radial keratotomy
Rotating slit delivery system, for keratectomies, 11
Rowsey, J. J.
on keratomileusis, 148
on keratoscopy, 21
Ruderman, Warren, on excimer laser, 2
Ruiz, L. A., on keratomileusis, 148

S

Safety issues, in corneal surgery, 71–72
St. Yves, on superficial keratectomy, 105
Salz, J. J., on radial keratotomy, 69–70
Sato, T., on radial keratotomy, 81
Sawusch, M. R., on astigmatism, 102
Scanning slit photorefractive keratectomy, 54–55
Scarring
corneal, 105
large-area PRK causing, 57–58
Scleral reinforcement, for high myopia, 91
Screening, preoperative, in photorefractive keratectomy, 33–34
Searles, Stuart, on rare gas dimers, 2
Seiler, Theo
on corneal ablation, 86
human studies by, 14–16
laser experimentation by, 6
on myopic PRK, 46, 47, 64, 70
Serdarevic, O. N.
animal studies by, 13–14
on infectious keratitis, 127
Setser, Donald, on rare gas dimers, 2
Sher, N. A., on photorefractive keratectomy, 16, 47, 70
Shock wave, in ablation, 140
Side effects, of corneal surgery, 71–72
Sighted eye studies, of myopia, 30–33
Sociological aspects, of high myopia, 80
Spectacles, for high myopia, 80
Srinivasan, R., on excimer laser, 2, 3
Stability, dioptric, in myopic photorefractive keratectomy, 48
Steinert, R. F., on laser keratotomy, 13
Stromal haze, in myopic photorefractive keratectomy, 49–50
Subsystems, of excimer laser, 8–10
Surface, corneal, *see* Cornea, surfaces of
Summit Technologies, laser experimentation by, 6, 31
Swinger, C. A., on keratomileusis, 82

T

Taboada, John, on argon fluoride laser, 2
Talamo, J. H., on corticosteroids, 138
Taunton Technologies
human studies by, 14, 16
laser experimentation by, 4–7, 47
Taylor, Daniel
human studies by, 14
laser experimentation by, 5
Tengroth, B., on large-area photorefractive keratectomy, 59, 60
Tenner, Alf, on excimer lasers, 63
Therapeutic keratectomy, *see* Phototherapeutic keratectomy (PTK)
Thompson, F. B., on myopia grading, 78
Thompson, K. P., on laser adjustable synthetic epikeratoplasty, 145
Tissue hydration, in corneal ablation, 140–141
Topographic Modeling System (TMS-1), 22–24
Topography, corneal, *see* Cornea, topography of
Trephination, corneal, 12, 131–135
Trokel, Stephen
on corneal ablation, 105
on corneal removal, 3–4
on laser-corneal interaction, 12
on myopic photorefractive keratectomy, 46, 53

Troutman, R. C., on keratomileusis, 82
Tuft, S. J., on corticosteroids, 138

U

Ulcer, astigmatism following, 101

V

Verzella, F., on clear lens extraction, 82
Villaseñor, Richard, on refractive surgery, 63
Visual acuity
  after large-area PRK, 57
  after phototherapeutic keratectomy, 108
Visual aspects, of high myopia, 80
VISX
  laser experimentation by, 7, 16
  myopia studies of, 37–38

W

Waring, G. O.
  on laser adjustable synthetic epikeratoplasty, 145
  on radial keratotomy, 64
Werblin, T. P., on epikeratophakia, 81
Wheel, astigmatism, in beam delivery, 9–10
Wilson, S. E., on preoperative myopia, 48
Wollensak, J.
  on excimer laser, 53
  keratectomies by, 64, 70
Wound healing
  in astigmatism, 98–99
  corneal, 107, 137–138
  inhibitors of, 138

Y

Yag laser, double, for high myopia, 90
Yerkes Regional Primate Research Center, collagen polymer research of, 145–147

Z

Zabel, R. W., on photorefractive keratectomy, 16
Zinn, Edward, on penetrating keratoplasty, 105